The Biliary Tract

CLINICAL SURGERY INTERNATIONAL

Volumes published

Vol. 1 **Large Bowel Cancer** *J. J. DeCosse*, New York

Vol. 2 **Nutrition and the Surgical Patient** *G. L. Hill*, Auckland

Vol. 3 **Tissue Transplantation** *P. J. Morris*, Oxford

Vol. 4 **Infection and the Surgical Patient** *H. C. Polk*, Louisville

Volumes in preparation

Vol. 6 **Surgery of the Thyroid and Parathyroids** *E. L. Kaplan*, Chicago

Vol. 7 **Arterial Surgery** *J. J. Bergan*, Chicago

Vol. 8 **Peptic Ulcer** *D. C. Carter*, Glasgow

Vol. 9 **Shock and Related Problems** *G. T. Shires*, New York

Vol. 10 **Liver Surgery** *S. Bengmark*, Lund

CLINICAL SURGERY INTERNATIONAL

VOL 5 *The Biliary Tract*

EDITED BY

L. H. BLUMGART BDS MD FRCS

Director and Professor of Surgery, Royal Postgraduate Medical School,
University of London, England

CHURCHILL LIVINGSTONE
EDINBURGH LONDON MELBOURNE AND NEW YORK 1982

CHURCHILL LIVINGSTONE
Medical Division of Longman Group Limited

Distributed in the United States of America by
Churchill Livingstone Inc., 1560 Broadway, New York,
N.Y. 10036, and by associated companies,
branches and representatives throughout
the world.

First published 1982

ISBN 0 443 02322 0

British Library Cataloguing in Publication Data
The biliary tract.—(Clinical surgery
    international; v. 5)
    1. Biliary tract—Surgery
    I. Blumgart, L. H.   II. Series
    617'.556059   RD546

Library of Congress Cataloging in Publication Data
Main entry under title:
The biliary tract.
    (Clinical surgery international; v. 5)
    Includes index.
    1. Biliary tract—Surgery. 2. Biliary tract—
Diseases. I. Blumgart, L. H. II. Series.
[DNLM: 1. Biliary tract—Surgery. 2. Biliary
tract diseases. W1 CL795U v.5/WI 700 B594]
RD546.B5 1982   617'.556059   82–4532
AACR2

Printed in Great Britain at The Pitman Press, Bath

Preface

Only one hundred years ago, Langenbuch carried out the first cholecystectomy and shortly afterwards choledochotomy was performed. While developments in anaesthesia, blood transfusion, and antibiotics have made surgical approaches to the abdominal viscera possible and safe, more specific advances and particularly in diagnostic radiology have opened the door to precise and ever-advancing approaches to diseases of the biliary tree.

This volume of Clinical Surgery International attempts to bring together the opinions of some of the world's leading authorities with a critical appraisal of established practice in the management of a wide range of disorders and an up-to-date assessment of new techniques in the diagnosis, management, and care of the patient with biliary disease. No attempt has been made to reconcile conflicting opinions but the contributing authors have been asked to place on record their current practice and those aspects of the problem which they consider to be of importance. I have been delighted with the results which reflect an international balance of views on many important aspects of the subject. The reader should find many things to agree with, a good deal to learn, and a great deal to debate.

I wish to record that I had invited the late Professor Clarence Schein of the Albert Einstein School of Medicine, New York City, to contribute the section on post-cholecystectomy problems. His untimely death has left a gap in the ranks of those particularly interested in biliary surgery. His contribution, which would undoubtedly have reflected the pragmatic personal and very practical views expressed in his book on the subject, is sorely missed.

London, 1982   L.H.B.

Contributors

D. J. Allison BSc, MD, FRCR
Consultant and Senior Lecturer, Department of Radiology, Royal
Postgraduate Medical School, Hammersmith Hospital, London, England

Stig Bengmark MD, PhD
Professor of Surgery and Director, Department of Surgery, University of
Lund; Chief Surgeon, Hospital of Lund, Sweden

Irving S. Benjamin BSc, FRCS
Lecturer in Surgery, Royal Postgraduate Medical School, Hammersmith
Hospital, London, England

George Berci MD, FACS
Associate Director of Surgery and Director, Division of Endoscopy,
Department of Surgery, Cedars-Sinai Medical Center; Associate Clinical
Professor of Surgery, UCLA Medical Center, Los Angeles, U.S.A.

Henri Bismuth MD
Professor of Surgery, Université Paris Sud; Director of the Hepato-biliary
Surgical Unit, Hôpital Paul Brousse, Villejuif, France

L. H. Blumgart BDS, MD, FRCS(Eng, Edin, Glas)
Professor of Surgery and Director, Department of Surgery, Royal
Postgraduate Medical School, Hammersmith Hospital, London, England

N. B. Bowley MB, BS, FRCR
Consultant Radiologist, Royal Postgraduate Medical School, Hammersmith
Hospital, London, England

Peter G. Jones MS(Melb), FRCS(Eng), FRACS, FACS, FAAP(Hon)
Surgeon, Head of Unit, Department of General Surgery, Royal Children's
Hospital, Melbourne, Australia

M. R. B. Keighley MS, FRCS
Consultant Surgeon and Reader in Surgery, General Hospital, Birmingham,
England

Björn Lindgren PhD
Lecturer, Department of Economics, University of Lund; Project Manager, Swedish Institute for Health Economics, Lund, Sweden

D. A. Lloyd MChir(Cantab), FRCS, FCS(S.A.)
Senior Paediatric Surgeon, King Edward VIII Hospital, Durban; Senior Lecturer in Paediatric Surgery, Faculty of Medicine, University of Natal, South Africa

N. J. Lygidakis MD
Honorary Consultant Surgeon, Hammersmith Hospital, London, England

Charles K. McSherry MD
Director of Surgery, Beth Israel Medical Center, New York; Professor of Surgery, Mount Sinai School of Medicine of the City University of New York, New York, U.S.A.

Frank G. Moody MD
Professor and Chairman, Department of Surgery, University of Utah School of Medicine, Salt Lake City, Utah, U.S.A.

Leon Morgenstern MD, FACS
Director of Surgery, Cedars-Sinai Medical Center; Clinical Professor of Surgery, UCLA School of Medicine, Los Angeles, U.S.A.

Roger W. Motson MS, FRCS
Senior Surgical Registrar, The London Hospital, London, England

J. M. A. Northover MS, FRCS
Senior Surgical Registrar, The Middlesex and St Mark's Hospitals, London, England; lately Arris and Gale Lecturer, Royal College of Surgeons of England

Erwin Seifert MD, FACG
Professor of Internal Medicine and Gastoenterology, 1st Medical Department, Städtisches Krankenhaus Kemperhof Koblenz, W. Germany

Ralph A. O. Sörbris MD, PhD
Assistant Professor of Surgery, University of Lund, Sweden

John Terblanche MB, ChB, ChM(Cape Town), FCS(S.A.), FRCS(Eng)
Professor of Surgery and Head of the Department of Surgery, University of Cape Town; Chief Surgeon, Groote Schuur and Somerset Hospitals, Cape Town; Co-Director of the South African Medical Research Council Liver Research Group, University of Cape Town Medical School, S. Africa

Ronald K. Tompkins MD, MSc, FACS
Professor of Surgery and Assistant Dean, Student Affairs, UCLA School of Medicine, Los Angeles, U.S.A.

James Toouli B(Med)Sci, PhD, MB, FRACS
Lecturer, Department of Surgery, Flinders University; Consultant Surgeon, Flinders Medical Centre, South Australia

James McK. Watts MB, BS, FRACS
Professor of Surgery, Flinders University of South Australia

Lawrence W. Way MD
Professor of Surgery, University of California; Chief, Surgical Service, San Francisco V.A. Medical Center, San Francisco, U.S.A.

J. A. M. White FRCS, FRCS(Edin)
Chief, Ambulance and Emergency Medical Services, Province of Natal; formerly Senior Lecturer in Surgery, University of Natal, South Africa

Malcolm J. Whiting BSc, PhD
Senior Hospital Scientist/Lecturer, Flinders Medical Centre and Flinders University of South Australia

Contents

1 Applied surgical anatomy of the biliary tree

J. M. A. NORTHOVER and JOHN TERBLANCHE

Biliary anatomy first became of practical importance to surgeons towards the end of the last century, following the first cholecystectomy by Carl Langenbuch in 1882 (Glenn & Grafe 1966). In 1900 George Emerson Brewer of the Mount Sinai Hospital, noting the 'many new and ingenious operative procedures' being carried out on the biliary tract, produced one of the first practical guides to the surgical anatomy of this region. Confronted with this developing surgical challenge, he performed 160 dissections 'to educate his tactile sense for recognition of structures which, during operation, are often concealed from view or rendered visible only with difficulty'. The modern surgeon, with excellent anaesthesia, muscle relaxation and good lighting at his command, enabling him to use direct vision rather than his sense of touch to demonstrate the biliary anatomy, must surely be grateful!

Following Brewer's work, the first half of this century saw the publication of many studies which amply demonstrated the enormous range of individual variation that so characterises this region (Flint 1923, Friend 1929, Michels 1955); indeed, the well-read surgeon of today can be forgiven if he remains baffled by the complexities reported in the literature. More recently, however, several surgeons have stressed the limited surgical usefulness of much of this data, preferring to emphasise the important major variations (Benson & Page 1976, Kune & Sali 1980).

In this chapter those aspects of *practical* importance and interest to the surgeon will be emphasised, for there are few areas of operative surgery in which accidents due to failed recognition of local anatomy can so easily lead to catastrophe. In addition, the blood supply of the bile duct will be carefully considered, as this previously neglected topic may well have clinical importance in the development of postoperative complications after various operative procedures.

Anatomical 'normality' in the biliary tree

Normality, in the sense of an anatomical pattern which is repeated in the majority of individuals, is a term which cannot be used in relation to the biliary tree (Dowdy 1969, Benson & Page 1976). Variation is such that less than 50% of individuals exhibit a pattern common in even major details. Any attempt to define the 'normal' anatomy of the biliary tree, therefore, would be artificial and misleading, so each major area of the extrahepatic biliary tree and its related vessels will be considered separately, and the more important variational groups described.

Bile ducts at the liver hilum

The ducts in the hilum may be encountered either deliberately during partial hepatectomy or when dealing with a tumour or stricture at the porta hepatis, or accidentally in the course of a difficult cholecystectomy! It is important to note that some portion of both the right and left hepatic ducts, and hence their confluence, *are always extrahepatic* and, therefore, accessible at the porta (Kune & Sali 1980). In some cases portions of the major tributaries of the right and left ducts are also outside the liver (Fig. 1.1).

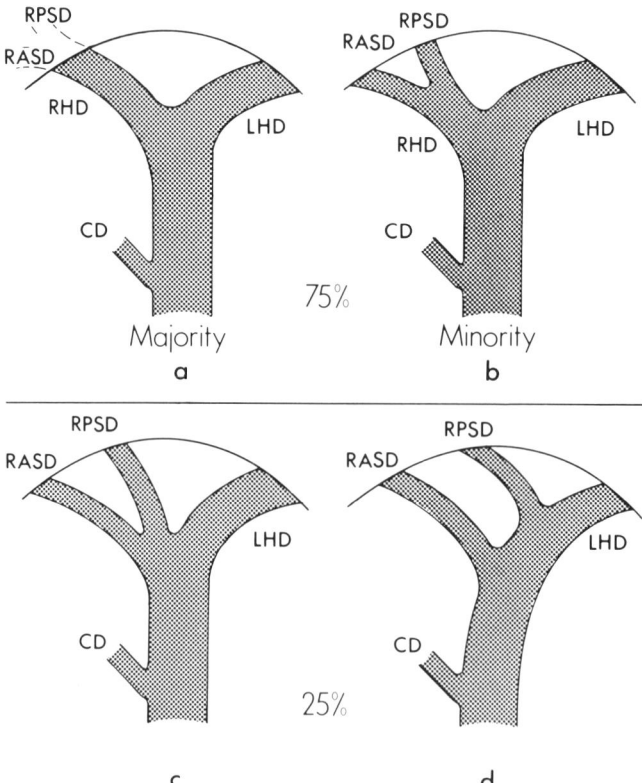

Fig. 1.1 Patterns of formation of hepatic ducts. A true right hepatic duct (RHD) is present in 75% of individuals, usually formed within the liver (a), but sometimes outside (b). In 25% no true RHD is found, the segmental ducts forming a triple confluence with the LHD (c) or joining it separately (d). In the latter instance, the RASD has in the past been wrongly designated an 'accessory' duct. RASD = right anterior segmental duct; RPSD = right posterior segmental duct; RHD = right hepatic duct; LHD = left hepatic duct; CD = cystic duct.

Right hepatic duct (RHD)

Just as the bronchial tree has a fairly constant pattern of branches, so have the intrahepatic bile ducts. Hjortsjo (1951) and later Healey & Schroy (1953) clearly demonstrated that each area of the liver has its own, nameable bile duct, and that the area ducts drain into major segmental ducts.

The functional right lobe (that part of the liver to the right of the lobar fissure, marked by the gallbladder fossa and the inferior vena cava) comprises two segments, anterior and posterior. In 75% of individuals the right anterior and posterior segmental ducts join to form a true right hepatic duct, i.e. a single channel carrying the whole bile output of the functional right lobe; *in the remaining 25% there is no true RHD*, the segmental ducts emptying into the left hepatic duct (LHD) separately (Fig. 1.1) (Healey & Schroy 1953, Balasegarem 1970, Kune & Sali 1980). This important point has bearing on the question of so-called 'accessory' bile ducts and will be referred to below.

Among those individuals (75%) in whom a true RHD is present, it is wholly extrahepatic in but a few. The extrahepatic segment is of variable length, being 1.0–2.5 cm long in 80% of cases, but may be up to 6 cm in length (Johnston & Anson 1952, Kune & Sali 1980).

The RHD is readily approached by dividing the peritoneum and fat overlying it in the porta hepatis. The right hepatic artery usually runs inferior to it, while the right branch of the portal vein lies posterior to these two structures.

'Accessory' bile ducts

Flint introduced the term 'accessory bile duct' in 1923 having found a structure in 15% of individuals which issued from the right lobe of the liver and entered the common hepatic duct (CHD) distal to the termination of the 'true' RHD. Since then many other authors have reported such 'accessory' ducts, usually in 10–30% of individuals, so that the term has become established in the nomenclature and minds of surgeons (Moosman & Coller 1951, Johnston & Anson 1952, Lichtenstein & Nicosia 1955, Michels 1955, Hayes et al 1958, Benson & Page 1976).

However, since the first description of the segmental pattern of liver drainage, several authors have shown that 'accessory' bile ducts occur in that group (approximately 25% of the population) in whom no true RHD exists — the 'extra' or 'accessory' duct and what was erroneously thought to have been the 'true' RHD in these individuals are, in fact, the two major segmental ducts from the right lobe draining separately into the LHD (Fig. 1.1c and 1.1d) (Healey & Schroy 1953, Hobsley 1958, Kune 1970). Damage to an 'accessory' duct will affect the bile drainage of a finite portion of the liver, while inadvertent, unnoticed division will lead to a sustained bile leak which may threaten the patient's life (Kune & Sali 1980).

In short, the term 'accessory' in this context (defined in Blakiston's *Gould Medical Dictionary* (1972) as pertaining to 'a lesser organ or part which supplements a similar organ or part') is both erroneous and dangerous, and should be dispensed with.

Left hepatic duct (LHD)

This structure is hardly ever seen during routine cholecystectomy, though it can be damaged during this procedure (Warren et al 1971). Unlike the right lobe, the left lobe of the liver is always drained by a single channel, the true left hepatic duct, and in most cases all its tributaries are intrahepatic (Healey & Schroy 1953, Kune & Sali 1980). The left hepatic artery usually runs below or behind the LHD, while the left branch of the portal vein may, unlike the right branch, partly spiral around the upper border of its hepatic duct to form an anterior relation of the latter as the two structures pass into the liver substance (Hobsley 1958).

The confluence of hepatic ducts

The point at which the right and left hepatic ducts join is often known to surgeons as 'the bifurcation'. From a functional standpoint, however, the term 'confluence' is more accurate; further, as 'bifurcation' suggests *two* 'branches', this term is especially inappropriate and misleading in those 25% of individuals in whom two right segmental ducts open separately into the left hepatic duct (Fig. 1.1c and 1.1d).

The confluence is always accessible in the normal individual, beneath the peritoneum in the porta hepatis; infrequently it is overlaid by the right hepatic artery. Sometimes the right and left hepatic ducts have a long extrahepatic course, so that the confluence may lie well down into the free edge of the lesser omentum where it is liable to damage during cholecystectomy.

Common hepatic duct (CHD)

This bile duct segment is of enormous surgical importance, being involved in two-thirds of postoperative strictures (Warren et al 1971). It is formed by the final confluence of all ducts issuing from the liver and ends when the lumen of the cystic duct opens into it to form the common bile duct (CBD). Its width does not differ significantly from the CBD (see below). In most individuals it is 2.5–3.5 cm in length (Flint 1923), but this is variable. In approximately 2% of cases, the CHD is non-existent, the cystic duct opening into the hepatic duct confluence (Benson & Page 1976), while in about 15–20% the CHD extends downwards behind the duodenum before the cystic duct opens into it (Flint 1923, Johnston & Anson 1952).

The major relations of the common hepatic duct are fairly constant; it lies in the right edge of the lesser omentum, with the common hepatic artery (CHA) to its left and the portal vein situated posteriorly. Its important variable neighbours are the right hepatic artery (RHA), cystic artery and cystic duct (Fig. 1.2). As the CHA normally bifurcates below the hepatic bile duct confluence, the RHA has to cross the CHD to reach the liver. In about 90% of cases, the RHA passes behind the duct, while in the rest it passes in front and is hence more prone to accidental injury (Daseler et al 1947, Michels 1955). The cystic artery usually arises in Calot's triangle and hence is not normally directly related to the CHD; in about 22%,

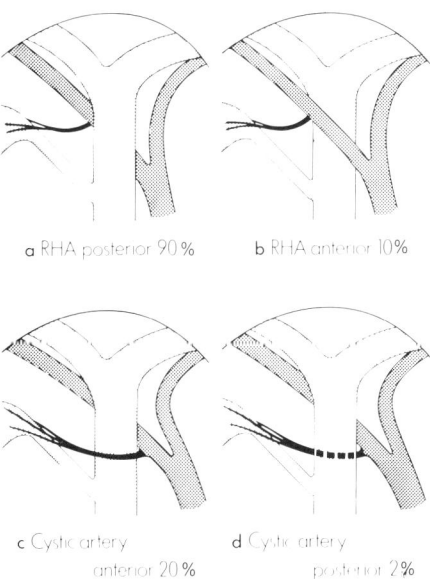

a RHA posterior 90%   b RHA anterior 10%

c Cystic artery
anterior 20%

d Cystic artery
posterior 2%

Fig. 1.2 Arterial relations of the common hepatic duct. The right hepatic artery normally passes behind the CHD (a); in the 10% in whom it passes in front of the duct (b), it is more vulnerable to operative damage. The cystic artery normally arises within Calot's triangle (a and b), but in about 22% it crosses the CHD from the left — anteriorly in 20% (c) and posteriorly in 2% (d). In these individuals hasty attempts to secure a bleeding cystic artery are particularly liable to damage the CHD.

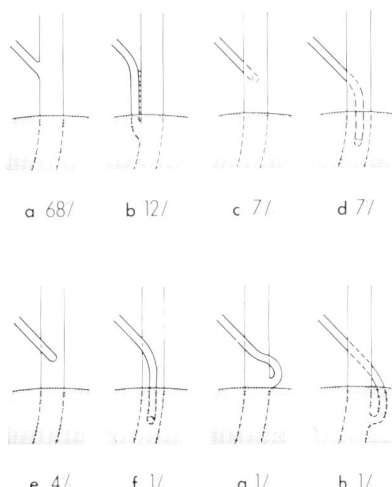

a 68/   b 12/   c 7/   d 7/

e 4/   f 1/   g 1/   h 1/

Fig. 1.3 Termination of the cystic duct (after Moosman & Coller 1951). In about two-thirds of individuals the cystic duct joins the common duct at an angle, entering its right side (a). In the remaining one-third (b–h) it either runs parallel with the duct, often incorporated in its wall, or spirals around it before entering the lumen. In all these situations, the dissection involved in an attempt to remove the *whole* cystic duct may damage the common duct or its blood supply.

however, it arises from the RHA to the left of the CHD, thence crossing it anteriorly in 20% and posteriorly in the remainder (Fig. 1.2c and 1.2d) (Daseler et al 1947). It is in these individuals that hurried attempts to secure a retracted, bleeding cystic artery are especially dangerous (Maingot 1980). The cystic duct normally joins the CHD at an angle, but in about 30% it is intimately bound to the right, anterior or posterior wall for a variable distance before the lumina join (Fig. 1.3). This is discussed further below.

The gallbladder

This least variable part of the biliary tree is usually globular, lying in its fossa on the undersurface of the liver. It is normally bound down to the liver surface by peritoneum except at its neck, where the origin of the cystic duct is enveloped in serosa. Rarely the whole gallbladder is on a mesentery, predisposing to torsion (Ashby 1965). The only common variant in form, occurring in up to 18%, is the Phrygian cap deformity, in which the distal fundus is folded upon itself (Boyden 1935). All other variants are rare, despite the exhaustive descriptions in some texts (Maingot 1980).

The arterial supply is via the cystic artery, which usually arises from the right hepatic artery in Calot's triangle (vide supra: CHD). In 15–20% of individuals an accessory cystic artery is present (Flint 1923, Michels 1955, Benson & Page 1976, Northover 1980) which also usually arises from the RHA. Venous drainage is via vessels running directly into the liver and several veins which join the pericholedochal venous plexus (vide infra: Bile duct blood supply — venous drainage).

Controversy surrounds the occurrence and clinical importance of the subvesical and cholecystohepatic ducts. The former is a duct which runs in the liver substance deep to the gallbladder fossa, and is present in about 50% of individuals (Moosman & Coller 1951, Healey & Schroy 1953, Hobsley 1958, Balasegarem 1970); it is liable to inadvertant damage during cholecystectomy, which may cause troublesome bile leakage (Kune & Sali 1980). Despite views to the contrary (Chilton & Mann 1980), this risk contributes to the need for routine use of a drain following cholecystectomy.

Bile ducts passing directly from the liver into the gallbladder (cholecystohepatic ducts), have been described by many authors (Neuhof & Bloomfield 1945, Williams & Williams 1955, Hayes et al 1958). Despite some reports of a high incidence, these ducts are probably rare (Hobsley 1958) and usually secondary to disease rather than congenital (Kune & Sali 1980).

The cystic duct

This structure is very variable in length and mode of union with the common hepatic duct. It arises from the neck of the gallbladder, usually rapidly narrowing to 1–3 mm internal diameter. In most people, the duct follows a straight oblique course to join the CHD. The junction is easily seen with minimal dissection in about 65%, while in the remainder, often deceptively, the duct runs a longer course, parallel with or spiralling around the CHD (Fig. 1.3) (Flint 1923, Moosman & Coller 1951, Johnston & Anson 1952). The distal part of the cystic duct in these circumstances is often incorporated into the wall of the CHD so that attempts to remove it entirely may lead to duct damage and stricture (Warren et al 1971, Kune & Sali 1980).

Absence of the cystic duct, with the gallbladder opening directly into the common duct, is almost certainly due to the inflammatory and erosive effect of the large gallstone always present when this 'anomaly' is found (Sutton & Sachatello 1967, Kune & Sali 1980), rather than a normal variant (Jackson & Kelly 1964).

Calot's triangle

This area, bounded by the cystic duct, common hepatic duct and the inferior surface of the liver, is the key to cholecystectomy. J-F. Calot (1861–1944), a Frenchman more noted in later life as an orthopaedic surgeon, first emphasised its importance in his MD thesis on cholecystectomy in 1890 (Wood 1979). The triangle includes the various structures to be sought or avoided when isolating the gallbladder (Fig. 1.4). Moosman & Coller (1951) highlighted the dangers in this area when they reported that, within the triangle and in accidental reach of a clamp placed on the cystic duct, are: the right hepatic artery in 83% of individuals, the aberrant right hepatic artery, when present, in 93% (i.e. in 16% of all individuals), and an 'accessory' bile duct, when present, in 85% (approximately

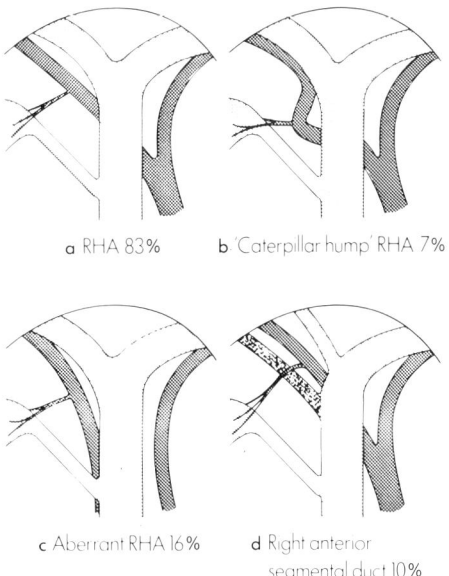

a RHA 83%   b 'Caterpillar hump' RHA 7%

c Aberrant RHA 16%   d Right anterior
segmental duct 10%

Fig. 1.4 Incidence of structures at risk in Calot's triangle. These structures all lie within range of a clamp carelessly applied to the cystic duct. The 'caterpillar hump' RHA (b) may be seen approaching the gallbladder and mistaken for the cystic artery, with serious results.

10% of all individuals). The RHA is in especial danger when it describes a loop to the right (the 'caterpillar hump') within the triangle, towards the neck of the gallbladder, as it does in about 7% (Benson & Page 1976); it may then be mistaken for the cystic artery and divided.

A thorough knowledge of the variations within Calot's triangle is surely a fundamental requirement for those embarking on biliary surgery.

Common bile duct (CBD)

Formed by the confluence of the common hepatic and cystic ducts, the CBD is normally located in the free edge of the lesser omentum, and subsequently passes behind the pancreas to enter the second part of the duodenum. In up to 20% of individuals, however, the CBD is not visible, as the confluence lies behind the duodenum or pancreas (Flint 1923, Moosman & Coller 1951, Johnston & Anson 1952).

The diameter of the CBD is variable; since the advent of operative cholangiography the individual importance of diameter as an indication for duct exploration has diminished. Sometimes, however, when the cholangiogram is difficult to interpret, duct diameter is a useful parameter in the decision to explore. Leslie (1968), in a useful practical study, found that ducts below 9 mm in diameter never contained stones, while those over 17 mm always had distal obstructive pathology, hence deserving exploration.

The CBD has several surgically important relations. The 'common duct lymph gland', located to the right of the duct as it disappears behind the duodenum, can be a useful pointer to the duct in a difficult dissection (Cattell & Braasch 1959). Crossing the duct anteriorly just below this point, behind the duodenum, is the retroduodenal artery (Fig. 1.5), a large vessel which supplies the duct and which can be the source of dangerous operative haemorrhage (Edwards 1941, Henley 1955). It arises from the gastroduodenal artery, which runs parallel to the duct behind the duodenum, about 1 cm to its left (Bradley 1973); this constant relation aids avoidance of the duct during gastrectomy.

The termination of the common duct at the duodenal papilla is normally found on the posteromedial wall of the descending duodenum. In about 5% the papilla is in the third part of the duodenum, but very rarely proximal to its normal position (Lindner et al 1976). When performing sphincterotomy or sphincteroplasty it is therefore best to begin the duodenotomy at the midpoint of the second part and proceed distally — the commonest error is to begin too proximally (Kune & Sali 1980).

Bile duct blood supply

Generally, failure to take account of the blood supply of an organ at operation can lead to disastrous complications (Michels 1955). However, the blood supply of the bile duct has received scant attention from surgeons and anatomists alike, almost certainly because the duct survives routine surgical intervention in the overwhelming majority of cases, despite this lack of surgical cognisance. Notwithstanding, is the bile duct really immune from damage to its blood supply? It is intriguing and clinically relevant to speculate on the possibility that the vessels supplying the duct can be damaged, and that such damage can sometimes lead to postoperative problems, including duct strictures. The largest recently published series of postoperative strictures (958 cases from the Lahey Clinic) included 648 (67%) patients in whom the lesion developed after apparently uneventful cholecystectomy (Warren et al 1971). Did the primary surgeons not notice direct duct trauma, or perhaps fail to record it, or was some occult factor responsible in at least some of the cases? Is it possible, for instance, that inadvertant damage to bile duct blood supply occurred sometimes with unexpected, though nonetheless disastrous, consequences?

While accepting that direct trauma to the ducts is the commonest cause of stricture, the present authors contend that the need to answer such questions requires a more general understanding of bile duct blood supply and further investigation of its clinical importance.

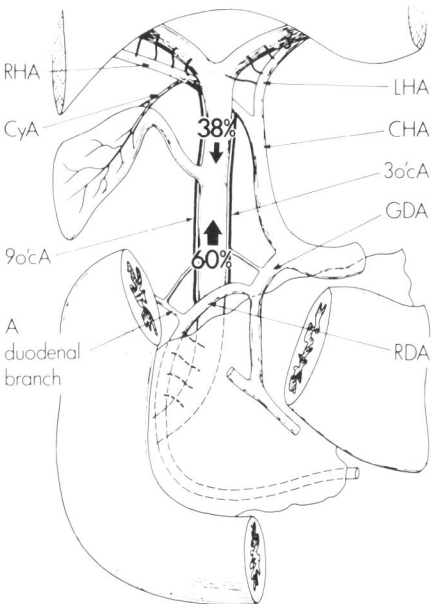

Fig. 1.5 Patterns of arterial supply of the extrahepatic bile ducts. This schematic drawing demonstrates the axial pattern of arterial supply of the supraduodenal common duct and the 'lateral' supply of the LHD, RHD and retropancreatic common duct. The 3 o'clock and 9 o'clock arteries (approx 0.3 mm diameter) form the skeleton of the pericholedochal plexus (not shown); these vessels usually arise from the RHA above and RDA below, with tributaries from other nearby vessels (e.g. GDA, CyA). The majority (approx 60%) of vessels supplying the supraduodenal duct reach it from below; in the occasional individual a vessel reaches the duct laterally from the CHA (2% of average total supply). The hilar and retropancreatic ducts have a more secure supply by short vessels arising from the nearby major trunks (N.B. The important retroportal artery behind the duct is not shown — see Figure 1.6). CHA = Common hepatic artery; GDA = Gastroduodenal artery. See Figure 1.6 for key to remaining abbreviations.

Arterial supply

Until recently, the basic pattern of bile duct arterial blood supply was ill-understood. Several authors had reported that the duct was supplied by end-arteries and was thus vulnerable to devascularisation (Shapiro & Robillard 1948, Michels 1955, Pforringer 1971), while others had suggested the presence of a dense plexus around the duct, making ischaemic injury unlikely after even the most vigorous dissection (Douglass & Cutter 1948, Munkacsi & Siklos 1960, Parke et al 1963). Recent studies have confirmed and more precisely described the pericholedochal arterial plexus, but the consequences of damage to it remain a matter for conjecture (Northover & Terblanche 1979, Northover 1980).

The pattern of supply of the supraduodenal duct (i.e. that segment between the hepatic duct confluence and the first part of the duodenum) is essentially axial (Fig. 1.5). On average, eight vessels, each about 0.3 mm diameter, arise from the major arteries related to the duct (mainly the retroduodenal artery below, and the right hepatic and cystic arteries above) and pass axially along the supraduodenal duct to join up with vessels coming from the opposite direction to form a freely anastomosing plexus. The most constant axial vessels run along the lateral borders of the duct, and have therefore been called the 3 o'clock and 9 o'clock arteries (Northover & Terblanche 1979). Another important axial vessel, the retroportal artery, runs along the posterior surface of the supraduodenal duct (Fig. 1.6). It arises from the coeliac axis or superior mesenteric artery and passes upwards behind the portal vein to reach the duct (Northover & Terblanche 1978; Northover & Terblanche 1979). In about one third of individuals it then runs up the duct to join the right hepatic artery, supplying the duct copiously en route (Fig. 1.6b), while in 50% it terminates by joining the retroduodenal artery, playing

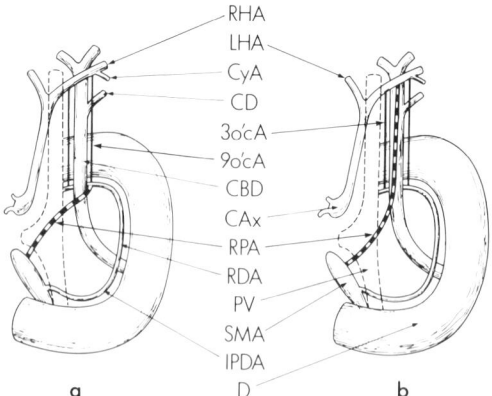

RHA
LHA
CyA
CD
3o'cA
9o'cA
CBD
CAx
RPA
RDA
PV
SMA
IPDA

a   D   b

Fig. 1.6 Main patterns of the retroportal artery (RPA). This constant vessel arises from the coeliac axis or superior mesenteric artery, passes behind the portal vein, and in 50% of individuals joins the retroduodenal artery, playing only a small part in bile duct blood supply (a). In one-third of individuals, the RPA runs up the back of the duct to join the RHA, supplying the duct copiously en route (b). In the remainder (not shown) combinations of these two patterns occur. RHA = right hepatic artery; LHA = left hepatic artery; CyA = cystic artery; CD = cystic duct; 3 o'c A = 3 o'clock artery; 9 o'c A = 9 o'clock artery; CBD = common bile duct; CAx = Coeliac axis; RPA = retroportal artery; RDA = retroduodenal artery; PV = portal vein; SMA = superior mesenteric artery; IPDA = inferior pancreatico duodenal artery; D = duodenum.

little part in supraduodenal duct blood supply (Fig. 1.6a). In other individuals a combination of these basic patterns is found.

The hilar and retropancreatic duct segments have a different pattern of supply (Fig. 1.5). These areas receive a series of short vessels which pass on to the duct surface from the major arteries running parallel with the duct; the pattern is thus lateral rather than axial.

Despite variations in the pattern of inflow into the pericholedochal plexus in the various duct segments, the plexus itself has the same conformation throughout the length of the extrahepatic duct system. The duct surface is covered by an interlacing network of arterioles approximately 0.1 mm in diameter which arises from the main axial vessels (Fig. 1.7). 'Windows' approximately 2–5 mm across lie between the vessels of the plexus. These spaces are filled by even finer vessels which arise from the plexus to pass through the wall to perfuse the mucosal capillary plexus.

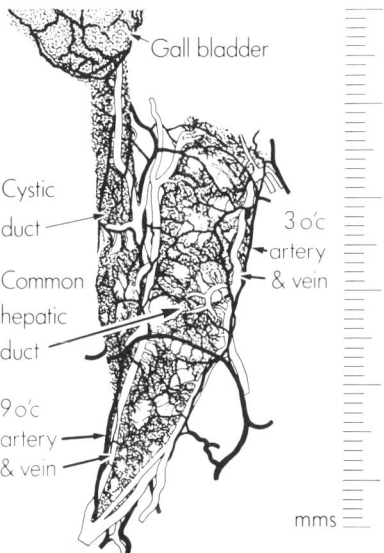

Fig. 1.7 The pericholedochal plexus. This anterior view of a resin cast of the blood vessels of the common duct and cystic duct shows the disposition of the main axial arteries and veins and their branches. Several arteries which have arisen from nearby major vessels can be seen joining the 3 o'clock and 9 o'clock arteries; the latter give rise every few millimetres to branches approximately 0.1 mm diameter which form a plexus surrounding the bile duct. In the 'windows' between these main vessels of the plexus, smaller arterioles run into the wall to perfuse the mucosal capillary plexus. Veins accompany all the arteries, although some have been omitted from this illustration for clarity.

The cystic duct is seen in this case to run parallel with the common duct in this specimen; attempts to flush-tie it would damage the 9 o'clock artery, and the large vessel joining it from the right.

Mucosal capillary plexus

A dense capillary plexus serves the pitted mucosa, made up of vessels 8–16 μm across, lying just below the surface (Fig. 1.8) (Northover et al 1980). The nature of

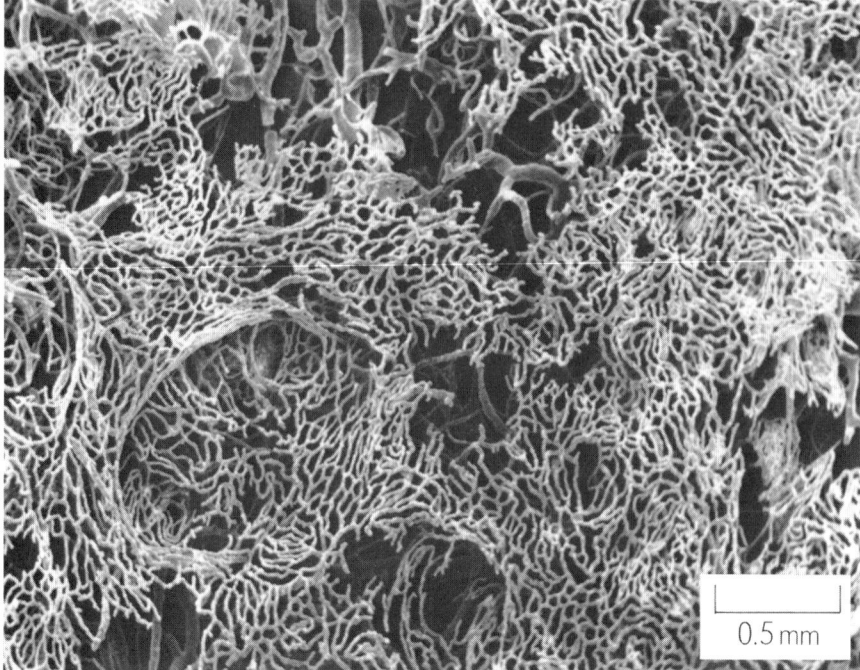

Fig. 1.8 The mucosal capillary plexus of the bile duct. This scanning electron micrograph of a resin cast of the plexus shows the dense network of capillaries in bile duct mucosa. Defects in the cast provide a view of arterioles and venules in the wall, serving the mucosal plexus.

the plexus raises the possibility that the mucosa has some dynamic function (Parke et al 1963). It has already been shown to play an active role in the secretion of bicarbonate and water into bile (Strasberg et al 1976). This remains an area for further investigation.

Venous drainage

The veins draining the bile duct correspond very closely in pattern to the arteries — each arteriole and artery is accompanied by a corresponding vein (Fig. 1.7). Recent studies (Northover & Terblanche 1981) confirm the findings of Saint, who first described an 'epicholedochal venous plexus' in 1961. The plexus drains into 3 o'clock and 9 o'clock veins which vary from 0.5–2 mm in diameter, running along the borders of the duct, separating the latter from the corresponding arteries. The veins draining the gallbladder normally empty into this venous system, (Douglas et al 1950, Saint 1961, Northover & Terblanche 1981) and not directly into the portal vein, as suggested by several standard texts (Last 1964, Kune & Sali 1980, Gray's Anatomy 1980).

Veins draining the first part of the duodenum can often be seen ramifying in front of the lower supraduodenal duct; the 3 o'clock and 9 o'clock veins connect with vessels below, while above they pass *directly into the liver at the hilum,* where they break up into capillaries (Petren 1932) and presumably contribute to portal triads near the hilum. It would appear, therefore, that the biliary tree has its own portal venous pathway into the liver; it is not known whether this has any hormone transport or other function.

Surgical implications

The most important surgical question relating to bile duct blood supply is: 'Can occult damage to bile duct blood supply sometimes lead to duct strictures?'

It is clear from the work of Warren and other notable biliary surgeons that, contrary to popular teaching, strictures may indeed follow uneventful cholecystectomy (Dragstedt et al 1943, Appleby 1959, Warren et al 1971, Thorbjarnarson 1975). Rarely, the whole extrahepatic biliary tree may 'disappear' after straightforward cholecystectomy (Dragstedt et al 1943, Appleby 1959), while in some cases of localised common hepatic duct strictures, intramural fibrosis develops *well below* the obvious narrowing (Kune & Sali 1980). In each of these circumstances factors other than localised, overt trauma to the duct wall must be involved. Moreover, an explanation is required for the fact that the common duct can be opened *vertically* and closed after exploration with impunity, while accidental, clean transection and reanastomosis may lead to stricture. Finally, why has liver transplantation been plagued until recently with major bile duct healing complications after simple duct-to-duct anastomosis (Starzl et al 1976, Calne 1976)?

There is now good laboratory evidence that bile can have a devastating effect on collagen in the bile duct wall (Carlson et al 1977) especially when the duct is ischaemic (McMaster 1979, Starzl & Koep 1980). It seems highly likely that a bile duct rendered ischaemic at operation will be damaged by the cytolytic and collogenolytic effects of bile.

The present authors have clearly shown that the supraduodenal duct has an axial blood supply via long, very narrow arteries (Northover & Terblanche 1979). Axial incision of the supraduodenal duct, i.e. standard exploratory choledochotomy, should have a minimal effect on bile duct blood supply (Fig. 1.9a). However, the axial pattern of supply renders the duct vulnerable to ischaemia if dissection around it, especially at its lateral borders, strips the pericholedochal plexus (Fig. 1.9d). High or low transection may well alter fundamentally the haemodynamics within the plexus (Fig. 1.9b and 1.9c), sometimes affecting the viability of the cut ends, especially in the presence of bile. This would explain the dangers involved in accidental duct transection and in duct-to-duct anastomosis after liver transplantation, or in duct-enteric anastomosis after pancreatic resection (Monge et al 1964, Gilsdorf & Spanos 1973). Alterations in the technique of biliary anastomosis after liver transplantation in an attempt to conserve bile duct blood supply have contributed to a major decrease in biliary complications (McMaster 1979, Terblanche et al 1979). Minimal mobilisation of the bile duct, especially when repairing the strictured duct, is now advocated on the basis of the new anatomical data (Bolton et al 1980), while the present authors recommend high CHD transection for duct-enteric anastomosis after pancreatic resection.

In summary, there is sufficient evidence to suggest that care should be taken at operation to preserve bile duct blood supply as one of the routine precautions to

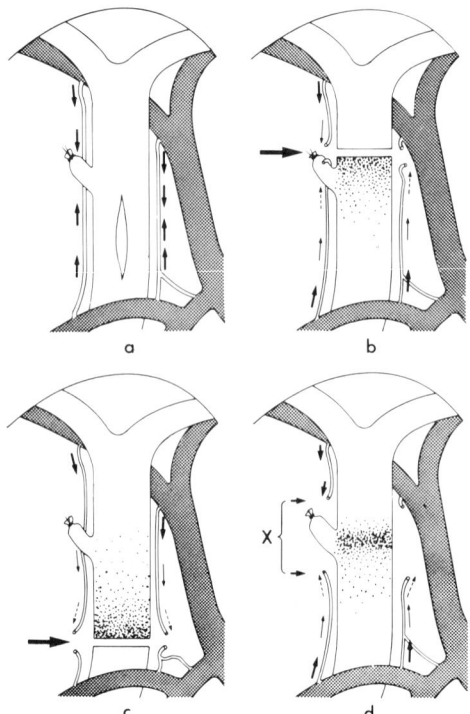

Fig. 1.9 Possible vascular consequences of (a) vertical choledochotomy (b) high, and (c) low common duct transection, and (d) vigorous dissection (in area X) around the common duct. By virtue of the axial pattern of arterial supply, vertical choledochotomy (a) should have little effect on perfusion of the duct wall, so that such an incision will heal without problems. On the other hand, division of the common duct and its axial blood supply at the sites shown in examples (b) and (c) will produce a long segment of duct supplied from one end only. Similarly, dissection sufficient to strip the axial vessels around the common hepatic duct (d) will have vascular consequences similar to example (b). Do these manoeuvres lead to relative ischaemia (stippled areas in Figure) with occasional failure of anastomotic healing, or stricture formation in some individuals? We can only speculate at present.

prevent damage to the duct. Fortuitously, the practice of many surgeons already includes such measures (minimal dissection around the common duct, no special attempts to flush-tie the cystic duct, which might strip the 9 o'clock artery, etc). It appears, however, that exhaustive display of the supraduodenal duct and flush-tying of the cystic duct remain key steps in the teaching of cholecystectomy in some surgical schools (Bolton et al 1980). There is no direct clinical evidence that such practice causes unexpected postoperative strictures, but in view of the anatomical data presented in this chapter, its continued use requires objective justification.

Acknowledgements

Financial support was received from the Medical Research Council and the Staff Research Fund of the University of Cape Town. J. M. A. Northover received a travel grant from the Ethicon Fund.

References

Appleby L H 1959 Indwelling common duct tubes. Journal of the International College of
   Surgeons 31: 631–643

Ashby B S 1965 Acute and recurrent torsion of the gallbladder. British Journal of Surgery
   52: 182–184

Balasegarem M 1970 Hepatic surgery: present and future. Annals of the Royal College of
   Surgeons of England 47: 139–157

Benson E A, Page R E 1976 A practical reappraisal of the extrahepatic bile ducts. British Journal
   of Surgery 63: 853–860

Blakiston's New Gould Medical Dictionary 1972 3rd edn. McGraw-Hill, New York

Bolton J S, Braasch J W, Rossi R L 1980 Management of benign biliary strictures. Surgical
   Clinics of North America 60: 313–332

Boyden E A 1935 Phrygian cap in cholecystography; congenital anomaly of the gallbladder.
   American Journal of Roentgenology 33: 589–602

Bradley R L 1973 Surgical anatomy of the gastroduodenal artery. International Surgery 58:
   393–396

Brewer G E 1900 Some observations upon the surgical anatomy of the gallbladder and bile ducts.
   In: Contributions to the science of medicine, dedicated by his pupils to William Henry Welch.
   Johns Hopkins Press, Baltimore, p 337–354

Calne R Y 1976 A new technique for biliary drainage in orthotopic liver transplantation utilising
   the gallbladder as a pedicle graft conduit between the donor and recipient common bile ducts.
   Annals of Surgery 184: 605–609

Carlson E, Zukoski C F, Campbell J, Chvapil M 1977 Morphologic, biophysical and biochemical
   consequences of ligation of the common biliary duct in the dog. American Journal of Pathology
   86: 301–312

Cattell R B, Braasch J W 1959 Primary repair of benign strictures of the bile duct. Surgery
   Gynecology and Obstetrics 109: 531–538

Chilton C P, Mann C V 1980 Drainage after cholecystectomy. Annals of the Royal College of
   Surgeons of England 62: 60–65

Daseler E H, Anson B J, Hambley W C, Reimann A F 1947 The cystic artery and constituents
   of the hepatic pedicle. A study of 500 specimens. Surgery Gynecology and Obstetrics 85: 47–63

Douglas B E, Baggenstoss H E, Hollinshead W H 1950 The anatomy of the portal vein and its
   tributaries. Surgery Gynecology and Obstetrics 91: 562–575

Douglass T C, Cutter W W 1948 Arterial blood supply of the common bile duct. Archives of
   Surgery 57: 599–612

Dowdy G 1969 The biliary tract. Lea and Febiger, Philadelphia

Dragstedt L R, Julian O C, Allen J G, Owens F M 1943 Implantation of the hepatic duct into
   the duodenum or stomach. Surgery Gynecology and Obstetrics 77: 126–129

Edwards L F 1941 The retroduodenal artery. Anatomy Record 81: 351–355

Flint E R 1923 Abnormalities of the right hepatic, cystic and gastroduodenal arteries, and of the
   bile ducts. British Journal of Surgery 10: 509–519

Friend E 1929 Abnormalities of the bile ducts and their blood vessels and their surgical
   significance. Illinois Medical Journal 56: 169–180

Gilsdorf R B and Spanos P 1973 Factors influencing morbidity and mortality in
   pancreaticoduodenectomy. Annals of Surgery 177: 332–337

Glenn F and Grafe W R 1966 Historical events in biliary tract surgery. Archives of Surgery
   93: 848–852

Gray's Anatomy 1980 Williams P L, Warwick R (eds) 36th edn. Churchill Livingstone,
   Edinburgh

Hayes M A, Goldenberg I S, Bischop C C 1958 The developmental basis of bile duct anomalies.
   Surgery Gynecology and Obstetrics 107: 447–456

Healey J E, Schroy P C 1953 Anatomy of the biliary ducts within the human liver. Archives of
   Surgery 66: 599–616

Henley F A 1955 The blood supply of the common bile duct and its relationship to the
   duodenum. British Journal of Surgery 43: 75–80

Hjortsjo C H 1951 The topography of the intrahepatic duct system. Acta Anatomica
   11: 599–615

Hobsley M 1958 Intrahepatic anatomy. A surgical evaluation. British Journal of Surgery
   45: 635–644

Jackson J B, Kelly T R 1964 Cholecystohepatic ducts: case report. Annals of Surgery
   150: 581–584

Johnston E V, Anson B J 1952 Variations in the formation and vascular relationships of the bile ducts. Surgery Gynecology and Obstetrics 94: 669–686

Kune G A 1970 The influence of structure and function in the surgery of the biliary tract. Annals of the Royal College of Surgeons of England 47: 78–91

Kune G A, Sali A 1980 The practice of biliary surgery. 2nd edn. Blackwell Scientific Publications, Oxford

Last R J 1964 In: Smith R, Sherlock S (eds) Surgery of the gallbladder and bile ducts. Butterworth, London

Leslie D R 1968 The width of the common bile duct. Surgery Gynecology and Obstetrics 126: 761–764

Lichtenstein M E, Nicosia A J 1955 The clinical significance of accessory hepatobiliary ducts. Annals of Surgery 141: 120–124

Lindner H H, Pena V A, Ruggeri R A 1976 A clinical and anatomical study of anomalous terminations of the common bile duct into the duodenum. Annals of Surgery 184: 626–632

McMaster P 1979 Bile studies after liver transplantation. Annals of the Royal College of Surgeons of England 61: 435–440

Maingot R 1980 Abdominal operations. 7th edn. Appleton-Century-Crofts, New York

Michels N A 1955 The blood supply and anatomy of the upper abdominal organs; with a descriptive atlas. J B Lippincott, Philadelphia

Monge J J, Judd E S, Gage R P 1964 Radical pancreaticoduodenectomy: a 22-year experience with complications, mortality rate and survival rate. Annals of Surgery 160: 711–722

Moosman D A, Coller F A 1951 Prevention of traumatic injury to the bile ducts. American Journal of Surgery 82: 132–143

Munkacsi I, Siklos I 1960 Blood supply of the common bile duct. Acta morphologica Academiae Scientiarum Hungaricae 10: 179–187

Neuhof H, Bloomfield S 1945 The surgical significance of an anomalous cholecystohepatic duct. Annals of Surgery 122: 260–265

Northover J M A 1980 The anatomy of bile duct arterial supply and its surgical implications. MS Thesis, University of London

Northover J M A, Terblanche J 1978 Bile duct blood supply — its importance in human liver transplantation. Transplantation 26: 67–69

Northover J M A, Terblanche J 1979 A new look at the arterial supply of the bile duct in man and its surgical implications. British Journal of Surgery 66: 379–384

Northover J M A, Terblanche J 1981 Unpublished data

Northover J M A, Williams E D F, Terblanche J 1980 The investigation of small vessel anatomy by scanning electron microscopy of resin casts. A description of the technique and examples of its use in the study of the microvasculature of the peritoneum and bile duct wall. Journal of Anatomy 130: 43–54

Parke W W, Michels N A, Ghosh G M 1963 Blood supply of the common bile duct. Surgery Gynecology and Obstetrics 117: 47–55

Petren T, Karlmark E 1932 Veins of the extrahepatic biliary system. Verhandlungen der anatomischen Gesellschaft 41: 139–143

Pforringer L 1971 Die arterielle versorgung des ductus choledochus. Acta anatomica 79: 389–408

Saint J H 1961 The epicholedochal venous plexus and its importance as a means of identifying the common duct during operations on the extrahepatic biliary tract. British Journal of Surgery 48: 489–498

Shapiro A L, Robillard G L 1948 The arterial supply of the common and hepatic bile ducts with reference to the problems of common duct injury and repair. Surgery 23: 1–11

Starzl T E, Koep L J 1980 Transplantation of the human liver. In: Maingot R (ed) Abdominal operations 7th edn. Appleton-Century-Crofts, New York

Starzl T E, Porter K A, Putnam C W et al 1976 Orthotopic liver transplantation in ninety-three patients. Surgery Gynecology and Obstetrics 142: 487–505

Sutton J P, Sachatello C R 1967 The confluence stone: A hazardous complication of biliary tract disease. American Journal of Surgery 113: 719–722

Terblanche J, Koep L J, Starzl T E 1979 Liver transplantation. Medical Clinics of North America 63: 507–521

Thorbjarnarson B 1975 Surgery of the biliary tract. Saunders, Philadelphia

Warren K W, Mountain J C and Midell A I 1971 Management of strictures of the biliary tract. Surgical Clinics of North America 51: 711–731

Williams C, Williams A M 1955 Abnormalities of the bile ducts. American Surgeon 141: 598–605

Wood McD 1979 Eponyms in biliary tract surgery. American Journal of Surgery 138: 746–754

2 Gallstone dissolution present and future

JAMES McK. WATTS, JAMES TOOULI
and MALCOLM J. WHITING

Introduction

The treatment of human gallstones by dissolution has fascinated medical practitioners, alchemists and charlatans for centuries. Claims of successful dissolution of gallstones by oral medication are found throughout recorded history (Rains 1964). Commonly used agents were purgatives, olive oil and mixed bile salts, usually given in large doses over short periods. There is no evidence that these methods were successful and it is likely that many patients in whom success was claimed did not have gallstones in the first place. Rewbridge in 1937 was first to document successful dissolution of human gallstones. He reported dissolution of gallstones in two out of five patients using prolonged administration of mixed bile salts and olive oil.

Modern interest in gallstone dissolution began in the early 1970s with reports of successful gallstone dissolution following prolonged treatment with the orally administered primary bile acid chenodeoxycholic acid (Danzinger et al 1972). At the same time, chemical techniques were also developed for dissolution of gallstones left in the common bile duct following biliary surgery (Way et al 1972).

Cholesterol solubility in bile

Most gallstones in patients from developed countries are composed principally of cholesterol (Sutor & Wooley 1971). Cholesterol is excreted by the liver into bile and is maintained in solution by the formation of soluble mixed micelles with phospholipid and bile salts (McBain 1913). In 1968 Admirand & Small defined the relationship between cholesterol, phospholipid and bile salts by expressing their relative molar proportions on triangular coordinates (Fig. 2.1). By estimation of the relative lipid composition of any bile sample (of between 5 and 15% solid content), it is possible to represent the bile sample as a point within the triangle. Studies have defined two lines at the base of the triangle which define the maximum relative molar concentration of cholesterol which remains in micellar solution at various concentrations of phospholipid and bile acids (Hegardt & Dam 1971, Holzbach et al 1971, Carey & Small 1978). At

17

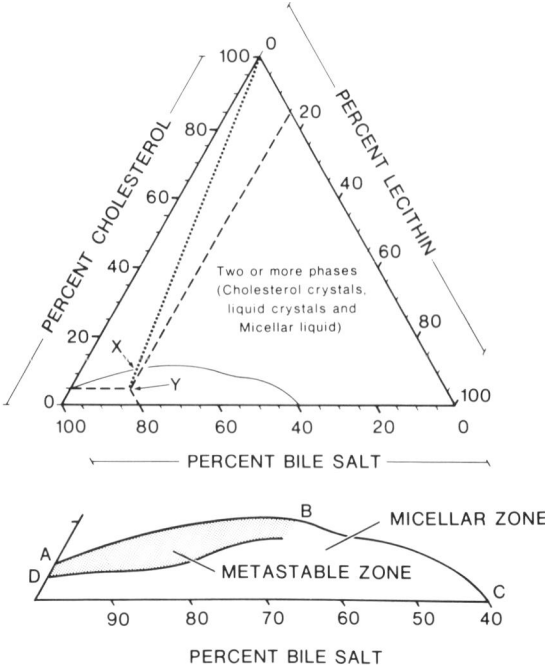

Fig. 2.1 The three biliary lipids plotted as mole percentages on triangular co-ordinates. On the upper diagram, point Y represents a bile with 15% phospholipid (lethicin), 80% bile salt and 5% cholesterol and is within the micellar zone. The dotted line connecting Y to the apex of the triangle intersects at point X the line of maximum solubility of cholesterol as defined by Admirand & Small (1968). To calculate the saturation index of the bile represented by Y, the actual mole percent cholesterol is divided by the mole percent cholesterol at point X, to give a value of 0.56.

The expanded lower diagram shows a line DBC which indicates the true equilibrium solubility line of bile (Hegart & Dam 1971, Holzbach et al 1971). Bile with a lipid composition represented by a point between ABC and DBC lies within a metastable zone where cholesterol may require nucleating factors to precipitate from solution. It is usual to calculate the saturation index using the line DBC and not ABC.

points above the upper line, the bile is supersaturated and cholesterol is likely to come out of solution, as free cholesterol crystals. At points below the lower line, cholesterol dissolves to form soluble micelles in combination with phospholipid and bile salt. The region between the two lines is known as the metastable zone (Carey & Small 1978). Cholesterol in bile with a lipid composition falling within this zone will precipitate slowly from solution and a nucleating agent may be required to initiate this process.

Cholesterol saturation in bile also may be mathematically expressed as a saturation index (Metzger et al 1978, Thomas & Hofmann 1973). This is a ratio of the actual amount of cholesterol in any bile sample to the maximum amount of cholesterol that can be dissolved in that sample. Therefore, bile samples which have a composition represented by a point which lies below the equilibrium line as drawn on the triangular co-ordinates have a saturation index of less than 1, a sample lying on the line has an index of 1 and a sample above the line has a saturation index of greater than 1.

Gallstone dissolution

Alterations in bile composition which reduce the relative molar proportion of cholesterol to phospholipid and bile salt should lead to stone dissolution. In vitro experiments of placing human cholesterol gallstones in bile salt and bile salt plus lecithin solutions have demonstrated that dissolution of cholesterol from gallstones occurs if the stone is immersed in solutions unsaturated with cholesterol (Toouli et al 1975a). Dissolution of cholesterol stones in the gallbladder has been achieved by oral administration of bile salts (Danzinger et al 1972). Cholesterol gallstones in the common bile duct have been dissolved both by oral ingestion of bile salts (Suc et al 1981) and by direct infusion of concentrated bile salt solutions (Way et al 1972, Toouli et al 1974).

Oral agents used for gallstone dissolution therapy

1. Chenodeoxycholic acid

Chenodeoxycholic acid (CDCA) was the first effective agent reported for oral gallstone dissolution therapy (Danzinger et al 1972). It is the established agent for medical treatment of gallstones and is available on prescription by the medical profession in Europe and Australia.

a. Mechanism of action

Patients with cholesterol gallstones have a smaller bile acid pool than normal people (Vlahcevic et al 1970). The effect of CDCA in dissolving gallstones was at first thought to be due to an expansion of the pool of this bile acid and a relative increase in the biliary secretion of bile acids and phospholipids over cholesterol, thereby desaturating bile and leading to conditions where dissolution may occur. Although this theory has been shown to be incorrect, the exact mechanism of action of CDCA in desaturating bile is still unclear (Andersen 1979). The current explanation for the observed reduction in biliary cholesterol secretion during CDCA treatment is that CDCA suppresses the activity of 3-hydroxy-3-methyl glutaryl CoA (HmGCoA) reductase, the rate limiting enzyme of hepatic cholesterol synthesis. Liver biopsies taken from gallstone patients show reduced activity of this enzyme after CDCA treatment (Coyne et al 1976, Maton et al 1980). However, it is doubtful whether secretion of cholesterol into bile is closely linked to the rate of hepatic synthesis (Andersen 1979) and other mechanisms of action of CDCA are still plausible. One postulated mechanism is alteration in cholesterol absorption from the intestine during CDCA therapy (Ponz de Leon et al 1979).

b. Treatment efficacy

Gallbladder stones. Since its introduction in 1970 (Danzinger et al 1972), chenodeoxycholic acid has been administered to thousands of patients around the world. A number of trials have been carried out to determine its efficacy (Table 2.1).

Table 2.1 Results of treatment with chenodeoxycholic acid.

Series	Number of patients	Dose	Complete dissolution	Partial dissolution	Total response
Maton et al 1982	125	13–15 mg/kg per d	47(38%)	7(6%)	54(43%)
Watts and Iser 1982	94	15 mg/kg per d	30(32%)	13(14%)	43(46%)
Schoenfield et al 1981	305	750 mg/d	41(14%)	83(27%)	124(41%)
	306	375 mg/d	15(5%)	56(18%)	72(24%)
	305	placebo	2(1%)	31(10%)	33(11%)

In a study by Maton et al (1982), 125 patients with radiolucent stones were treated with CDCA (13–15 mg/kg per d). The diameter of the stones was less than 15 mm in most patients. In 47 patients (38%), complete dissolution of the stones was recorded. Considering the results in retrospect, the success rate for dissolution was better than at first apparent, as 21 patients withdrew from the study before completing six months treatment. If these 21 patients are excluded from the analysis the complete dissolution rate was 45%. Furthermore, if patients whose bile did not become unsaturated during treatment also are excluded from the analysis, then the complete dissolution rate was 78%. The median duration of treatment for complete dissolution was 7.5 months for stones <5 mm in diameter, 12 months for stones 5–10 mm in diameter and 22 months for stones 10–15 mm in diameter.

In a similar study carried out at two centres in Australia (Watts & Iser 1982), 94 patients with radiolucent gallstones were treated with CDCA (15 mg/kg per d) for 6 months or more. The complete dissolution rate in all patients was 32%. In patients with stones less than 15 mm in diameter the dissolution rate was 42% and in patients with stones less than 5 mm in diameter, the complete dissolution rate was 66%.

Results from the large American National Co-operative gallstone study have been published recently (Schoenfield et al 1981). This multicentre study involved 916 patients with radiolucent stones. Patients were allocated randomly to three treatment groups; CDCA 750 mg/d, CDCA 375 mg/d and placebo. After two years treatment, complete dissolution for each treatment group was as follows: 14% (750 mg/d), 5% (375 mg/d) and 1% (placebo). Included in the analysis were 15% of the total group who for various reasons failed to complete the course of treatment. Dissolution occurred more frequently in women, thin patients, patients with small or floating gallstones and patients with serum cholesterol greater than 227 mg/dl. When compared to the studies done in England and Australia, the American results appear to suggest a lower dissolution efficacy for CDCA. Two possible explanations may account for the lower efficacy. In the American trial, the daily dose of CDCA was fixed so that most of the patients did not receive the larger doses of 13–15 mg/kg per d employed in the other trials. In addition, females under the age of 40 years were excluded from the American study but not from either the English or Australian trials. From our experience, younger women have a high prevalence of small radiolucent stones which are very amenable to dissolution.

The results in these three studies indicate that even in carefully selected patients, prolonged therapy with CDCA is often unsuccessful in achieving complete gallstone dissolution. Nevertheless, with careful selection of patients an acceptable rate of dissolution can be achieved.

Common duct stones. There is little information about the efficacy of CDCA for the treatment of radiolucent stones in the common bile duct. In a recently reported study by Sue et al (1981) 13 patients with radiolucent stones in the common bile duct were randomized into two groups of CDCA 750 mg/d or placebo. After four months treatment those patients given placebo were then changed to CDCA 750 mg/d. Five of the 13 patients did not complete the study and required surgery for acute symptoms. Of the eight patients who completed the study, two of the three who received CDCA initially for six to eight months showed complete dissolution of the stones; all five patients who took the placebo failed to show dissolution. One of these patients subsequently had dissolution of the stones following eight months of CDCA. From this study it is clear that common duct stones can dissolve during therapy with CDCA. However, the high incidence of obstructive symptoms due to stones in the common duct often prevents prolonged treatment with CDCA. Dissolution therapy may be employed usefully in a patient with recurrent intrahepatic cholesterol stones as an alternative to multiple and hazardous surgical procedures. We have treated one such man for over 10 years. In that time, the radiolucent intrahepatic stones have dissolved and there has been no recurrence of symptoms.

c. Factors influencing the efficacy of treatment

Stone composition. Stones rich in cholesterol content are most suitable for dissolution therapy with CDCA. These stones appear radiolucent on oral cholecystograms. However, a potential error exists in assuming that all radiolucent stones are rich in cholesterol. This error has been estimated to be between 14 and 20% (Bell et al 1975, Trotman et al 1975), and must account for some of the treatment failures. In a study of the gallstones of 14 patients who had been unsuccessfully treated with CDCA for at least six months, we found that the stones of two patients were pigment in type (Whiting et al 1980). While there is at present no completely accurate way of distinguishing patients with cholesterol stones from those with pigment stones, careful analysis of radiographic features (Dolgin et al 1981), and microscopic examination of duodenal bile for cholesterol crystals or pigment granules (Sedaghat & Grundy 1980, Whiting et al 1982), may solve this problem in the future.

Apart from pigment stones, it is possible that some radiolucent gallstones of high cholesterol content will not respond to treatment due to the presence of calcium salts on their surface (Whiting et al 1980), forming a thin dissolution-resistant covering.

Stone size. In all reported studies (Maton et al 1982, Watts & Iser 1982, Schoenfield et al 1981, Toouli et al 1980, Iser et al 1975), it has been shown that stone size influences the dissolution rate. The larger the stone, the smaller the surface available for dissolution in relation to stone volume. Small radiolucent stones which float in the gallbladder when visualized by oral cholecystography are usually composed of cholesterol. These stones because of their small size and high cholesterol content, have a higher dissolution rate than other stones (Schoenfield et al 1981).

The efficacy of CDCA in stones greater than 15 mm in diameter is so poor and the time taken for dissolution so long that, except in very unusual circumstances, dissolution therapy should not be contemplated. Furthermore, large stones are probably older than small stones, the cholesterol is tightly packed and they are more likely to contain calcium-rich rings inhibiting dissolution (Wolpers 1974).

CDCA dose. Although there may be individual variations in response to CDCA, the overall response is dose-related (Maton et al 1982, Watts & Iser 1982, Schoenfield et al 1981, Iser et al 1975). The optimal dose appears to be in the range of 13–15 mg/kg per d. At this dose, a small proportion of patients have troublesome diarrhoea.

Treatment duration. Provided that the stones are capable of being dissolved, a response to therapy is almost always observed after six to nine months (Maton et al 1982, Schoenfield et al 1981) of treatment. Therefore, treatment should not be prolonged unless there is a definite reduction in stone volume after nine months (Schoenfield et al 1981).

Obesity. Most reported studies (Maton et al 1982, Watts & Iser 1982, Schoenfield et al 1981, Iser et al 1978) have shown that obesity may lead to difficulty with bile desaturation and dissolution of stones. Dosage schedules which are based on body weight have recognised this 'resistance' to chenodeoxycholic acid therapy in the overweight patient and some patients greater than 130% of ideal body weight had supersaturated bile even if chenodeoxycholic acid was given at 15 mg/kg per d (Iser et al 1978). Higher doses are probably necessary in obese patients.

d. Side effects due to treatment with chenodeoxycholic acid

Diarrhoea. This is by far the most common side effect of oral CDCA treatment and occurs in more than one half of the treated patients (Maton et al 1982). It is dose related and always responds to temporary cessation of treatment. The severity of diarrhoea is rarely sufficient to stop treatment and with continuation of treatment ultimately adaptation usually occurs after two to three months. The diarrhoea may cease altogether or may occur episodically perhaps every 10–14 days for a few hours.

The cause of diarrhoea is unabsorbed bile acid in the colon and this occurs when the ability of the small intestine to absorb bile acid is exceeded. Presumably, improvement in the diarrhoea after a time is related to more efficient bile acid absorption in the terminal ileum.

Liver transaminase abnormalities. When chenodeoxycholic acid therapy was first introduced, there was considerable anxiety that this bile acid or its bacterial metabolite, lithocholic acid, might cause liver damage in man. However, these fears have been largely unfounded. Lithocholic acid is toxic to the liver in many animal species (Hunt et al 1964), but in man the lithocholic acid undergoes sulphation (Palmer & Bolt 1971, Cowen et al 1975) and this is probably responsible for its lack of toxicity.

Up to one-third of patients undergoing CDCA treatment show transient rises in the serum levels of hepatic transaminases. In the US National Co-operative study (Schoenfield et al 1981), clinically significant hepatotoxicity occurred in 3% of patients treated with 750 mg/d CDCA. The mechanisms for these abnormalities are unknown and histologic and electron-microscopic studies have not revealed specific CDCA related disease (Coyne et al 1975, Bouma et al 1980, Hartmann et al 1980, Koch et al 1980). It is usual for hepatic enzyme elevations to return towards normal despite continuation of the drug. Occasionally, the elevated level persists and the drug should then be discontinued. Under these circumstances, it is important to remember that biliary obstruction may be responsible for these biochemical abnormalities.

The effect of CDCA on the liver of the human foetus is unknown and therefore CDCA is contraindicated in women capable of becoming pregnant. Studies in pregnant rhesus monkeys receiving high doses of CDCA demonstrated that this bile acid, or lithocholic acid, may cross the placenta and produce severe damage to the foetal monkey liver (Palmer & Heywood 1974).

Changes in fasting serum lipids. Since CDCA suppresses the catabolism of cholesterol to bile acids, it was predicted that prolonged administration might lead to hypercholesterolaemia and increased atherosclerosis (Small 1971). This has not proved to be the case and fasting levels of serum cholesterol and the cholesterol pool size and rate of turnover are either unchanged (Hoffman et al 1974) or serum cholesterol levels only show slight elevation (Schoenfield et al 1981). Fasting levels of serum triglyceride are lowered during CDCA therapy (Schoenfield et al 1981, Miller & Nestel 1973, Angelin et al 1978, Camarri et al 1978).

Carcinogenic potential. CDCA has now been used in man for more than ten years and no serious longterm side effects have been encountered. There is no evidence that the frequency of gastrointestinal or hepatobiliary cancer is increased in patients who have had prolonged treatment with CDCA.

Symptom response during CDCA therapy. Many patients undergoing dissolution treatment with CDCA report improvement in their symptoms. There is usually a reduction in the frequency of biliary pain and also a reduction in the frequency of the common minor gastrointestinal symptoms (e.g., bloating, flatulence and intolerance of fatty foods) which are commonly ascribed by the patient to gallstones. However, when this effect of CDCA was prospectively appraised in the US National Co-operative Study no differences in the frequency of biliary pain, dyspepsia or nausea between patients treated with CDCA and placebo were found (Schoenfield et al 1981). It is likely therefore that the symptomatic improvement during CDCA treatment is simply a placebo effect.

f. Gallstone recurrence after CDCA therapy

Recurrence of gallstones following therapy has been reported in most series (Maton et al 1982, Beker 1977, Thistle et al 1978, Iser et al 1975) (Table 2.2).

Table 2.2 Recurrence of gallstones after dissolution with CDCA.

Series	Duration of follow-up (months)	Number of patients studied	Number of patients with recurrence
Iser et al 1975	12	10	5 (50%)
Becker 1977	6	9	2 (22%)
Thistle et al 1978	6–48	15	3 (20%)
Maton et al 1982	0–60	47	14 (30%)

However, these studies must all be viewed with extreme caution, as dissolution was judged by oral cholecystography. Our experience is that oral cholecysto-graphy is quite unreliable and that ultrasound should always be employed to check complete dissolution. It is not surprising that gallstones should recur after CDCA treatment as nothing has been done to influence the abnormal mechanism leading to their formation. These recurrent stones may be redissolved by further treatment with CDCA. In this event, treatment is required in full therapeutic doses as intermittent and low dose therapy is ineffective in maintaining bile unsaturated (Iser et al 1977). Dietary modification including decreased caloric intake or the addition of bran to the diet may be useful in the prevention of recurrence, but the effect of these measures is unproven (Pomare et al 1974, Watts et al 1978). Lifelong treatment with chenodeoxycholic acid cannot be justified on economic grounds and unless simpler measures such as dietary manipulation can be shown to be effective in preventing recurrence, the usefulness of oral dissolution therapy must be limited to aged or unfit patients.

g. Protocol for CDCA therapy

For dissolution therapy to be contemplated several conditions should apply. Firstly, patients of any age or sex can be treated, but females capable of becoming pregnant must have adequate contraception. Many young patients especially females have small cholesterol stones which dissolve readily, so that further studies on this group are justified. Secondly, the patient must not have severe and persistent symptoms. This requirement is not absolute, as after taking CDCA the patient's symptoms are often improved. Thirdly, the patient must comply with treatment and be prepared to take tablets for a minimum of six to nine months when response to treatment is first assessed. Finally, the stones must be radiolucent and the largest stone must not exceed 1.5 cm. The gallbladder must opacify on oral cholecystography indicating a patent cystic duct and the ability of the gallbladder mucosa to concentrate its contents.

Patients on dissolution therapy are treated in the outpatient clinic and treatment supervision may be confined to an initial monthly and subsequent two monthly visit. An investigation plan for a patient undergoing dissolution is shown in Table 2.3. Before treatment is started, liver function tests are performed, and the patient is instructed to increase the dose gradually to the prescribed level over several days. If diarrhoea occurs, one or more doses of the drug are omitted. At one month, liver function tests are repeated. If transaminase levels are raised to more than twice normal values these tests are repeated after a further two weeks and treatment discontinued if the elevated transaminase level is still present.

Table 2.3 Recommended protocol for investigations of patients undergoing dissolution therapy
$\oplus$ = Investigation is optional

Investigation	Before treatment	4–6 weeks	6 months	12 months
Oral cholegram	+	−	+	$\oplus$
Ultrasound of gallbladder	+	−	+	+
Liver function tests	+	+	+	+
Bile sampling	$\oplus$	$\oplus$	−	−

Most treatment centres consider it valuable to be able to monitor the effectiveness of treatment by obtaining pre- and post-treatment samples of fasting gallbladder bile. The bile is obtained by duodenal intubation and stimulation of the gallbladder by intravenous cholecystokinin. The pre-treatment sample of fasting gallbladder bile also may be analysed microscopically in order to exclude some patients who are likely to have pigment stones. If pigment granules are found on microscopy and the bile saturation index is less than unity, the chances of the stones being composed of cholesterol are less than 50% (Whiting et al 1982, Bruusgaard et al 1977). Conversely, the finding of cholesterol crystals in the bile indicates a 99% probability that the stones are cholesterol in type (Whiting et al 1982). The finding of a saturation index of less than unity in the presence of multiple small radiolucent stones indicates that these stones are more likely to be composed of pigment (Bruusgaard et al 1977). Estimation of the saturation index of fasting duodenal bile after several weeks of CDCA treatment may indicate an inadequate dose of bile acid, especially in an obese patient (Iser et al 1978). However, the saturation index is subject to considerable biological variation (Whiting et al 1981), and this must be born in mind in interpreting changes in saturation index values. Furthermore, most patients do not readily tolerate repeated duodenal intubations to obtain bile.

A novel way of monitoring patient compliance during CDCA treatment has been developed by analysing serum for its CDCA content relative to the other bile acids, and predicting the percentage of CDCA present in gallbladder bile (Whiting & Watts 1980). When bile contains greater than 70% CDCA, it is usually unsaturated with cholesterol. This method has the advantage of not requiring the patient to undergo duodenal intubation, but it does require a specialised laboratory to perform the bile acid analysis.

2. Ursodeoxycholic acid

Ursodeoxycholic acid (UDCA) is the 7ß-epimer of CDCA and normally occurs in low concentrations in human bile (Fromm et al 1976). The proportion of UDCA in human bile often increases in some patients during CDCA therapy, sometimes up to 51% of the bile acid pool (Fromm et al 1976). Ursodeoxycholic acid was first isolated in the bile of polar bears (Hammarsten 1902) (Latin *ursus* = bear). Bear bile has been used in Japanese folk medicine for the cure of various gastrointestinal and hepatic ailments and was credited with making gallstones disappear. The first therapeutic trial of UDCA in man was done in Japan by Makino in 1975 (Table 2.4). He reported successful dissolution of radiolucent gallstones in five of nine patients treated with ursodeoxycholic acid for 4–12 months (Makino et al 1975).

a. Mechanism of action

Experimental studies with UDCA in the rhesus monkey indicate that its mechanism of action on bile cholesterol saturation is the same as that of CDCA (Fedorowski et al 1978). There was a similar suppresion of hepatic HMGCoA reductase after both UDCA and CDCA indicating a reduction of cholesterol synthesis and excretion into bile. UDCA, unlike CDCA, is not hepatotoxic in this species and did not produce a rise in biliary lithocholic acid.

Administration of UDCA in man was found also to suppress HMGCoA reductase (Maton et al 1977, Maton et al 1980) and produce a rise in biliary and plasma UDCA without any increase in biliary lithocholic acid (Stiehl et al 1980, Makino & Nakagowa 1978).

UDCA is a poor detergent in terms of cholesterol solubility capacity (Carey 1978), and the dissolution rate of cholesterol in vitro is significantly faster in CDCA solutions than in UDCA solutions (Igimi & Carey 1981). However, results of clinical trials with UDCA indicate this bile acid to be comparable to CDCA with respect to cholesterol gallstone dissolution in vivo (Thistle et al 1978). An explanation of this apparent paradox has recently been proposed from in vitro studies (Corrigan et al 1980), comparing cholesterol gallstone dissolution in bile acid-lecithin-solutions. Cholesterol release from the gallstones into a lecithin-UDCA containing medium continued far beyond the apparent equilibrium solubility in the isotropic phase by formation of a turbid, liquid crystalline phase (mesophase). In comparison, cholesterol release from stones in the lecithin-CDCA medium stopped once the apparent equilibrium solubility was reached.

b. UDCA dose

The dose of UDCA at which bile is consistently desaturated with cholesterol is approximately 5 mg/kg per d (Maton et al 1977, Thistle et al 1978), although desaturation may occur with a dose as low as 1.9 mg/kg per d (Nakagawa et al 1977). The optimal dose of UDCA for gallstone dissolution is unknown but it is unlikely to be very much less than the optimal dose of CDCA (15 mg/kg per d). However, definite dissolution responses have been observed at a dose of UDCA as low as 150 mg/d (2.8 mg/kg per d) (Nakagawa et al 1977).

c. Treatment efficacy

Clinical experience with the use of UDCA to treat cholesterol gallstones has been limited (Table 2.4). The largest single study was that of Ashizawa et al (1977) who treated 55 patients with radiolucent gallstones in a multicentre double blind trial for an average period of five months. Complete gallstone dissolution occurred in 29% of 24 patients on 600 mg/d, 13% of 16 patients on 500 mg/d and 7% of 15

Table 2.4 Results of treatment with UDCA

Series	Number of patients	Dose mg/d	Complete dissolution	Partial dissolution	Total response
Makino et al 1975	9	450–2000	5	0	5
Ashizawa et al 1977	24	600	7 (29%)	3 (13%)	10 (42%)
	16	150	2 (13%)	1 (6%)	3 (19%)
	15	placebo	1 (7%)	0	1 (7%)
Nakagawa et al 1977	15	600	2 (13%)	0	2 (13%)
	16	150	3 (19%)	3 (19%)	6 (38%)
	13	placebo	0	0	0
Nakayama 1980 Combined Japanese Trial	287	150–2000	53 (19%)	63 (22%)	116 (40%)
Tint et al 1981	18	1000	–	–	15 (85%)
	18	500	–	–	12 (69%)
	17	250	–	–	11 (62%)

patients on placebo. Similar results were obtained by Nakagawa et al (1977) in a separate Japanese study. The combined Japanese experience with UDCA at varying doses was summarised by Nakayama in 1980. A total of 287 patients were treated with UDCA for varying lengths of time. In 53 patients, there was complete dissolution of the stones and in 63 patients, partial dissolution was achieved, giving an overall response rate of 116 out of 287 patients (40%). The best response has been reported recently by Tint et al (1981) who treated 53 patients with doses ranging from 250–1000 mg/kg per d. A response rate of 70% was achieved where a response was defined as at least 50% decrease in stone size.

The results of treatment with UDCA are similar to those obtained with CDCA therapy, at comparable or slightly lower doses. However, a study directly comparing the two agents has not been done.

d. Side effects due to treatment with UDCA
Side effects of UDCA are uncommon. Infrequently, diarrhoea may occur when using high doses (Nakayama 1980). However, this is much less of a problem when compared to similar doses of CDCA. A study by Debougnie & Phillips (1977) demonstrated that, unlike CDCA, UDCA does not exert a secretory effect on the colon. Abnormalities in liver transaminases, serum cholesterol or serum triglyceride have not been reported during UDCA therapy (Nakagawa et al 1977, Aschizawa et al 1977, Nakayama 1980). For these reasons, UDCA is likely to replace CDCA as the drug of choice for treating cholesterol gallstones. A disadvantage is that treatment with UDCA is more expensive than CDCA at comparable doses. The reason for the difference in cost is because UDCA is synthesized from CDCA.

3. Other agents employed to dissolve gallstones
A number of other chemicals have been tried as cholesterol gallstone dissolving agents. Some of these substances have met with limited success and others with no success. However, none of these agents have been found to be as effective as either CDCA or UDCA. Clinical reports are available for the following agents: Rowachol (Bell & Doran 1979), glycerophosphate (Linscheer & Raheja 1974, Holan et al 1979), lecithin (Tompkins et al 1970), cholic acid (Thistle et al 1978), cholic acid plus lecithin (Toouli et al 1975b), phenobarbitone (Coyne et al 1975), choline (Thistle et al 1978), ß sitosterol (Thistle et al 1978) (Tangedahl et al 1977), clofibrate (Pertsemlidis et al 1974) (Thistle & Schoenfield 1971) and thyroid hormones (Faloon 1974).

Infused solutions used to promote dissolution of common bile duct stones

Retained or recurrent stones in the common bile duct may be treated by chemical solutions infused directly into the bile duct via a T-tube (Way et al 1972, Toouli et al 1974), or via a long nasobiliary tube introduced into the common bile duct in a retrograde direction through an endoscope (Witzel et al 1980). A number of solutions have been used. The most successful solutions in dissolving common duct stones have been cholic acid (Way et al 1972, Toouli et al 1974) and mono-octanoin solutions (Thistle et al 1980).

1. Cholic acid

Successful treatment of radiolucent gallstones retained in the common bile duct by infusion of 100mM sodium cholate solution was first reported in 1972 (Way et al 1972). Since that time, there have been numerous other studies demonstrating the effect of cholate infusion in treating retained stones (Toouli et al 1974, Lansford et al 1974, Britton et al 1975) (Table 2.5). The technique is simple and the prepared bile salt solution easy to administer through the T-tube by slow infusion either by an infusion pump or by gravity flow. The major side effect of this treatment is diarrhoea which is produced by concentrated bile salt entering the intestine. This symptom may be partly controlled by oral ingestion of cholestyramine (Toouli et al 1974). However, in some patients adequate control of the diarrhoea is not achieved and the treatment has to be abandoned. Most studies have demonstrated that the overall success rate in treating retained stones with cholate solutions is approximately 60%. The length of treatment is usually 7–21 days, and the treatment is usually given with the patient in hospital.

Table 2.5 Experience with cholic acid solutions for the dissolution of common bile duct stones

Series	Number of patients	Complete dissolution	Partial dissolution	Total response
Way et al 1972	22	12 (55%)	–	12 (55%)
Toouli et al 1974	30	17 (57%)	5 (17%)	22 (73%)
Lansford et al 1974	6	5 (83%)	–	5 (83%)
Britton et al 1975	7	4 (57%)	1 (14%)	5 (71%)

2. Mono-octanoin

Mono-octanoin (Capmul 8210) is a commercial emulsifying agent consisting largely of glyceryl-1-mono-octanoate and glyceryl di-octanoate. In vitro studies (Thistle et al 1980) showed that mono-octanoin rapidly dissolved cholesterol gallstones and the rate of dissolution was faster than for cholate solutions. A summary of the reported experience with mono-octanoin is presented in Table 2.6. Thistle et al (1980) successfully treated radiolucent gallstones in 10 out of 12 patients with stones retained in the common bile duct. Six of the stones were totally dissolved and four partially dissolved. Retrieval of the two stones that could not be dissolved showed that these stones were black in colour, consistent with bilirubinate stone appearance and thus not expected to dissolve.

In a larger group of patients, Jarrett et al (1981) reported complete stone dissolution in 15 of 24 patients and partial reduction in stone size in a further five patients. Although the length of treatment was not appreciably different to other studies, a reduction in time spent in hospital was achieved in nine patients by the use of portable battery-operated syringe pumps. Therefore the treatment could be administered on an outpatient basis.

Table 2.6 Experience with mono-octanoin for the dissolution of common bile duct stones

Series	Number of patients	Complete dissolution	Partial dissolution	Total response
Thistle et al 1980	12	6 (50%)	4 (33%)	10 (83%)
Witzel et al 1980	11	9	0	9 (82%)
Jarrett et al 1981	24	15 (63%)	5 (21%)	20 (83%)
Uribe et al 1981	12	6 (50%)	1 (8%)	7 (58%)

Side effects during infusion with mono-octanoin are few and appear to be related to the rate of infusion and the occurrence of transient obstruction of the common bile duct by the stone (Thistle et al 1980, Jarrett et al 1981). The main side effects consist of nausea, biliary pain and diarrhoea (Thistle et al 1980). In all reported series these side effects responded to temporary cessation of the infusion. One death has been reported (Uribe et al 1981) due to persistent diarrhoea despite cessation of the infusion.

3. Other solutions used for treating stones retained in the common bile duct

A number of other solutions have been used in attempts to treat stones retained in the common bile duct. Tissue corrosive solutions of ether (Pribrom 1939) and chloroform (Semb et al 1974) were used in early studies. However, the potentially harmful effects to the biliary tree of these solutions has precluded their further use (Best et al 1953). Heparin alone (Gardner 1973) or in combination with cholate (Christiansen et al 1977) has been advocated by a number of investigators. However, there is no good evidence that heparin actually dissolves or fragments stones. On the contrary, numerous studies have shown that stone dissolution or fragmentation does not occur when stones are immersed in heparin solutions in vitro (Hardie et al 1977, Toouli et al 1979). A simple method for eliminating small stones from the distal common bile duct has been reported by Catt et al (1974). The method consists of rapid flushing of the stones with saline. The method is successful in approximately 50% of patients with small stones situated distal to the T-tube insertion in the common bile duct. Our approach to the problem of a stone retained in the common bile duct, discovered on T-tube cholegraphy, is to attempt flushing of the stone with an infusion of normal saline. This method may succeed if the stone is less than 1 cm in diameter and situated caudad to the T-tube.

If flushing fails, the treatment options are dissolution therapy, manipulative methods for removing the stone, surgical re-exploration of the duct, or doing nothing. The latter option is unacceptable in most patients as the chances of complications from a stone retained in the common bile duct warrant its removal. If dissolution of the stone is chosen as the method of treatment, then infusion with mono-octanoin appears to be the most effective and acceptable form of treatment currently available. The use of portable infusion pumps will eliminate a long stay in hospital. However, careful monitoring is required by an intelligent patient to avoid the complications of cholangitis and/or diarrhoea.

The impact and future of dissolution therapy

Gallstone dissolution therapy has only a limited place in the management of patients with cholelithiasis or choledocholithiasis. Its place in cholelithiasis may best be illustrated by an analysis of 406 consecutive patients who presented to Flinders Medical Centre, a community general hospital in South Australia, during a 30-month period. Only 43 patients of the 406 (11%) had radiolucent stones 1 cm or less in size in a functioning gallbladder and could therefore be considered suitable for dissolution therapy. The other 363 patients were unsuitable for dissolution therapy either because the stones were radioopaque, or radiolucent but larger than 1 cm, or present in a nonfunctioning gallbladder. 35 of the 43 patients assessed to have stones suitable for dissolution underwent cholecystectomy, and in 33 of these patients the stones removed from the gallbladder were chemically analysed. Only 25 of the 33 stones were found to be high in cholesterol content and hence expected to respond to treatment. Therefore using the usually accepted clinical and radiological criteria for selecting patients for dissolution therapy a 25% error exists in predicting the suitability of stones for dissolution. From our experience we believe that only approximately 10% of gallstone patients have functioning gallbladders which contain stones that exhibit the physical and chemical characteristics required for successful dissolution treatment. These figures are probably representative of what can be achieved with gallstone dissolution therapy in Western communities given our present state of knowledge, and in countries where pigment stones are more common, oral dissolution therapy is likely to be even less rewarding.

Most of the effort in research should be directed at the detection of those patients at high risk from developing gallstones and the development of effective methods of prevention. It seems unlikely that the cost of bile acid therapy will allow it to be used for preventive treatment. Elective biliary tract surgery is now so safe that for any method of prevention to be justified, it must be cheap and effective; this is simply not the case with CDCA or UDCA at present.

Dissolution therapy will become very much more attractive if the time taken for successful dissolution can be reduced. Additives of various types to bile acid therapy are under investigation and the most promising approach is the use of accelerating substances which decrease the interfacial resistance to dissolution. There are no known dissolving agents for pigment stones, but this is not surprising as there is very little known about their chemical composition or why they occur.

The place of dissolution therapy in choledocholithiasis also is limited. Increasingly, successful techniques such as stone extraction through the T-tube tract (Mazzariello 1973) or per-endoscopic stone extraction following sphincterotomy (Safrany 1977) allow for rapid treatment of retained or recurrent common duct stones with only a short stay in hospital. Dissolution therapy for common duct stones may continue to be useful in institutions where the newer invasive techniques are not readily available and the use of portable infusion pumps in selected patients may reduce the length of hospital stay. In addition, stones of large diameter that cannot be removed through either a T-tube tract or a standard size endoscopic sphincterotomy could be reduced in diameter by infusion with mono-octanoin either through the T-tube or via a nasobiliary catheter. When the stones have reached a suitable size (less than 1.5 cm) then extraction, or crushing followed by extraction, can be attempted.

References

Admirand W H, Small D M 1968 The physiochemical basis of cholesterol gallstone formation in man. Journal of Clinical Investigation 47: 1043–1050

Andersen J M 1979 Chenodeoxycholic acid desaturates bile — but how? Gastroenterology 77: 1146–1151

Angelin B, Einarsson K, Leud B 1978 Effects of chenodeoxycholic acid on serum and biliary lipids in patients with hyperlipoproteinaemia. Clinical Science 54: 451–455

Ashizawa S, Ishii N, Ishihara F, Ito Y, Ueno Y, Osawa H, Osuga T et al 1977 A clinical study of gallstone dissolution with ursodeoxycholic acid. A controlled double blind trial. Igaku no Ayumi 101: 922–936

Beker S 1977 Treatment of cholesterol gallstones with chenic acid. A follow-up study of 25 patients. American Journal of Gastroenterology 68 (5): 456–460

Bell G D, Doran J 1979 Gallstone dissolution in man using an essential oil preparation Rowachol. British Medical Journal 1: 24

Bell G D, Dowling R H, Whitney B et al 1975 The value of radiology in predicting gallstone type when selecting patients for medical treatment. Gut 16 (5): 359–364

Best R R, Rusmussen J A, Wilson C E 1963 An evalution of solutions for fragmentation and dissolution of gallstones and their effect on liver ductal tissue. Annals of Surgery 138: 570–580

Bouma M E, Levy V G, Infante R 1980 Liver ultrastructure in cholesterolic gallstone patients before and after treatment with chenodeoxycholic acid. Gastroenterology and Clinical Biology 4: 569–576

Britton D C, Gill B S, Taylor M R, James O 1975 The removal of retained gallstones from the common bile duct; experience with sodium cholate infusion and the Burhenne catheter. British Journal of Surgery 62: 520–523

Bruusgaard A, Malver E, Pedersen L R et al 1977 Criteria for selection of patients for medical treatment (chenodeoxycholic acid therapy) of gallstones. Scandinavian Journal of Gastroenterology 12(1): 97–102

Camarri E, Fici F, Marcolongo F 1978 Influence of chenodeoxycholic acid on serum triglycerides in patients with primary hypertriglyceridaemia. International Journal of Clinical Pharmacology and Biopharmacy 16: 523–526

Carey M C 1978 Critical tables for calculating the cholesterol saturation of native bile. Journal of Lipid Research 19: 945–957

Carey M C, Small D M 1978 The physical chemistry of cholesterol solubility in bile. Journal of Clinical Investigation 61: 998–1002

Catt P, Hogg D F, Hardie I R et al 1974 Retained biliary calculi: removal by a simple non-operative technique. Annals of Surgery 180: 247–249

Christiansen L A, Scherston T, Burcharth et al 1977 Treatment of retained bile duct calculi with T tube infusion of sodium cholate and heparin. Scandinavian Journal of Gastroenterology 12: 337–339

Corrigan O L, Su C C, Higuchi W I et al 1980 Mesophase formation during cholesterol dissolution in ursodeoxycholate-lecithin solution: a new mechanism for gallstone dissolution in humans. Journal of Pharmaceutical Science 69: 869–874

Cowen A E, Korman M G, Hofmann A F et al 1975 Metabolism of lithocholate in healthy man. I Biotransformation and biliary excretion of intravenously administered lithocholate, lithocholylglycine and their sulphates. Gastroenterology 69 (1): 59–66

Coyne M J, Bonorris G G, Chunt A et al 1975 Treatment of gallstones with chenodeoxycholic acid and phenobarbital. New England Journal of Medicine 292 (12): 604–607

Coyne M J, Bonorris G G, Goldstein L I et al 1976 Effect of chenodeoxycholic acid and phenobarbital on the rate-limiting enzymes of hepatic cholesterol and bile acid synthesis in patients with gallstones. Journal of Laboratory and Clinical Medicine 87: 281–291

Danzinger R G, Hofmann A F, Schoenfield L J et al 1972 Dissolution of cholesterol gallstones by chenodeoxycholic acid. New England Journal of Medicine 286: 1–5

Debougnie J C, Phillips S F 1977 Colonic function and diarrhoea. Gastroenterology 72: 1046 (Abstract)

Dolgin S M, Schwartz J S, Kressel H Y et al 1981 Identification of patients with cholesterol or pigment gallstones by discriminant analysis of radiographic features. New England Journal of Medicine 304: 808–811

Faloon W W 1974 Gallstone prophylaxis and therapy. American Journal of Digestive Diseases 19: 81–87

Fedorowski T, Salen G, Zaki F G et al 1978 Comparative effects of ursodeoxycholic acid and chenodeoxycholic acid in the Rhesus monkey: Biochemical and ultrastructural studies. Gastroenterology 74 (1): 75–81

Fromm H, Erbler H C, Eschler A, Schmidt F W 1976 Alterations of bile acid metabolism during treatment with chenodeoxycholic acid. Studies of the role of the appearance of ursodeoxycholic acid in the dissolution of gallstones. Klinische Wochenschrift 54: 1125–1131

Gardner B 1973 Experiences with the use of intracholedochal heparinized saline for the treatment of retained common duct stones. Annals of Surgery 177: 240–244

Hammersten O 1902 Untersuchungen Über die Galle einiger Polar-Thiere. 1 Ueber die Galle des Eisbären. Zeitschrift für Physiologische Chemie 36: 525–555

Hardie I R, Green M K, Burnett W et al 1977 In vitro studies of gallstone dissolution using bile salt solutions and heparinized saline. British Journal of Surgery 64: 572–576

Hartmann W, Paulini K, Goebell H 1980 Light and electron microscopy of human liver before and during chenodeoxycholic acid therapy. Hepatogastroenterology 27: 91–98

Hegardt F G, Dam H 1971 The solubility of cholesterol in aqueous solutions of bile salts and lecithin. Zeitschrift für Ernahrungswissenschaft 10: 233–241

Hoffman H E, Hofmann A F, Thistle J L 1974 Effect of bile acid feeding on cholesterol metabolism in gallstone patients. Mayo Clinic Proceedings 49: 236–9

Holan K R, Holzbach R T, Hsieh J Y et al 1979 Effect of administration of 'essential' phospholipid, ß-glycerophosphate and linoleic acid on biliary lipids in patients with cholelithiasis. Digestion 19: 251–262

Holzbach R E, Marsh M, Holan K 1971 Cholesterol solubilizing capacity: A direct assessment of lithogenic potential in bile. Gastroenterology 60 (4): 777 (Abstract)

Hunt R D, Leveille G A, Sauberlich H E 1964 Dietary bile acids and lipid metabolism. III. Effects of lithocholic acid in mammalian species. Proceedings of the Society of Experimental Biology and Medicine 115: 277–280

Igimi H, Carey M C 1981 Cholesterol gallstone dissolution in bile: dissolution kinetics of crystalline (anhydrate and monohydrate) cholesterol with chenodeoxycholate, ursodeoxycholate and their glycine and taurine conjugates. Journal of Lipid Research 22: 254–263

Iser J H, Dowling H, Mok H Y et al 1975 Chenodeoxycholic acid treatment of gallstones. A follow-up analysis of factors influencing response to therapy. New England Journal of Medicine 293 (8): 378–382

Iser J H, Maton P N, Murphy G M, Dowling R H 1978 Resistance to chenodeoxycholic acid (CDCA) treatment in obese patients with gallstones. British Medical Journal 1: 1509–1512

Iser J H, Murphy G M, Dowling R H 1977 Speed of change in biliary lipids and bile acids with chenodeoxycholic acid —is intermittent therapy feasible? Gut 18 (1): 7–15

Jarrett L N, Balfour T W, Bell G D, Knapp D R, Rose D H 1981 Intraductal infusion of mono octanoin experience in 24 patients with retained common ductal stones. Lancet 1: 68–90

Koch M M, Giampiere M P, Lorenzini I, Jezequel A M, Orlandi F 1980 Effect of chenodeoxycholic acid on liver structure and function in man. A stereological and biochemical study. Digestion 20: 8–21

Lansford C, Mehta S, Kern F 1974 The treatment of retained stones in the common bile duct with sodium cholate infusion. Gut 15: 48–51

Linscheer W G, Raheja K L 1974 Effect of glycerophosphate on lithogenic bile. A new approach to treatment of cholelithiasis. Lancet 2: 551–553

McBain J W 1913 Mobility of highly charged micelles. Transactions of the Faraday Society 9: 99

Makino I, Nakagawa S 1978 Changes in biliary lipid and biliary bile acid composition in patients after administration of ursodeoxycholic acid. Journal of Lipid Research 19: 945–951

Makino I, Shinozaki K, Yoshinok, Nakagawa S 1975 Dissolution of cholesterol gallstones by ursodeoxycholic acid. Japanese Journal of Gastroenterology 72: 690–702

Maton P N, Ellis H J, Higgin M J et al 1980 Hepatic HMGCoA reductase in human cholelithiasis: effects of chenodeoxycholic and ursodeoxycholic acids. European Journal of Clinical Investigation 10: 325–332

Maton P N, Iser J H, Reuben A, Saxton H M, Murphy G M, Dowling R H 1982 Personal communication

Maton P N, Murphy G M, Dowling R H 1977 ursodeoxycholic acid treatment of gallstones. Dose-response study and possible mechanism of action. Lancet 2: 1297–1301

Mazzariello R 1973 Review of 220 cases of residual biliary tract calculi treated without reoperation: an eight year study. Surgery 3: 299–306

Metzger A L, Heymsfield S, Grundy S M 1972 The lithogenic index — a numerical expression for the relative lithogenicity of bile. Gastroenterology 62: 449

Miller N E, Nestel P J 1974 Triglyceride-lowering effect of chenodeoxycholic acid in patients with endogenous hypertriglyceridemia. Lancet 2: 929–931

Nakagawa S, Makino I, Ishizaki T et al 1977 Dissolution of cholesterol gallstones by ursodeoxycholic acid. Lancet 2: 367–369

Nakayama F 1980 Oral cholelitholysis —Cheno versus urso. Japanese experience. Digestive Disease and Science 25: 129–132

Palmer A K, Heywood R 1974 Pathological changes in the rhesus fetus associated with the oral administration of chenodeoxycholic acid. Toxicology 2: 239–246

Palmer R H, Bolt M G 1971 Bile acid sulphates I Synthesis of lithocholic acid sulphates and their identification in human bile. Journal of Lipid Research 12: 671–679

Pertsemlidis D, Panvelwalla D, Ahrens E H Jr 1974 Effects of clofibrate and of an estrogen-progestin combination on fasting biliary lipids and cholic acid kinetics in man. Gastroenterology 66: 565–573

Pomare E W, Heaton K W, Low-Beer T S et al 1974 Effect of wheat bran on bile salt metabolism and bile composition. Gut 15 (10): 824–825

Ponz de Leon M, Carulli N, Laric P et al 1979 The effect of chenodeoxycholic acid on cholesterol absorption in man. Gastroenterology 77: 223–230

Pribrom B O C 1939 Ether treatment of gallstones impacted in the common bile duct. Lancet 1311–1313

Rains A J H 1964 Gallstones: causes and treatment. London Heinemann Medical

Rewbridge A G 1937 Disappearance of gallstone shadows following prolonged administration of bile salts. Surgery 1: 395

Safrany L 1977 Duodenoscopic sphincterotomy and gallstone removal. Gastroenterology 72: 338–343

Schoenfield L J, Lachin J M et al 1981 Chenodiol (chenodeoxycholic acid) for dissolution of gallstones: the National Cooperative Gallstone Study. Annals of Internal Medicine 95: 257–282

Sedaghat A, Grundy S M 1980 Cholesterol crystals and the formation of cholesterol gallstones. New England Journal of Medicine 302: 1274–1277

Semb B K H, Norderral Y, Holvorsen J F 1974 The non-operative removal of retained common duct stones after biliary surgery. Acta chirurgico, Scandinavica 140: 469–474

Small D M 1971 Prestone gallstone disease — Is therapy safe? New England Journal of Medicine 284: 214–215

Stiehl A, Raedsch R, Czygan P ct al 1980 Effects of biliary bile acid composition on biliary cholesterol saturation in gallstone patients treated with chenodeoxycholic acid and/or ursodeoxycholic acid Gastroenterology 79: 1192

Sue S O, Taub M, Pearlman B J, Marks J W, Bonorris G G, Schoenfield L J 1981 Treatment of choledocholithiasis with oral chenodeoxycholic acid. Surgery 90: 32–34

Sutor D J, Wooley S E 1971 A statistical survey of the composition of gallstones in eight countries. Gut 12: 55

Tangedahl T N, Matseshe J W, Thistle J L, Hofmann A F 1977 Plant sterols increase effectiveness of chenodeoxycholic acid therapy in lowering cholesterol saturation of fasting state bile in patients with radiolucent gallstones. Gastroenterology 72 (5): A115 (Abstract)

Thistle J L, Schoenfield L J 1971 Induced alterations in composition of bile of persons having cholelithiasis. Gastroenterology 61: 488–496

Thistle J L, Carlson G L, Hofmann A F et al 1980 Monooctanoin, a dissolution agent for retained cholesterol bile duct stones: Physical properties and clinical application. Gastroenterology 78: 1016–1022

Thistle J L, Carlson G L, Larusso N F, Hofmann A F 1978 Comparison of the effects of 5 and 10 mg/kg/day of ursoedeoxycholic acid and chenodeoxycholic acid on cholesterol saturation of bile in patients with gallstones. Proceedings of V Bile Acid Meeting Falk Symposium Nr 26,14 (Abstract)

Thistle J L, Hofmann A F, Otto B J et al 1978 Chenotherapy for gallstone dissolution 1 efficacy and safety. JAMA 239 (11): 1041–1046

Thomas P J, Hofmann A F 1973 Letter: A simple calculation of lithogenic index of bile; expressing biliary lipid composition on rectangular coordinates. Gastroenterology 65: 698

Tint G S, Collallilo A, Salen G, Graber D, Shefer S 1981 Ursodeoxycholic acid is a safe and effective gallstone dissolving agent in humans. Gastroenterology 80: 1304 (Abstract)

Tompkins R K, Burk L G, Zollinger R M et al 1970 Relationship of biliary phospholipid and cholesterol concentrations to the occurrence and dissolution of human gallstones. Annals of Surgery 172: 36–45

Toouli J, Jablonski P, Watts J M 1974 Dissolution of stones in the common bile duct with bile salt solution. Australian and New Zealand Journal of Surgery 44: 334–340

Toouli J, Jablonski P, Watts J M 1975a Dissolution of human gallstones: the efficacy of bile salts plus lecithin and heparin solutions. Journal of Surgical Research 19: 47–53

Toouli J, Jablonski P, Watts J M 1975b Gallstone dissolution in man using cholic acid and lecithin. Lancet 2: 1124–1126

Toouli J, Jablonski P, Watts J M 1980 Treatment of gallstones by chenodeoxycholic acid. Medical Journal of Australia 1: 478–479

Toouli J, Williamson B W A, Gooszen H, Blumgart L H 1979 In vitro dissolution of human gallstones: the efficacy of heparinized solutions. British Journal of Surgery 66: 770–771

Trotman B W, Petrella E J, Soloway R D et al 1975 Evaluation of radiographic lucency or opaqueness of gallstones as a means of identifying cholesterol or pigment stones. Correlation of lucency or opaqueness with calcium and mineral. Gastroenterology 68 (6): 1563

Uribe M, Uscanza L, Farcer S, Sanjurio J L, Lagarrica J, Oritz J H 1981 Dissolution of cholesterol ductal stones in the biliary tree with medium chain glycerides. Digestive Disease and Sciences 26: 636–640

Vlahcevic Z R, Bell C C Jr, Buhac I et al 1970 Diminished bile acid pool size in patients with gallstones. Gastroenterology 59: 165

Watts J M, Iser J H 1982 Chenodeoxycholic acid for gallstone dissolution. Unpublished observations

Watts J M, Jablinski P, Toouli J 1978 The effect of added bran to the diet on the saturation of bile in people without gallstones. American Journal of Surgery 135: 321–324

Way L, Admirand W H, Dunphy J E 1972 Management of choledocholithiasis. Annals of Surgery 176: 347–354

Whiting M J, Watts J M 1980 Prediction of the bile acid composition of bile from serum bile acid analysis during gallstone dissolution therapy. Gastroenterology 78: 220

Whiting M J, Down R H L, Watts J M 1982 Biliary crystals and granules, the cholesterol saturation index, and the prediction of gallstone type. Surgical Gastroenterology (in press)

Whiting M J, Down R H, Watts J M 1981 Precision and accuracy in the measurement of the cholesterol saturation index of duodenal bile. Gastroenterology 80: 533–535

Whiting M J, Jarvinen V, Watts J M 1980 Chemical composition of gallstones resistant to dissolution therapy with chenodeoxycholic acid. Gut 21: 1077–1081

Witzel I, Widerholt J, Wolbergs E 1980 Dissolution of gallstones by perfusion with monooctanoin via a teflon catheter introduced endoscopically into the bile duct. Acta Hepato Gastroenterologica Suppl Abstracts of the XI International Congress of Gastroenterology Hamburg June 3–13: 276

Wolpers C 1974 Morphologie der gallenstein. Leber Magen Darm 4: 43–57

3

Diagnostic approaches in the biliary tract

N. B. BOWLEY and I. S. BENJAMIN

Introduction

Approaches to the diagnosis of biliary tract disorders have undergone considerable change during the last decade. Improvements in radiological imaging techniques have been accompanied by changes in our approach to the management of many biliary conditions. In addition, advances in the new discipline of interventional radiology have made a major impact. The aim of this chapter is to outline the currently available methods of diagnosis, and to review the way in which these methods are applied to specific clinical problems in the biliary tract.

Methods of investigation

Non-imaging methods

History and examination

A careful history and thorough physical examination may suggest the diagnosis in a large proportion of patients with biliary tract disease, and may also usefully direct the sequence of radiological investigations. The signs and symptoms of the classical syndromes of biliary and pancreatic disease have been well described. In the post-cholecystectomy case a history is particularly important, and should be directed not only to the present symptoms and their relation to the timing of previous surgery, but also to the course of events at the time of the previous operation. Previous hospital notes are valuable in this respect but are not always available, and patients' memories are unreliable. Important questions relate to whether external drainage tubes were present after the operation, whether any biliary fistula was of large volume or prolonged, and whether there was associated major infection. It must be remembered, however, that operative injury to the bile duct is recognised in only some 15–25% of patients (Maingot 1964, Way et al 1981).

Examination of the patient is important, and if repeated at frequent intervals may elicit transient or intermittent signs of value, such as the intermittently palpable gallbladder associated with periampullary carcinoma (Blumgart & Kennedy 1973). Stigmata of hepatocellular insufficiency should be sought, as these suggest either intrinsic parenchymal liver disease or the secondary effects of prolonged biliary obstruction.

Biochemical tests of liver function
The standard laboratory liver function tests will be performed as a routine in all cases of suspected biliary disease. Most of the available tests, however, are non-specific, and are more valuable in following the course of the disease in an individual patient than in providing diagnostic information. Minor changes in liver function tests should not be ignored, however, and in particular an isolated elevation in alkaline phosphatase in the absence of other evidence of liver dysfunction may be indicative of biliary obstruction. Many of the non-invasive radiological techniques, including intravenous and oral contrast studies and some forms of scintigraphy will be unsuccessful in the jaundiced patient. Thus with a bilirubin value of 70 μmol/l the diagnostic yield of intravenous cholangiography becomes negligible (Blumgart et al 1974). Dynamic tests such as the clearance of bromsulphthalein or indocyanine green may be of more value in estimating defects in hepatocellular function, but again are usually invalidated in the patient with biliary obstruction. Tests of drug metabolism are not universally available, but there is evidence that they may have predictive value in patients undergoing major biliary surgery, and are applicable in the jaundiced patient (McPherson et al 1982). Similarly, tests of reticuloendothelial function are infrequently used in routine practice but may have a specific prognostic value (see Chapter 10).

The use of computers in diagnosis
A combination of history, examination and readily available laboratory tests yields a high rate of crude diagnosis in diseases of the biliary tract. Application of Bayesian theory to the results of such tests has allowed the use of computers as so called 'expert systems' in diagnosis. Computer analysis of a range of clinical and laboratory data was able to give a correct diagnostic rate of 90% between intra- and extrahepatic obstruction, a figure which compared reasonably with results from a specialist unit, and probably represents an improvement on results obtainable in a general unit (Knill-Jones et al 1975). However, it has been shown that to a large degree the improvements obtainable by the use of computers over routine clinical questioning arise from the completeness of the data base which is elicited, rather than from superior interpretation of the data (DeDombal, personal communication). Thus the introduction of specific disease-orientated questionnaires for routine investigation of patients may direct the clinician and prevent the omission of important data, so improving clinical diagnosis.

Functional disorders of the biliary tract
This term and its various synonyms (biliary dyskinesia, Odditis) is open to wide abuse, and covers a multitude of ill defined syndromes. At its least precise this is a diagnosis of exclusion, following completely normal radiological examination of the biliary tract. Now that such examination is possible in great detail with advances in radiological technique, the syndrome must be more precisely defined. Since the common bile duct is known to have no motor role in relation to bile flow, disorders of motility must be localised to the papilla of Vater. The anatomy and

physiology of this region have now been fairly well defined (Boyden 1957, Caroli et al 1960). If one excludes congenital anomalies and neoplasms of the papilla and secondary inflammation and stenosing papillitis due to the passage of stones, the diagnosis of biliary dyskinesia resulting from spasm of the sphincter remains open to question (Moody 1981).

As far as it may be characterised the syndrome affects women more than men, and consists of episodes of upper abdominal pain which have proved refractory to biliary investigation. Such investigation must include ERCP or PTC or both, and it is important to note that small stones and debris in the biliary tract can be masked by the use of too dense a contrast medium during such cholangiography. Barium studies and upper gastrointestinal endoscopy must be performed to exclude other gastrointestinal lesions. Positive diagnosis is more difficult. The use of the morphine-prostigmine provocation test produces unreliable and non-specific results. Attempts to carry out clinically relevant manometry of the bile duct via the cannulated papilla have met with little success. Many such patients may come to laparotomy, and in these cases manometric studies are also sometimes recommended. Bismuth (1981) carried out manometric studies in an unselected series of patients undergoing operative exploration of the bile duct. Abnormal pressure-flow results were obtained in a proportion of patients, but long term follow-up demonstrated no difference in subsequent symptoms or operative results between these patients and those who had normal manometric findings. This vital piece of work casts considerable doubt on the value of such procedures. Sphincteroplasty and transampullary septectomy have been performed for such cases, following a thorough and otherwise negative abdominal exploration (Moody 1981).

The advent of endoscopic papillotomy has placed in the hands of endoscopists a technique which may be a fine instrument for some indications, but is a blunt weapon for the ill-defined syndrome of primary papillitis. The diagnosis is made with an unaccountably higher frequency on the continent of Europe than in the United Kingdom or the United States. Indications for papillotomy are difficult to define, and the long-term results uncertain.

Imaging techniques

The plain abdominal radiograph

It is customary to obtain a plain radiograph when searching for gallstones, over 10% of which are radioopaque. This is often obtained at the time the patient attends to make an appointment and receive the drugs for his oral cholecystogram, and serves as a defence against the possibility of an opaque stone being masked by contrast medium.

The advent of ultrasound has to some extent superceded the use of the plain film. There are nevertheless reasons for its retention even when ultrasound is the primary investigation of choice, and it may be of specific value when the gallbladder is not definitely identified by ultrasound.

The plain abdominal radiograph is also important in other hepatobiliary diseases. Pancreatic calcification should be carefully sought, since it is virtually diagnostic of chronic pancreatitis, and its presence may save some patients from further invasive investigations. Air in the bile ducts may be the result of many processes: its presence in a patient with dilated small bowel loops will indicate gallstone ileus, a condition which in the elderly is a common cause of small bowel obstruction. Air in the bile ducts may also be the result of a biliary-enteric anastomosis, sphincteroplasty or sphincterotomy, but its presence should not be taken to indicate adequate drainage of the biliary tree. Air or gas may also be demonstrated within the liver or subphrenic space as an indicator of abscess formation.

The oral cholecystogram

Oral cholecystography has long been held sacrosanct as a biliary investigation. There are, however, a number of problems associated with it apart from radiation and side-effects of the contrast media (Burhenne 1975). Earlier reports indicating an accuracy of over 95% for oral cholecystography were misleading since only patients with a positive study were submitted to surgery. Neverthless, such studies did indicate that false positive results were rare. What was not known was how many patients with a cholecystogram interpreted as normal had gallstones. With the availability of ultrasound we are closer to knowing this figure and studies indicate that the accuracy of oral cholecystography is closer to 85–90% (Burhenne 1975). There is therefore good reason to consider other imaging modalities in patients with symptoms highly suggestive of gallbladder disease in whom the oral cholecystogram is negative.

A second problem is impaired visualisation of the gallbladder. Gallbladder examinations are not always optimal on the first occasion and may be improved by a second study (Berk 1971). Second dose examinations are required rather too frequently, depending to some extent upon the willingness of an individual radiologist to accept a particular degree of opacification as adequate for diagnosis and to some extent on the competence with which the oral cholecystogram is performed. Reported series indicate a frequency of second dose studies ranging from 15–50% (Berk 1970, Rosenbaum 1959, Mujahed et al 1974, Stanley et al 1974).

Non-visualisation of the gallbladder occurs with an obstructed cystic duct, and some surgeons are still prepared to act on this information if the symptomatology is strongly suggestive of gallbladder disease and other situations known to cause non-visualisation are excluded. However, the causes are not completely defined and patients are seen in whom initial studies do not visualise the gallbladder but in whom second studies reveal an apparently normal gallbladder. Mujahed (1974, 1976) has reviewed the subject of the non-opacified gallbladder and lists the following extrinsic causes:

1. Faulty instructions given to the patient.
2. Failure of transfer, e.g. achalasia, gastric diverticula
3. Excessive diarrhoea and vomiting as a result of the contrast medium
4. Small intestinal resection and gastrointestinal anastomoses
5. Diseases of the small intestine (doubtful)
6. Liver disease (bilirubin over 3.5 mg/100 ml)
7. Biliary-enteric anastomoses or fistulae

8. Poor timing — radiographs are usually done 14 hours after ingestion, but this gives optimum opacification in only 15%, most patients taking longer (even up to 21 hours)
9. Cholestasis: patients on a fat-free diet have their gallbladder distended with thick bile and this is not receptive to the inflow of contrast
10. Acute pancreatitis

Most of the causes listed above are infrequent, but as Mujahed points out, together they make a significant contribution to the non-visualised gallbladder. Malabsorptive diseases of the small intestine are often quoted as causes of non-opacification, but Low-Beer & Heaton (1972) found satisfactory visualisation in 80 of 84 patients with various diseases of the small intestine: three of the remaining four had cholecystitis and cholelithiasis and the fourth was jaundiced.

A number of approaches have been suggested for an unsatisfactory oral cholecystogram apart from a second study. If during intravenous cholangiography the common duct opacifies without opacification of the gallbladder after four hours then this is said to be direct evidence of gallbladder disease (Berk 1973). However, the intravenous route is more hazardous than an oral study, very time-consuming for both X-ray department and patient, and a normal study does not reliably exclude gallstones (Mujahed et al 1974). Other approaches to the problem centre upon techniques to obviate a second study. These include double-dose studies (Burhenne & Obata 1975), administering the contrast over a six hour period rather than as a single dose (Koehler & Kyaw, 1973), and administering calcium ipodate as a reinforcement in poor studies (Besemann 1970, Crummy 1976). This last method has the advantage that the contrast is concentrated by the liver and opacifies the bile ducts. Failure to opacify the gallbladder is thus highly suggestive of disease if the bile ducts are seen (Stephens et al 1976).

Intravenous cholangiogram
With the advent of ERCP and the Chiba needle for PTC together with less invasive techniques such as ultrasound and CAT scanning, intravenous cholangiography has lost its previous eminent position. Its limitations in the jaundiced patient are well-known. In the post-cholecystectomy patient it can be very misleading and is only useful if it demonstrates a stone unequivocally. Since most surgeons with an interest in biliary surgery would in any case perform an ERCP there seems little place for intravenous cholangiography in the post-cholecystectomy patient; indeed in a specialist biliary practice we have used this investigation in only two patients in the last two years.

Ultrasound
As a method of examining the gallbladder, ultrasound has considerable appeal. It is non-invasive, non-hazardous, not affected by liver disease, may be performed at short notice, requires usually only one visit by the patient and may provide additional information about the liver, biliary tree and pancreas. Claims are made that it is expensive of highly trained personnel. However, when a broader view is taken of the savings in visits and hours lost from work by the patient these criticisms become weaker. Additionally, it appears that satisfactory results may be

obtained by non-medically qualified personnel providing equipment is good and motivation high (Russell & Davies 1981).

The overall accuracy of gallbladder ultrasound is said to be about 90% (Arnon & Rosenquist 1976) but is highly operator-dependent. Using real-time grey-scale scanning, Cooperberg & Burhenne (1980) reported a sensitivity and specificity of 98% in detecting gallstones.

Good studies may be impossible in fat patients, if bowel gas prevents an adequate acoustic window to the gallbladder or if the gallbladder is shrunken or contracted. Experience, however, can reduce the last problem since it is still possible sometimes to identify a shrunken or empty gallbladder (Marchal et al 1980) and failure to visualise at a second visit is strong evidence of gallbladder disease. Similarly, if the gallbladder is packed with stones no fluid will be seen and the acoustic shadow may be difficult to differentiate from bowel gas (Crow 1976).

Another feature sometimes seen in chronic cholecystitis is a thickened gallbladder wall. Whilst this may be seen in patients with acute or chronic cholelithiasis it may also be seen in hypoalbuminaemic patients, especially cirrhotics with ascites (Fiske et al 1980, Saunders 1980). Moreover, the normal gallbladder in its undistended or incompletely distended state will exhibit a thick wall and since the size of the gall bladder is so variable from individual to individual it becomes an unreliable sign if taken in isolation.

Many observers have noted the presence of layered bile in which the lower or more dependent layer is diffusely and homogeneously echogenic. This has been termed 'biliary sludge' (Fig. 3.1). It is frequently seen in patients not only with chronic cholecystitis but also acute cholecystitis, extrahepatic biliary obstruction and those undergoing prolonged fasts (Gosink & Leopold 1976). The unifying feature in all of these conditions is stasis. However, since it disappears when fasting patients resume eating, it does not necessarily indicate an organic lesion. The origin of these echoes has been ascribed to the presence of cholesterol crystals which are known to produce echoes in fluid structures at other sites, notably the spleen. It has also been ascribed to increased viscosity. Recently, experiments have been carried out in which 'echogenic bile' was passed through a sequence of millipore filters until it became echolucent. The filtration residue was then examined microscopically and revealed the echoes to be due to small particles predominantly consisting of pigment granules. Partial chemical characterisation revealed this sludge to be mainly calcium bilirubinate (Filly et al 1980). In these experiments viscosity did not appear to be important. Such granules are known to occur in bile from patients with hepatic or pancreatic disease and those with unrelated disorders in the absence of gallstones (Juniper & Burson 1957), and as noted above sludge may be seen in fasting patients. It is therefore inappropriate to suggest a diagnosis of gallbladder disease on the basis of an isolated finding of biliary sludge without additional features.

Ultrasound in the investigation of jaundice
Ultrasound is now the investigation of choice in jaundiced patients in whom laboratory and clinical assessment has failed to give a clear answer to the question 'Is the jaundice medical?'. The answer depends upon the ability of ultrasound to identify the bile ducts and demonstrate dilatation.

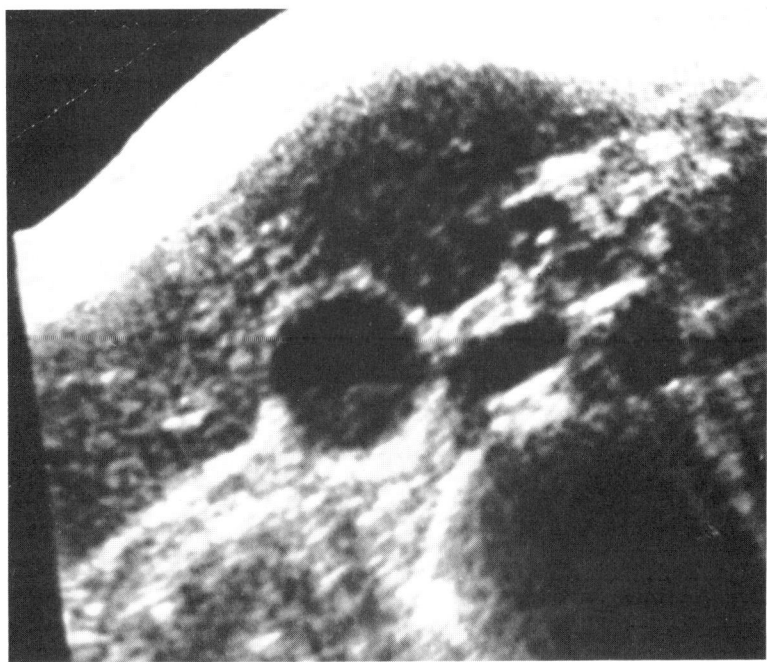

Fig. 3.1 Transverse ultrasound section of gallbladder demonstrating a layer of low level echoes in the dependent portion due to biliary sludge.

In the past the distinction between medical and surgical jaundice was made by assessing the intrahepatic biliary tree. It is clear, however, that some patients with biliary tract obstruction do not have a dilated intrahepatic tree, and this is particularly so in patients with intermittent obstruction. Conversely, obstruction at the porta hepatis will result in a dilated intrahepatic biliary tree and non-dilated extrahepatic ducts. Both subsystems may therefore need to be examined.

The extrahepatic bile ducts can be demonstrated in most patients either using a static B scanner (Dewbury 1980) or a real-time scanner (Cooperberg, 1978) irrespective of whether the ducts are dilated or not (Fig. 3.2). It is possible therefore not only to report that 'the ducts are dilated' but also to make a positive identification of a normal duct. Choledocho-enteric anastomoses represent the most difficult challenge since bowel gas may obscure visualisation of the porta and gas in the biliary tree may make duct identification in the liver difficult.

The patient with a grossly distended duct and the one with a barely visible lumen are not a problem. One is probably obstructed, the other probably not. In between there exists a grey borderline area. Dewbury (1980) found the normal duct to measure 2–5 mm. Cooperberg (1978) in 98 normal patients found a range of 1–4 mm. However, somewhat higher figures have been given by other authors: Behan & Kazam (1978) and Koenigsberg et al (1979) found the maximum duct size in normal subjects to be 8 mm. Parulekar (1979) found that 11% of normal subjects had a duct diameter of more than 6 mm, and 4% more than 7 mm. It

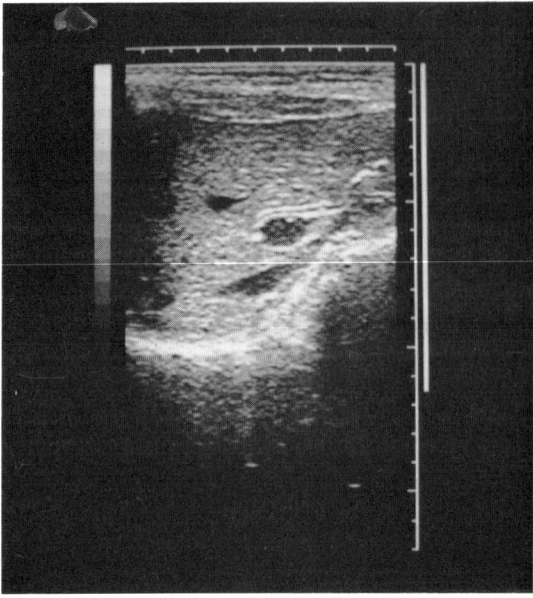

Fig. 3.2 Ultrasound examination demonstrating a normal calibre common duct coursing in front of the portal vein.

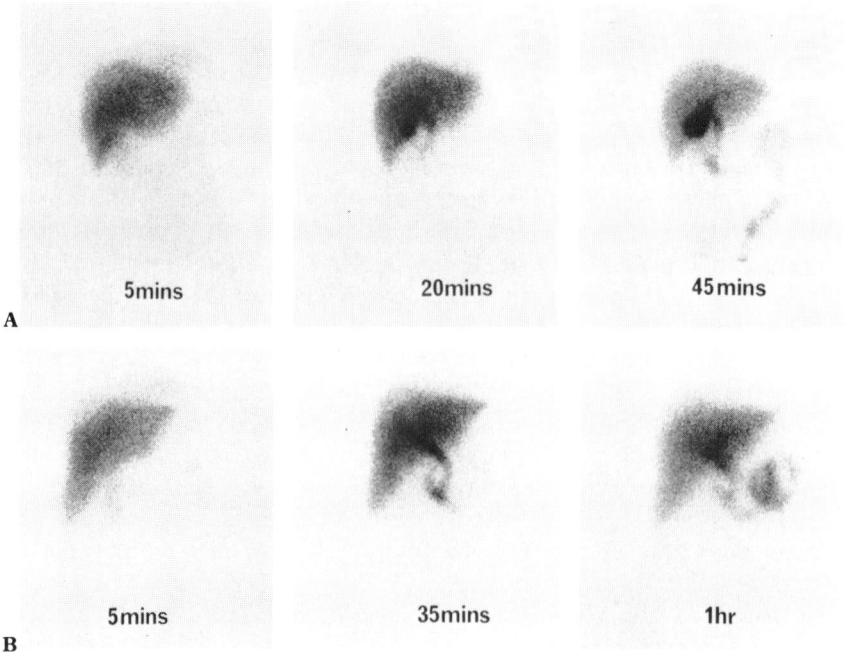

Fig. 3.3A Normal HIDA scan demonstrating progressive filling of gallbladder and free passage of radioisotope down the common duct and into the intestine. **3.3B** HIDA scan in a patient with an obstructed cystic duct. No filling of gallbladder is seen.

would seem that the 6–8 mm region is the grey area where cases of surgical and medical jaundice overlap (Sample et al 1978). Those patients therefore with measurements of 6–8 mm require confirmation by other modalities if a lesion likely to cause obstruction is not sonographically identified (e.g. stones, pancreatic mass). There will of course be the occasional patient with obstruction who has a duct smaller than this (Dewbury 1980, Cooperberg 1978, Graham et al 1981), and where the history is strong further, more invasive studies may be required. Similarly, a few patients, for example those with previous obstruction, will have ducts greater than 6 mm and not be obstructed. Fortunately, in this latter situation the problem is usually historically evident.

When there is a high obstruction, as may occur for example in cholangio-carcinoma, assessment of the intrahepatic biliary tree must be made. The right and left main hepatic ducts can be identified ventral to the branches of the portal venous system. Conrad et al (1978) suggested that the ability to visualise these intrahepatic ducts in itself indicated obstruction, but with improvements in ultrasound equipment this no longer holds true. Dewbury (1980) was prospectively able to identify the right or left hepatic ducts in 41 of 100 normal patients (41%) and second-order branches in four (12%). Measurements would indicate that a right or left duct measuring 1–2 mm is within normal limits, but further work is required.

Whereas ultrasound is extremely accurate at distinguishing medical from surgical jaundice it is somewhat less accurate at determining the site and cause, though Koenigsberg et al (1979) determined the site and aetiology correctly in 81%. Pancreatic masses and pancreatitis (acute or chronic) can often be identified. Small tumours, however, are more elusive, particularly tumours of the ampulla of Vater. Similarly, only about 55–58% of common duct stones are identified (Graham & Lees 1980, Dewbury et al 1979).

High bile duct tumours and benign strictures are also difficult to diagnose with ultrasound. Dillon et al (1981) have suggested that attenuation of the ultrasound beam in the bile duct area, especially if multiple and/or from intrahepatic ducts, is a helpful clue to the diagnosis of cholangiocarcinoma. This sign was present in 10 of their 12 patients. It remains to be seen how helpful this sign will be prospectively, since there are many other causes of intrahepatic shadowing on ultrasound (Weeks et al 1978).

Computerised axial tomography (CAT)

As a primary imaging tool for the investigation of jaundice CAT is reasonably accurate. Levitt et al (1977) distinguished medical from surgical jaundice in 90% of 91 patients and the site of obstruction in 80%. Morris et al (1978) were able to assess the site or cause of obstruction in 84% of their patients. More recently even better results have been obtained. Pedrosa et al (1981 a,b) report a 97% overall accuracy in determining the level of obstruction, and the correct cause was determined in 94%. These workers have also reported good results using multisection reconstruction in coronal and sagittal planes (Pedrosa et al 1981c).

However, CAT is much more expensive and time-consuming than ultrasound and is not so widely available. It has particular use in those patients in whom ultrasonography is difficult, e.g. obese patients or those with excessive bowel gas.

It is also useful in detecting the presence of metastases, abscesses, atrophy or local extension of tumour in the liver if hepatic resection is planned, although ultrasound can provide much of this information (Fig. 3.7).

CAT is rather disappointing in gallstone disease. Although rarely it may show thickening of the gallbladder wall (Havrilla et al 1977), it is poor at demonstrating gallstones (Levitt et al 1977).

Percutaneous transhepatic cholangiography (PTC)
Although this is an invasive procedure, the majority of complications and hazards of this technique are avoidable with careful attention to detail. The advent of the Chiba needle has added greatly to its safety (Okuda et al 1974), and in expert hands over 98% of dilated ducts and 80% of non-dilated ducts can be punctured.

The patient is fasted for 8 hours and generally antibiotic cover is given immediately before and after the procedure. If coagulation studies are abnormal the patient is given parenteral vitamin K, 10 mg daily prior to PTC. If there is no improvement in these studies after vitamin K, then consideration should be given to using ERCP, or if this is not possible the patient can be transfused with fresh frozen plasma and platelets and the number of punctures limited.

Sedation is usually given but this should be prescribed on an individual basis: the most important factor in this respect is control of respiration in order to avoid liver trauma. The injection into the bile duct should be slow. Rapid injection may acutely raise the intrabiliary pressure, which increases the likelihood of bacteraemia if the bile is infected. It may also cause biliary colic which, if severe and associated with vomiting, may necessitate premature termination of PTC to prevent the needle causing liver laceration. The aim should be to opacify the whole intra- and extra hepatic biliary system by injecting enough contrast medium. However, if pain occurs despite slow injection then it may be possible to demonstrate the whole system by utilising gravity and altering the position of the patient.

During injection there is often a period of time when the contrast medium does not appear to be progressing beyond the hilus, and mistakes will be made if PTC is terminated too early in the belief that the hilus is the site of obstruction. This delay is partly due to layering of the contrast medium in a dependent position, and partly due to inadequate mixing of viscid bile. Further injection, rotating the patient on to his left side or raising the head of the fluoroscopic table, usually clarifies the situation. When the obstruction is indeed hilar it is important to inspect the radiographs carefully before finishing. Quite commonly segments or a lobe of the liver may not have opacified, either because the patient has not been rotated to allow the contrast to enter all segments (particularly of the left lobe) or because a segment or lobe is separately obstructed. Full assessment is necessary, and if major biliary surgery is being considered, multiple punctures may be required in order to demonstrate the non-opacified segments or lobe. This may mean anterior puncture if the left lobe needs to be shown and the patient is too large for the needle to reach across from the right side.

Although not always possible, an attempt should be made to persuade contrast past the site of obstruction (Fig. 3.4). This allows assessment of the extent of the

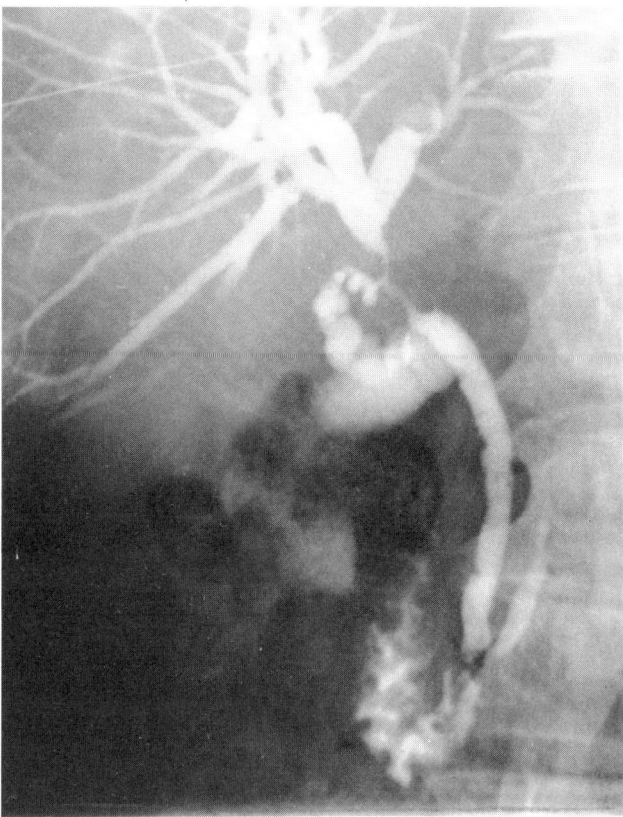

Fig. 3.4 PTC: relatively undistended ducts in a patient with a cholangiocarcinoma: a short stricture involves the junction of common hepatic and common bile ducts.

lesion, the presence of multiple strictures and the possibility of a second more distal lesion. In this context it is worth remembering that stones and/or fibrinous or mucinous debris not uncommonly collect above a malignant stricture. Where an 'apparent stone' is seen at the lower end of the common bile duct and contrast does not pass beyond, an ERCP should be performed since tumours of the papilla may give an identical appearance.

Before the needle is finally withdrawn, an attempt should be made to aspirate some of the contrast and bile. This may not be possible if the bile is very viscid but will temporarily decrease intrabiliary pressure, reducing the likelihood of leaks and bacteraemia. It will also provide a sample of bile for bacteriological examination; contrast medium mixed with it does not appear to inhibit growth of the culture.

PTC with a sheathed needle carries a mortality of about 0.5% and a complication rate of at least 5%, due to major leaks of bile or blood, septicaemia, pneumothorax and haemobilia. PTC with a Chiba needle carries a complication rate of about 2%, primarily due to septic complications.

Endoscopic retrograde choledocho-pancreatography (ERCP)
ERCP was the first precise and direct method of contrast imaging of the biliary tract which could be safely and non-invasively used as a diagnostic procedure, and its widespread use followed the development of new fibre-optic duodenoscopes in the 1970s. As a diagnostic tool it has several clear advantages. Firstly, in a large percentage of cases, in expert hands, it can outline both the biliary and pancreatic ducts. Secondly, it allows at the same time inspection of the stomach and duodenum for other lesions. Thirdly, it allows visualisation and, where appropriate, biopsy or cytological studies of the papilla of Vater. Finally, it carries the potential for therapeutic techniques, such as retrograde intubation for distal obstructing lesions (Laurence & Cotton 1980) and endoscopic sphincterotomy (Cotton 1979, Safrany 1978).

ERCP has been compared in a randomised fashion with PTC as a means of diagnosis in jaundice (Elias et al 1976). This type of comparison is probably not valid, since both ERCP and PTC have a place, and selection can be made according to clinical criteria. ERCP has probably now given pride of place to PTC as the procedure of choice for diagnosis of obstructive jaundice. ERCP however remains the procedure of first choice for the post-cholecystectomy patient, largely because of its ability to provide information in addition to cholangiography, and partly because of its success rate in the patient with non-dilated ducts (Blumgart et al 1977). This investigation is particularly valuable in patients in whom sphincteroplasty or choledochoduodenostomy has been performed. It is possible to cannulate the orifices and obtain a cholangiogram, and also obtain information regarding peristomal inflammation, patency and competence.

ERCP is probably the best method of diagnosing carcinoma of the papilla of Vater, and in many cases after endoscopic biopsy it is still possible to obtain a cholangiogram. Some workers have recommended endoscopic papillotomy in this situation as a means of preliminary decompression of the biliary tract, to be followed later by definitive treatment of the tumour.

ERCP carries a low morbidity (less than 3%) and a mortality of about 0.2% (Bilbao et al 1976), mainly due to septicaemia following cholangitis or pancreatitis. This risk is greatest in those with tight duct strictures or pancreatic pseudocysts, and patients should be screened by ultrasonography for cyst formation before being subjected to ERCP.

Vascular radiology
The majority of cholangiocarcinomas and many gallbladder carcinomas are relatively avascular, but cause strictures and/or displacement of arteries (Voyles et al 1982, Williamson et al 1980). In the patient with obstruction due to tumour therefore, vascular studies are of value to assess irresectability and also to act as a surgical 'road map'.

Hepatic arterial anatomy is highly variable and many of the variants have surgical implications. The superior mesenteric artery gives rise to segmental or total arterial flow in 18.5% and 2.5% of individuals respectively (Fig. 3.5). Such an artery passes behind the portal vein and frequently lies lateral to the common bile duct in the hepato-duodenal ligament, where it may be susceptible to operative injury if not recognised. Part, or rarely all, of the hepatic arterial supply may arise

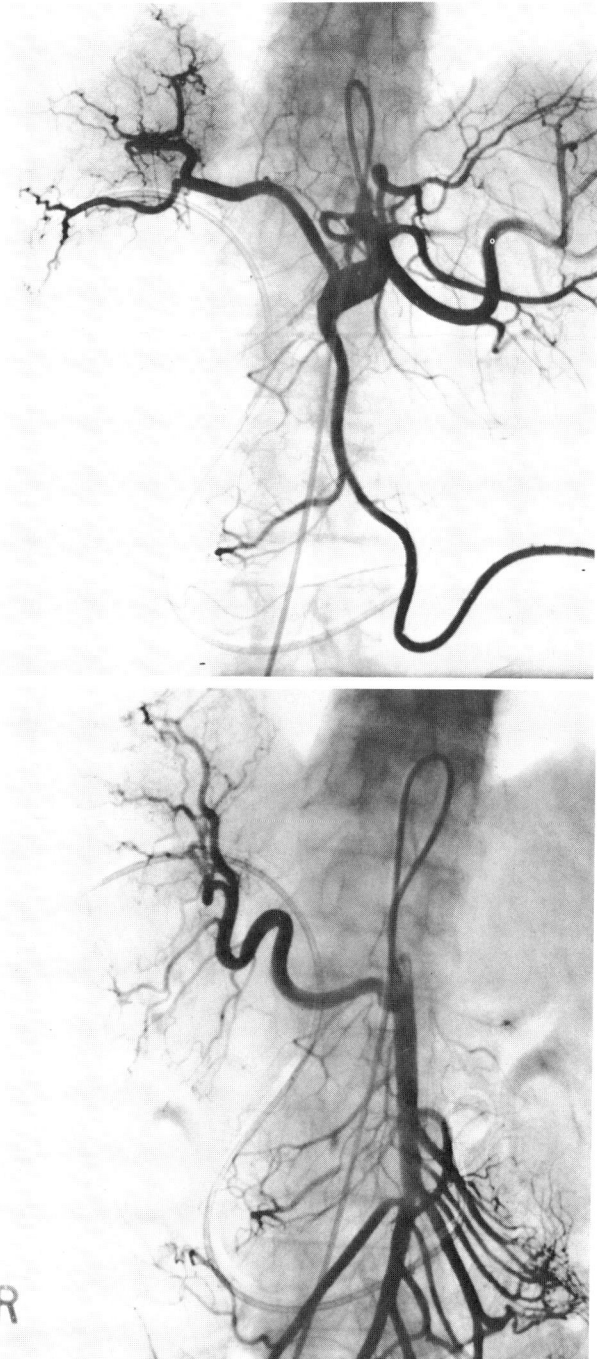

Fig. 3.5 Angiographic studies in a patient with obstructive jaundice due to a hilar cholangiocarcinoma. A percutaneous drainage tube is seen in place. (Above) Coeliac arteriogram: part of the arterial supply to the right lobe of the liver is demonstrated. (Below) Superior mesenteric arteriogram: there is also a large supply to the right lobe of the liver arising from an accessory right hepatic artery.

from the left gastric artery (25% of individuals); such a supply enters the liver medial to the confluence at the base of the umbilical fissure. The main hepatic artery may divide early, or even trifurcate with the gastroduodenal artery. If this happens the two branches of the hepatic artery may course together to the hilus in a common vascular bundle making dissection difficult, or they may separate and the right branch pass behind the portal vein to lie lateral in the hepatoduodenal ligament. When the right hepatic artery crosses the common hepatic duct anteriorly (rather than its normal posterior course) dissection at the hilus is more difficult. This variant however is not easily recognised unless the common bile duct is indicated by a trans-hepatic drain during arteriography.

The portal system may be opacified by several routes: arterioportography — contrast medium injected into the splenic artery or superior mesenteric artery; direct splenoportography — contrast medium injected into the splenic pulp; or transhepatic portography — contrast medium injected directly into the portal system. Each method has its merits and disadvantages, and sometimes more than one method may be necessary before an adequate assessment is made.

The portal system may be encased, displaced, impressed, occluded or invaded by tumour thrombus (Fig. 3.6). As with the arterial system some care is needed in interpretation. A haematoma may be present in the hepatoduodenal ligament following PTC or drainage procedures and cause compression or displacement of the portal vein, as may undrained dilated bile ducts. These problems apart, the

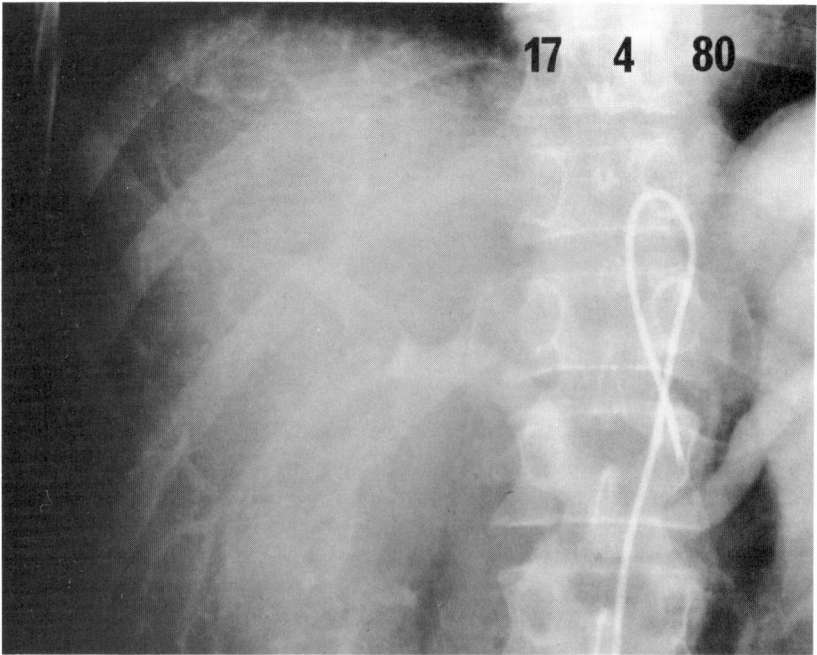

Fig. 3.6 Arterioportography in a patient with cholangiocarcinoma: the left portal vein is occluded by tumour and tumour thrombus is invading the right portal vein.

slightest impression or displacement is probably equivalent to infiltration by tumour (Hoevels & Ihse 1979). Even allowing for these rigid criteria portography underestimates vascular involvement. Only a positive result therefore is helpful since it may exclude that patient from an extensive exploratory laparotomy.

Operative mortality for partial hepactectomy is largely related to haemorrhage especially from the vena cava, hepatic veins and major hilar vessels (Williamson et al 1980). In cases of hilar malignancy where surgery is contemplated, and ultrasound or CAT scanning indicate a large mass extending back near to the cava, then an inferior vena cavagram may be required.

Unfortunately with the possible exception of periampullary tumours most pancreatic tumours causing jaundice are not resectable for cure. There has however been a renewed interest in total pancreatectomy for carcinoma, but such radical surgery is not possible once the tumour has grown outside the pancreas (Reichardt & Ihse 1980). There may be evidence on CAT or ultrasound studies that a carcinoma has spread either locally or distally. In those where such spread is not obvious vascular studies may be required to assess irresectability and also provide an anatomical 'road map' (vide supra).

There is a strong correlation between the extent of arterial involvement shown by angiography and the operability and survival time (Suzuki et al 1972, Tylen & Arnesjo 1973). Pancreatic tumours involving the common hepatic artery, coeliac trunk, superior mesenteric artery, splenic artery and gastroduodenal artery are rarely resectable with clear margins and where attempts to extirpate the tumour have been made the operation has almost always been exceedingly difficult and the survival very poor.

The importance of the venous phase of coeliac and superior mesenteric arteriograms in assessment of pancreatic carcinoma was recognised by Buranasiri & Baum (1972). Involvement of major veins — splenic, portal or superior mesenteric — indicates irresectability for cure. The criteria of involvement of these major veins are circular stenosis, irregular vessel walls or tumour thrombus. A smooth local impression on the veins does not necessarily indicate invasion but does warn that surgery is likely to be difficult. (Reichardt & Ihse 1980). Direct or transhepatic portography may be used in those patients in whom the arterial and venous phases of angiography do not give unequivocal information about non-resectability.

Radioisotope scanning
Like computerised axial tomography, radioisotope techniques are not as widely available as the oral cholecystogram and ultrasound. With the availability of the newer Technetium-99m labelled imino-diacetic acid (IDA) derivatives which are rapidly taken up by hepatocytes and excreted into the biliary tract the place of radioisotope studies of the gallbladder and biliary tract has changed (Loberg et al 1976, Wistow et al 1977, 1978). Nevertheless, its anatomical detail remains inferior to the oral cholecystogram or ultrasound and like the oral cholecystogram it is dependent on liver function.

The various agents available differ in hepatocyte extraction, rate of transport from hepatocyte and the fraction removed by the kidneys. Moreover, these aspects change more with some agents than others as liver damage increases. A number of clinical evaluations and comparisons have been made (Klingensmith et al 1980, Reichelt & Popescu 1979, Hernandez & Rosenthall 1980, Rosenthall et al 1978).

Because of its poor anatomical detail the use of isotope scanning in acute and chronic cholecystitis is confined to the demonstration of patency of the cystic duct (Fig. 3.3). It possibly has a place in suspected chronic cholecystitis when oral cholecystography has failed to visualise the gallbladder yet ultrasound examination is normal. However, the conclusion of Nicholson et al (1980) was that it offered no advantage over the oral cholecystogram. Its place in the investigation of acute cholecystitis is less controversial (vide infra).

Radioisotope scanning has only a minor role in investigating the rest of the biliary tree, but may be of value in two circumstances: firstly, in patients with a suspected biliary leak, and secondly, in assessing the function of a biliary-enteric anastomosis, particularly in the patient who presents with episodes of fever and pain but is not jaundiced and has a normal or only marginally raised alkaline phosphatase.

Fistulography and trans-tubal cholangiography
In patients with a biliary fistula following previous surgery, or rarely in patients with post-traumatic or spontaneous biliary fistulae, examination by injection of contrast down the track may provide valuable anatomical information regarding the site of origin of the fistula. Frequently, however, the fistula track communicates with a rather diffuse cavity and it is not possible to fill the biliary tract from this cavity. If there is a biliary-enteric fistula as well as an external fistula, as may occur with a major leak from a biliary-enteric anastomosis, the contrast may preferentially enter the gut and fail to produce a cholangiogram. Nevertheless, this relatively non-invasive test should be the first examination in patients of this type, in preference to the alternatives of ERCP or PTC.

In patients whose biliary tract has been intubated therapeutically, either as definitive palliation for bile duct tumours and strictures, as a temporary drainage measure pending definitive surgery, or as a splintage tube through a biliary-enteric anastomosis, biliary tubography is a most valuable procedure. T-tubograms are of course performed as a routine following exploration of the common bile duct with T-tube drainage, to determine adequate clearance of the bile duct and to demonstrate free flow into the duodenum. This is normally performed 7–10 days after operation, although some surgeons prefer an earlier examination. It is our practice to perform a tubogram at 7–10 days in patients who have trans-anastomotic splintage tubes, either of the U-tube variety or a straight tube passing via the transhepatic or the trans-jejunal route. This examination will demonstrate the patency and calibre of the anastomosis or anastomoses, and any significant leakage will be disclosed.

Following insertion of a percutaneously placed biliary endoprosthesis, it is our practice to leave a biliary drainage tube in the intrahepatic ducts above the endoprosthesis for 24 hours, and then to perform a tubogram to check the position of tube and endoprosthesis. If the position is satisfactory, the external drainage tube is then removed.

Barium studies

Barium studies are unhelpful in the patient with jaundice. They are unreliable as an indicator of pancreatic masses and generally have a very limited role in biliary practice. They are sometimes used to assess duodenal obstruction in pancreatic carcinoma, but many surgeons perform gastric drainage as a routine during palliative bypass in such cases. An effervescent drink may be used, particularly in children, to assess bilioduodenal anastomoses and may provide useful information if an abnormality is identified. On the other hand patency of the anastomosis does not exclude the biliary tree as the seat of symptoms, and intrahepatic strictures and stones causing intermittent obstruction are easily missed.

General approach to diagnosis

A variety of specific clinical situations are considered below, but it may be useful firstly to comment on the general approach to the diagnosis of two of the major clinical syndromes in the biliary tract: the patient with jaundice, and the patient with acute or chronic cholecystitis.

Jaundice

In the majority of patients presenting with jaundice a combination of clinical history and physical examination will yield a diagnosis. Although much attention is concentrated on the techniques for distinguishing 'medical' from 'surgical', this distinction may be obvious in a large percentage of cases. The relevance of laboratory investigation in this problem has already been discussed. In the problem case, however, an ordered approach must be adopted. Numerous algorithmic schemes for diagnosis have been described, and these may require adaptation to suit a particular clinical environment.

Ultrasonography is the technique of choice for distinguishing patients with dilated and non-dilated bile ducts, and in the majority of cases this distinction will serve to differentiate obstructive from non-obstructive jaundice. There are important exceptions which have already been noted, and the clinician must be aware of these. If ultrasound fails to reveal ducts in the presence of a high clinical suspicion of biliary obstruction, then contrast imaging should still be performed before embarking on a prolonged and expensive search for intrahepatic causes of jaundice. However, if the clinician is prepared to accept the evidence for non-surgical jaundice, then it is appropriate to perform percutaneous liver biopsy, and to pursue further biochemical and serological investigations.

Percutaneous transhepatic cholangiography and endoscopic retrograde cholangiography each have advantages and drawbacks. The choice of technique may depend in part upon availability of expertise, but it is preferable to select the most appropriate investigation. We have preferred to use percutaneous cholangiography in the majority of patients with dilated ducts. ERCP is preferred in postcholecystectomy patients with jaundice, when ultrasound suggests a low obstruction, and in patients in whom PTC raises suspicion of a periampullary tumour. It is important to appreciate that if one technique fails the other may be performed, and that in some cases a combination of both routes may be necessary to provide a complete diagnosis.

Once the diagnosis of obstructive jaundice has been made and the site and probable nature of the obstructing lesion demonstrated, other investigations may be required for diagnostic reasons (such as cytology) or to help with the planning of therapy (such as angiography).

Acute cholecystitis

The pace of investigation for patients with the clinical diagnosis of acute cholecystitis has been altered by the increasing practice of early cholecystectomy for this syndrome. If early cholecystectomy is to be considered, then a clinical diagnosis is insufficient. The choice of technique lies between ultrasound and radioisotope (HIDA) scanning, and these techniques have already been described. It must be remembered that demonstration of gallstones on ultrasound does not constitute proof of acute cholecystitis. The most valuable ultrasonographic sign is that of precisely localised tenderness over the gallbladder during the scanning procedure, and in this respect the test is more sensitive than clinical examination. Conversely, a HIDA scan which fails to outline the gallbladder may be indicative of chronic cholecystitis, while the origin of the patient's acute symptoms may lie elsewhere. Nevertheless, the use of one or both of these techniques will improve the diagnostic rate for acute cholecystitis, and may allow safe early operation when indicated.

Chronic cholecystitis

The choice for this syndrome lies between ultrasound, HIDA scanning and oral cholecystography. It has been noted above that the value of ultrasound lies in the diagnosis of gallstones, while HIDA scanning will demonstrate an obstructed cystic duct. While the oral cholecystogram may have the benefit of providing both of these items of information, sensitivity and specificity are both very variable. The caveats discussed in relation to acute cholecystitis apply to the chronic syndrome also, and the results of these examinations must be taken carefully in conjunction with clinical assessment.

Specific clinical problems

Post-cholecystectomy syndromes

A proportion of patients return with significant symptoms following chole-cystectomy. Ultrasound or intravenous cholangiography and upper gastro-intestinal contrast studies or endoscopy are frequently used as first line investigations for such patients. There remains however a group of patients who are refractory to diagnosis by these simple techniques. In this group we have found ERCP the technique of choice (Blumgart et al 1977).

In patients in whom iatrogenic biliary stricture has been demonstrated at ERCP, it may be necessary in some instances to perform PTC in addition in order to delineate the intrahepatic ducts.

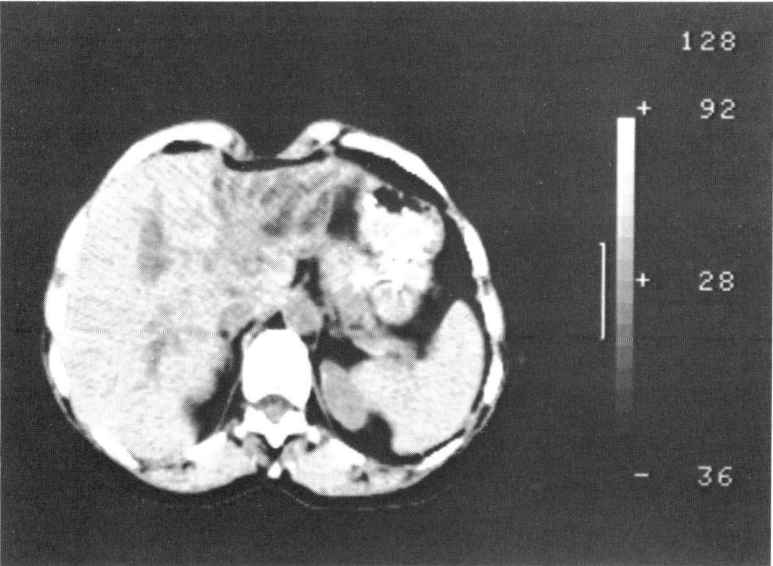

Fig. 3.7 CAT scan in a patient with hilar cholangiocarcinoma. The scan reveals markedly dilated bile ducts crowded together in a shrunken left lobe: atrophy of the left lobe was confirmed at surgery.

Hilar cholangiocarcinoma

Cholangiocarcinoma of the hilus of the liver was until recently usually diagnosed at laparotomy or at autopsy. In 9 of the 13 cases reported by Klatskin (1965) and 8 of 25 cases reported by Longmire et al (1973), an operative procedure was performed for obstructive jaundice and no lesion identified. The advent of improved methods of biliary imaging has changed this situation. Following ultrasound, PTC is the method of choice for delineation of the biliary tract when this condition is suspected (Figs. 3.4, 3.8). Full assessment of a carcinoma at the confluence of the bile ducts (the commonest site) may require several separate punctures in order to ensure visualisation of all of the intrahepatic segmental ducts. ERCP may be required to demonstrate the full extent of the lesion if no contrast material can be persuaded through the stricture. Except in post-cholecystectomy patients and those with appearances consistent with sclerosing cholangitis, the diagnosis is usually clear following these contrast examinations, and may be confirmed by bile cytology or percutaneous needle aspiration.

Determination of the appropriate therapy for patients with hilar cholangio-carcinoma may be difficult, and it is important to pursue radiological investigations to determine whether curative resection may be possible, and if not to delineate the biliary anatomy accurately and plan the best palliative approach. We have employed a combination of cholangiography, arteriography, and late-phase arterial or direct portography in order to assess resectability in such patients (Fig. 3.6) and have found these techniques valuable and accurate (Voyles et al 1982).

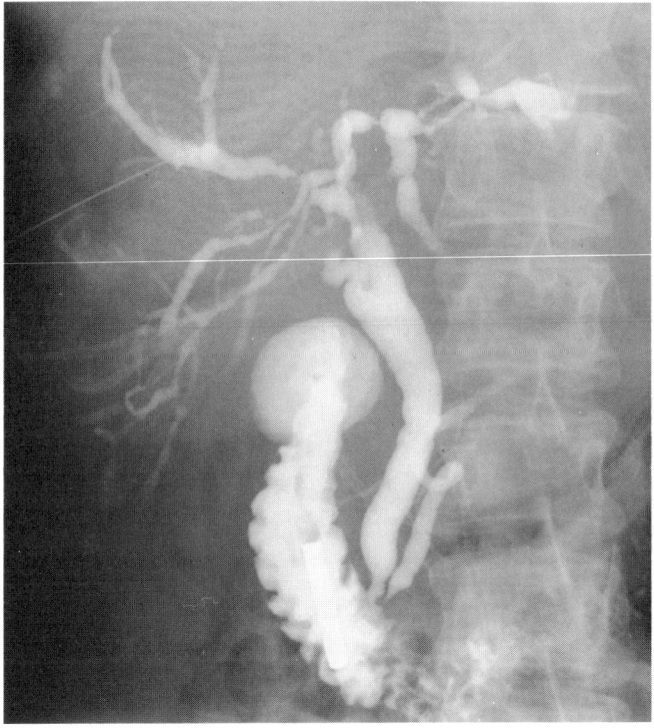

Fig. 3.8 PTC: multiple strictures are seen throughout the intrahepatic biliary tree suggesting sclerosing cholangitis. A liver biopsy however revealed a minute focus of adenocarcinoma.

Benign strictures

The vast majority are the result of previous surgery, a few are due to other forms of trauma, and some the result of various inflammatory conditions such as pancreatitis, inflammation secondary to stones, TB and presumed inflammatory conditions such as Asiatic cholangitis and primary sclerosing cholangitis. Those resulting from previous surgery fall into two groups, the low and the high.

Low strictures are commonly associated with iatrogenic choledochoduodenal fistulae. These are important to identify and if ultrasound or other studies suggest the obstruction is low ERCP is the investigation of choice. If the strictured sphincter is difficult to cannulate such a fistula can often be cannulated and a cholangiogram obtained.

High strictures may be delineated well by ERCP but not uncommonly strictures involve first or second order branches, and for this reason if it is known from ultrasound that a stricture is high PTC should be performed and all separately obstructed segments identified. Those cases of strictured biliary-enteric anastomoses where a long jejunal Roux loop has been brought up to the hilus can of course only be delineated by PTC.

Apart from those secondary effects on the biliary tree and liver seen with any biliary obstruction (cholangitis, communicating abscesses and atrophy), in patients with long-standing benign strictures there may in addition be severe fibrosis or cirrhosis leading to portal hypertension and varices. Such patients may require delineation of the portal system by indirect or direct portography.

Some patients with benign strictures require anatomical delineation of the hepatic arterial tree. Occasionally hepatic arterial aneurysms form at the site of damage to the vessel and may result in haemobilia.

Primary sclerosing cholangitis is a diffuse fibrosis of the bile ducts resulting in irregular compression and narrowing of the lumen. The aetiology of this condition is unknown, and it is designated 'primary' in order to distinguish it from the secondary changes associated with biliary tract obstruction, gallstones or previous surgery. The presentation may be vague and non-specific, and includes episodes of jaundice with abdominal discomfort and pruritus. Investigation must include detailed cholangiography, liver function studies, and a liver biopsy to exclude other forms of intrinsic liver disease. There is a strong association with inflammatory bowel disease and barium enema and/or colonoscopy is mandatory.

While sclerosing cholangitis is usually diffusely distributed, in some cases the disease is highly localised within the biliary tract. In such cases differentiation from a benign iatrogenic stricture or from cholangiocarcinoma may be difficult. It is particularly difficult to distinguish between the diffuse form of cholangio-carcinoma and sclerosing cholangitis, either preoperatively or at operation (Fig. 3.8). Choledochoscopy and biopsy are recommended, but are not always easy, and by no means always diagnostic. Moreover, since sclerosing cholangitis may itself predispose to malignant change, there must be a high index of suspicion, and long follow-up and an open verdict must be maintained. This difficult area remains one of the unsolved diagnostic problems of biliary surgery.

Cholangitis

Cholangitis is invasive sepsis of the normally sterile biliary tract. Bacteria are found frequently in the bile in the presence of gallstones, but also occur in malignant biliary obstruction (McPherson et al 1982a). The highest incidence is seen in patients with benign biliary strictures, particularly after multiple surgical procedures (Jackaman et al 1980).

The syndrome is seen in its most florid form as acute suppurative cholangitis. The diagnosis is essentially clinical, and urgent treatment is required with little further investigation since the mortality may be as high as 50% in patients with a 24–72 hour delay in treatment (Welch & Donaldson 1976). The conventional treatment is early laparotomy with wide bore T-tube drainage of the bile duct. Percutaneous transhepatic tube drainage of the biliary tree in this condition appears an attractive alternative. The fine-bore tubes which are used for this purpose may, however, fail to drain dilated ducts containing thick purulent bile, and we have had to operate on one patient 24 hours after 'successful' percutaneous drainage for this reason. There may also be a place for endoscopic papillotomy in this syndrome, especially for elderly patients.

Acute suppurative cholangitis is uncommon, even in patients with gallstone obstruction (Boey & Way 1980). However, chronic cholangitis, with its more subtle presentation of occasional fever with or without transient jaundice or pruritus, is an important syndrome. Chronic incomplete obstruction of the biliary tract produces cholangiolitis as a result of bile salt stasis, and this in turn leads to the deposition of collagen fibres in the periductular region. The lobular architecture of the liver usually remains well preserved, and the perilobular fibrosis produced rarely proceeds to a true cirrhotic pattern. These secondary changes may be an important cause of failure of the intrahepatic biliary tree to dilate above an obstruction. These changes are reflected in the appearances at PTC or ERCP, and consist of irregularity of the small ducts with segments of narrowing and dilatation, giving a flame-shaped or rat-tailed appearance. In less chronic cases, small intrahepatic abscesses may be opacified. The larger ducts may also be affected and show a 'shaggy' appearance of the mucosa on cholangiography. These changes may be uniformly distributed throughout the biliary tree, or may be segmental.

Periampullary tumours
The periampullary tumour provides a clinical pitfall of great importance, since these lesions have a high resectability rate and the potential for curative surgery. All patients with obstructive jaundice, including those with transient attacks, must arouse a suspicion of this lesion.

In patients who present with jaundice due to this cause, PTC will demonstrate dilatation of the biliary tree with a distally placed obstruction. It may be difficult to distinguish between tumours of the periampullary region and other filling defects, such as small stones, particularly when the tumours are of the intraductal papillary variety. It is therefore important to follow up such a radiological finding with endoscopy or ERCP. We have seen such tumours associated with stones in the common bile duct. Choledochoscopy may be valuable for examination of the lower end of the common bile duct in cases where there is no flow into the duodenum on operative cholangiography, or in which the distal end of the bile duct shows distortion or is not clearly seen.

The value of biopsy and cytology for this lesion has already been discussed. Tumours of the papillary variety have a significantly greater resectability rate and also a better prognosis than the flat ulcerating lesions, and these visual appearances correlate well with histological characteristics (Blumgart & Kennedy 1973).

Choledochal cyst
Jaundice, cholangitis or an abdominal mass are the usual presenting features of choledochal cysts. While ultrasound is the first examination of choice, contrast studies such as PTC or ERCP should also be performed.

An important diagnostic goal is the detection of malignancy (Fig. 3.9). Echogenic material at ultrasound or filling defects at cholangiography may be misinterpreted as stones or debris but it should be remembered that there is a greatly increased incidence of malignant change in choledochal cysts in adults. These tumours are usually papillary in type, appearing much like stones and debris to the radiologist and like chronic inflammatory changes to the surgeon at laparotomy.

Jaundice in infancy
Prolonged jaundice in the infant is usually due to biliary atresia, the neonatal hepatitis syndrome or more rarely a choledochal cyst. The cause of neonatal

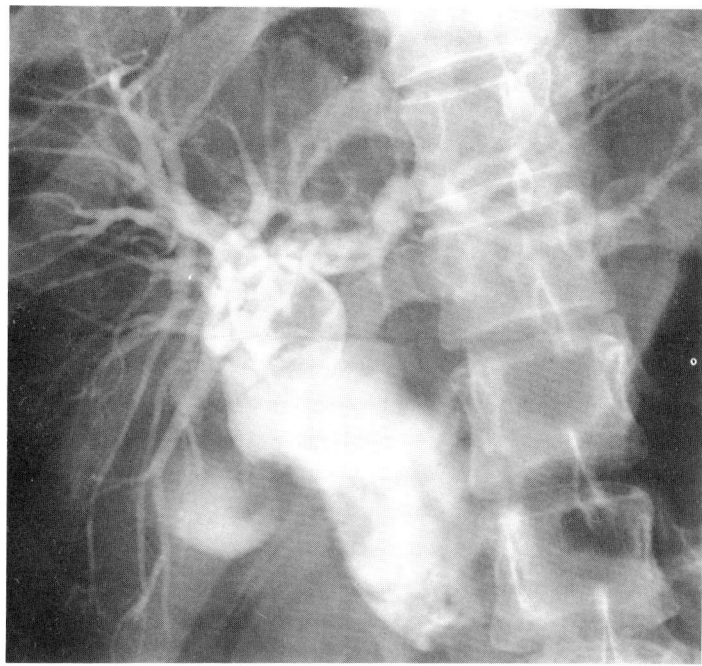

Fig. 3.9 Known case of choledochal cyst referred for further management. PTC reveals a hugely dilated common duct. Multiple ill-defined filling defects are seen which could easily be misinterpreted as inflammatory debris and stones. Tumour was suggested however, and confirmed at laparotomy.

hepatitis remains obscure in about 70% of cases and such cases must be differentiated within a few months of birth from biliary atresia and choledochal cyst. Late recognition of biliary atresia is associated with a lower operative success rate (Kasai et al 1968).

Ultrasonography should be performed to identify those with choledochal cysts. In those without such cysts, if liver biopsy is equivocal or suggests biliary atresia, PTC can be performed using a modified Chiba needle immediately before laparotomy under the same general anaesthetic (Howard & Nunnerley 1979). Failure to identify ducts does not preclude laparotomy, however.

References

Arnon S, Rosenquist C 1976 Gray scale cholecystosonography: an evaluation of accuracy. American Journal of Roentgenology 127: 817–818
Behan M, Kazam 1978 Sonography of the common bile duct: value of the right anterior oblique view. American Journal of Roentgenology 130: 701–709
Benjamin I S, Allison M E M, Moule B, Blumgart L H 1978 The early use of fine needle percutaneous transhepatic cholangiography in an approach to the diagnosis of jaundice in a surgical unit British Journal of Surgery 65: 92–98
Benjamin I S, Blumgart L H 1979 Biliary bypass and reconstruction. In: Liver and biliary disease: pathophysiology, diagnosis, management: Eds Wright R, Alberti K G M M, Karran S and Millward-Sadler G D T. Saunders, London, Chapter 54

Benjamin I S, Imrie C W, Blumgart L H 1977 Liver biopsy in 'difficult' jaundice. British Medical Journal (ii) 578

Berk R N 1970 The consecutive dose phenomenon in oral cholecystography. American Journal of Roentgenology 110: 230–234

Berk R N 1971 The problem of impaired first-dose visualization of the gallbladder. American Journal of Roentgenology 113: 186–188

Berk R N 1973 Radiology of the gallbaldder and bile ducts. Surgical Clinics of North America 53: 973–1005

Besemann E F 1970 Can ipodate calcium save the patient one day in hospitalisation? American Journal of Roentgenology 110: 226–229

Bilbao M K, Dotter C T, Lee T G, Katon R M 1976 Complications of ERCP. A study of 1000 cases. Gastroenterology 70: 314–320

Bismuth H 1981 Data presented to American Gastroenterological Association, New York, June 1981

Blumgart L H, Kennedy A 1973 Carcinoma of the ampulla of Vater and duodenum. British Journal of Surgery 60: 33–40

Blumgart L H, Salmon P R, Cotton P B 1974 Endoscopy and retrograde choledochopancreatography in the diagnosis of the patient with jaundice. Surgery, Gynecology and Obstetrics 138: 565–570

Blumgart L H, Carachi R, Imrie C W, Benjamin I S, Duncan J G 1977 Diagnosis and management of post-cholecystectomy symptoms: the place of endoscopy and retrograde choledochopancreatography. British Journal of Surgery 64: 809–816

Boey J H, Way L W 1980 Acute cholangitis. Annals of Surgery 191: 264

Boyden E A 1957 The anatomy of the choledochuduodenal junction in man. Surgery Gynecology and Obstetrics 104: 641

Buranasiri S, Baum S 1972 The significance of the venous phase of coeliac and superior mesenteric arteriography in evaluating pancreatic carcinoma. Radiology 102: 11–20

Burhenne H J 1975 Problem areas in the biliary tract. Current Problems in Radiology 5

Burhenne H J, Obata W G 1975 Single-visit oral cholecystography. New England Journal of Medicine 292: 627–628

Caroli J, Porcher P, Peqvignot G, Delatre M 1960 Contributions of cineradiography to the study of function of the human biliary tract. American Journal of Digestive Diseases 5: 677–696

Conrad M R, Landay M J, Janes J O 1978 Songraphic 'parallel channel' sign of biliary tree enlargement in mild to moderate obstructive jaundice. American Journal of Roentgenology 130: 279–286

Cooperberg P L 1978 High-resolution real-time ultrasound in the evaluation of the normal and obstructed biliary tract. Radiology 129: 477–480

Cooperberg P L, Burhenne H J 1980 Real time ultrasonography. Diagnostic technique of choice in calculous gallbladder disease. New England Journal of Medicine 302: 1277–9

Cooperman A M 1981 Cancer of the ampulla of Vater, bile duct and duodenum. Surgical Clinics of North America 61: 99–106

Cotton P B 1979 Endoscopic treatment of biliary tract diseases. The Lancet 1: 150

Crow H C, Bartrum R J Jr, Foote S R 1976 Expanded criteria for the ultrasonic diagnosis of gallstones. Journal of Clinical Ultrasound 4: 289–292

Crummy A B 1976 Five hour reinforcement cholecystography. Gastrointestinal Radiology 1: 91–92

Dewbury K C 1980 Visualisation of normal biliary ducts with ultrasound. British Journal of Radiology 53: 774–780

Dewbury K C, Joseph A E A, Hayes S, Murray C 1979 Ultrasound in the evaluation and diagnosis of Jaundice. The British Journal of Radiology 52: 276–280

Dillon E, Peel A L G, Parkin G J S 1981 The diagnosis of primary bile duct carcinoma (cholangiocarcinoma) in the jaundice patient. Clinical Radiology 32: 311–317

Elias E, Hamlyn A N, Jain S, Long R G, Summerfield J A, Dick R, Sherlock S 1976 A randomised trial of percutaneous transhepatic cholangiography with the Chiba needle versus endoscopic retrograde cholangiography for bile duct visualisation in jaundice. Gastroenterology 71: 439–443

Filly R A, Allen B, Minton M J, Bernhoft R, Way L W 1980 In vitro investigation of the origin of echoes within biliary sludge. Journal of Clinical Ultrasound 8: 193–200

Fiske C E, Laing F C, Brown T W 1980 Ultrasonographic evidence of gallbladder wall thickening in association with hypoalbuminaemia. Radiology 135: 713–716

Gosbink B B, Leopold G R 1976 Ultrasound and the gallbladder. Seminars in Roentgenology 11: 185–189

Graham M F, Cooperberg P L, Cohen M M, Burhenne H J 1981 Ultrasonographic screening of the common hepatic duct in symptomatic patients after cholecystectomy. Radiology 138: 137–139

Graham N, Lees W R 1980 The problem of gallstones in the ultrasonographic diagnosis of jaundice. British Journal of Radiology 53: 617–628

Havrilla T R, Haaga J R, Alfidi R J, Reich N E 1977 Computed tomography and obstructive biliary disease. American Journal of Roentgenology 128: 765–768

Hernandez M, Rosenthall L 1980 A cross-over study comparing the kinetics of 99m Tc-labelled diisopropyl and p-butyl IDA analogues in patients. Clinics in Nuclear Medicine 5: 159–165

Hoevels J, Ihse I 1979 Percutaneous transhepatic portography in bile duct carcinoma — correlation with percutaneous transhepatic cholangiography and angiography. Fortschritte auf dem Gebiete der Röntgenstrahlen 131: 140–150

Howard E R, Nunnerley H B 1979 Percutaneous cholangiography in prolonged jaundice of childhood. Journal of Royal Society of Medicine 72: 495–502

Jackaman F R, Hilson G R F, Lord Smith of Marlow 1980 Bile bacteria in patients with benign bile duct stricture. British Journal of Surgery 67: 329–332

Juniper K, Burson E N 1957 Biliary tract studies II. The significance of biliary crystals. Gastroenterology 32: 175

Kasai M, Kimura S, Asakura Y, Susuki H, Taira Y, Ohashi E 1968 Surgical treatment of biliary atresia. Journal of Paediatric Surgery 3: 665–675

Klatskin G 1965 Adenocarcinoma of the hepatic duct at its bifurcation within the porta hepatis. American Journal of Medicine 38: 241–256

Klingensmith W C, Fritzberg A R, Spitzer V M, Koep L J 1980 Clinical comparison of 99m Tc-diethyl IDA and 99m Tc PIPDA for evaluation of the hepatobiliary system. Radiology 134: 195–199

Knill-Jones R P, Cochrane K M, Sokhi G S, Russell R I, Blumgart L H 1975 Early diagnosis of jaundice. A computer and clinical study. British Journal of Surgery 62: 654–655

Koehler, Kyaw M M 1973 Effect of fractionated administration of telepaque on gallbladder visualisation. Radiology 108: 517–519

Koenigsberg M, Wiener S W, Walzer A 1979 The accuracy of sonography in the differential diagnosis of obstructive jaundice: a comparison with cholangiography. Radiology 133: 157–165

Lance P, Bevan P G, Hoult J G, Paton A 1977 Liver biopsy in 'difficult jaundice'. British Medical Journal (ii) 236

Laurence B H and Cotton P B 1980 Decompression of biliary obstruction by duodenoscopic intubation of bile duct. British Medical Journal 280: 522–523

Levitt R G, Sagel S S, Stanely R J 1977 Accuracy of computed tomography of the liver and biliary tract. Radiology 124: 123–128

Loberg M D, Cooper M, Harvey E 1976 Development of new radio pharmaceuticals based on N-substitution of iminodiacetic acid. Journal of Nuclear Medicine 17: 633–638

Longmire W P Jr, McArthur M S, Bastounis E A, Hiatt J 1973 Carcinoma of the extrahepatic biliary tract. Annals of Surgery 178: 333–345

Low-Beer T S and Heaton K Y 1972 Oral cholecystography in patients with small bowel disease. British Journal of Radiology 45: 427–428

McPherson G A D, Benjamin I S, Boobis A R, Brodie M J, Hampden C, Blumgart L H 1982 Antipyrine elimination as a dynamic test of hepatic functional integrity in obstructive jaundice. Gut (in press)

Maingot R 1964 Injuries of the biliary tract. In: Smith R, Sherlock S (eds) Surgery of the Gallbladder and Bile Ducts, Butterworth, London

Marchal G, Van de Voorde P, Van Dooren W, Ponette E, Baert A 1980 Ultrasonic Appearance of the filled and contracted normal gallbladder. Journal of Clinical Ultrasound 8: 439–442

Moody F G 1981 Surgical applications of sphincteroplasty and choledochoduodenostomy. Surgical Clinics of North America 61: 909–922

Morris A I, Fawcett R A, Wood R, Forbes W S C, Isherwood I, Marsh M N 1978 Computed tomography, ultrasound and cholestatic jaundice. Gut 19: 685–688

Morris J S, Gallo G A, Scheuer P J, Sherlock S 1975 Percutaneous liver biopsy in patients with large bile duct obstruction. Gastroenterology 68: 750–754

Mujahed Z, Evans J A, Whalen J P 1974 The non-opacified gallbladder on cholecystography. Radiology 112: 1–4

Mujahed Z 1976 Factors interfering with the opacification of a normal gallbladder. Gastrointestinal Radiology 1: 183–185

Nicholson R W, Hastings D L 1980 HIDA scanning in gallbladder disease. British Journal of Radiology 53: 877–882

Okuda K, Tanikawa K, Emura T, Kuratomi S, Jinnouchi S, Urabe K, Sumikoshi T, Kanda Y, Fukuyama Y, Musha H, Mori H, Shimokawa Y, Yaku Shiji F, Matsuura Y 1974 Non surgical, percutaneous transhepatic cholangiography — diagnostic significance in medical problems of the liver. American Journal of Digestive Diseases 19: 21–36

Parulekar S G 1979 Ultrasound evaluation of common bile duct size. Radiology 133: 703–707

Pedrosa D S, Casanova R, Rodriguez R 1981a Computed tomography in obstructive jaundice. Part I: The level of obstruction. Radiology 139: 627–634

Pedrosa C S, Casanova R, Lezana A H, Fernandez M C 1981b Computed tomography in obstructive jaundice. Part II: The cause of obstruction. Radiology 139: 635–645

Pedrosa C S, Casanova R, Rodriguez R 1981c CT Cholangiography: Multiplanar reconstruction in obstructive jaundice. Journal of Computer Assisted Tomography 5: 503–508

Riechelt H G, Popescu H I 1979 The importance of liver uptake and retention indices in assessment of clinical usefulness of hepatobiliary imaging agents. Journal of Nuclear Medicine 20: 171–172

Rosenthall L, Shaffer E A, Lisbona R, Pare P 1978 Diagnosis of hepatobiliary disease by 99m Tc Cholescintigraphy. Radiology 126: 467–474

Rosenbaum H D 1959 The value of re-examination in patients with inadequate visualisation of the gallbladder following single dose of Telepaque. American Journal of Roentgenology 82: 1011

Russell J G B, Davies J M 1981 Letter to the Editor. Ultrasound of the gallbladder. British Medical Journal 282 p. 1794

Safrany L 1978 Endoscopic treatment of biliary-tract diseases. An International study. Lancet 2 983–985

Sample W F, Sarti D A, Goldstein L I, Weiner M, Kadell B M 1978 Gray-scale ultrasonography of the jaundiced patient. Radiology 128: 719–725

Saunders R C 1980 The significance of sonographic gallbladder wall thickening. Journal of Clinical Ultrasound 8: 143–146

Stanley R J, Melson G L, Cubillo E et al 1974 A comparison of three cholecystographic agents: a double blind study with and without a prior fatty meal. Radiology 112: 513–517

Stephens D H, Gisvold J J, Carlson H C 1976 Tomography of the gallbadder in oral cholecystography. Gastrointestinal Radiology 1: 93–98

Suzuki T, Kawabe K, Imamura M, Honjo I 1972 Survival of patients with cancer of the pancreas in relation to findings on arteriography. Annals of Surgery 176: 37–41

Tylen U, Arnesjo B 1973 Resectability and prognosis of carcinoma of the pancreas evaluated by angiography. Scandinavian Journal of Gastroenterology 8: 691–697

Voyles C R, Bowley N B, Allison D J, Benjamin I S, Blumgart L H 1982 Carcinoma of the proximal extrahepatic biliary tree. Radiological assessment and therapeutic alternatives. Annals of Surgery (in press)

Way L W, Bernhoft R A, Thomas J M 1981 Biliary stricture. Surgical Clinics of North America 61: 963–972

Weeks L E, McCune B R, Martin J F, O'Brien T F Jr 1978 Differential diagnosis of intrahepatic shadowing on ultrasound examination. Journal of Clinical Ultrasound 6: 399–401

Welch J P, Donaldson G A 1976 The urgency of diagnosis and surgical treatment of acute suppurative cholangitis. American Journal of Surgery 131: 527

Williamson B W A, Blumgart L H, McKellar N J 1980 Management of tumours of the liver. Combined use of arteriography and venography in the assessment of resectability, especially in hilar tumours. American Journal of Surgery 139: 210–215

Wilson R L, Shaub M 1978 The use of ultrasound in suspected cholecystitis. Applied Radiology 7: 119–121

Wistow B W, Subramanian G, Van Heertum R L, Henderson R W, Gagne G M, Hall R C, McAfee J 1977 An evaluation of 99m Tc-labelled hepatobiliary agents. Journal of Nuclear Medicine 18: 455–461

Wistow B W, Subramanian G, Gagne G M 1978 Experimental and clinical trials of new 99m Tc-labelled hepatobiliary agents. Radiology 128: 793–794

4 Endoscopy and biliary disease

E. SEIFERT

Duodenoscopy and endoscopic cannulation of the papilla of Vater have added a new dimension in the diagnosis and management of biliary and pancreatic disease. Precise diagnosis, especially in the jaundiced patient, is now possible and biopsy and cytology of lesions suspected to be malignant is feasible.

Operative endoscopic procedures have been developed and offer new methods for the management of some biliary tract diseases. Techniques of endoscopic sphincterotomy, biliary drainage, implantation of endoprosthesis and methods for dissolving stones by agents applied via a nasobiliary tube have evolved.

The techniques are complex and require the co-operation of a skilled endoscopist and an interested radiologist, both using optimal equipment.

Diagnostic procedures

Techniques

Cannulation is usually performed with a special side-viewing duodenoscope (Anacker et al 1977, Blumgart & Salmon 1973, Classen 1976, Classen 1977, Cotton 1977b, Demling et al 1974, Demling 1976). Forward-viewing endoscopes cannot be used except after Billroth II partial gastrectomy. Catheters for papillary cannulation are simple teflon tubes with a smooth or metal tip and a single end-hole. Fine-tipped catheters may occasionally facilitate cannulation of an abnormal papilla or of the accessory papilla (Cotton & Williams 1980).

Patients are starved for at least 8 hours. The patient is placed in the left lateral position with the left arm behind the back. An intravenous line is placed in the right arm or hand. Immediately prior to examination the patient is sedated with a combination of pethidine and diazepam. ERCP requires suppression of duodenal peristalsis. After entering the duodenum this is achieved with an intravenous injection of Buscopan (hyoscine N-butylbromide 40 mg) or of Glucagon (Cotton 1972, Cotton & Kizu 1977).

With the patient in the left lateral position, the duodenoscope passes through the pylorus. Passage into the descending duodenum is partially blind. The tip of the instrument is first advanced to a position over the superior duodenal angle and then is deflected downwards to slide into the second part of the duodenum. As the instrument passes downwards the tip is deflected and rotated to follow the duodenal axis. When the papilla is visible it is necessary to bring it en face ready for cannulation (Blumgart & Salmon 1973, Cotton & Williams 1980).

To achieve this, two methods are available; to straighten the endoscope by rotating hand and body 90° to the right, moving the instrument upwards and withdrawing the shaft to about 60 cm or, alternatively, to advance the instrument instead of withdrawing it (Cotton & Williams 1980).

When the papilla is seen face-on, cannulation can be attempted (Demling & Classen 1978a). The great majority of patients have a single orifice for the pancreatic and biliary system with a variable length of common channel. Both ducts may opacify simultaneously if contrast is injected when the catheter tip has only barely entered the orifice. When in the correct axis, the tip usually slides more deeply and selectively into one or other duct. Pancreatography is more likely to result if the catheter enters the orifice perpendicular to the duodenal wall or points only slightly upwards. For the bile duct, the papillary orifice should be approached from below and slightly from the right. Water soluble contrast materials are used. Dense contrast agents (50–70%) give best definition of small ducts (Cotton & Kizu 1977). The correct amount is judged solely by fluoroscopy and intermittent radiographs. Opacification of the pancreatic parenchyma should be avoided (Ohto et al 1978, Stewart et al 1977).

ERCP is rarely performed in children and there are no special paediatric instruments. The standard duodenoscope is applicable from the age of 3 years, but success has been claimed even in the neonatal period (Becker et al 1980). Duct cannulation may be easier with a fine-tipped catheter. Usually general anaesthesia is needed (Cotton & Williams 1980).

Where there is disease of the duodenal loop and papilla ERCP has special problems and the cannulation rate falls. The most common lesion involving the descending duodenum is cancer of the pancreas. Bleeding malignancies give characteristic endoscopic appearances and tissue specimens will confirm the diagnosis. In such cases, the orifice of the common bile duct is sometimes not visible and cannulation is impossible. While pancreatic cancer often remains submucosal, the endoscopic appearances of oedema and irregularity are similar to those seen in patients with advanced chronic pancreatitis. A large tumour may cause duodenal stenosis near the papilla and prevent access for cannulation (Cotton & Williams 1980). Prolonged probing is unnecessary and may be hazardous. Most primary tumours of the papilla are obvious endoscopically and the diagnosis can be confirmed by biopsy. The actual orifice may be obscured by tumour and cannulation may be difficult but is, in any event, usually unnecessary.

The papilla may appear oedematous, lumpy and congested even in the absence of tumour or previous surgery. These changes are often associated with calculus biliary tract disease and the orifice may be lax and ragged soon after the passage of a stone.

Duodenal diverticulae virtually all occur close to the papilla. They are most frequently above the papilla or in the immediate peripapillary region and a large diverticulum may override the papillary area or completely envelop it so that the orifice lies in the floor or anterior wall. Cannulation is then more difficult but seldom fails.

Following papillary, pancreatic or biliary surgery there are special problems. Papillary appearances after surgical sphincterotomy vary from normality to complete disorganisation. Standard surgical sphincteroplasty usually results in a groove-like opening and the pancreatic duct orifice is often visible. Cannulation is usually simple unless stenosis has occurred. A traumatic fistula is sometimes seen above the true orifice and results either from the passage of a dilator forced through the duodenal wall above the papilla during surgical exploration, or as a result of a false passage being created in error during attempted sphincteroplasty (Hunt & Blumgart 1980). A choledochoduodenostomy stoma is usually easily visualised in the right superolateral region of the duodenum and cannulation is not difficult. Most operations on the pancreas do not involve the papillary region and cannulation is not affected. The standard Whipple's procedure with pancreaticojejunal reconstruction, however, takes the pancreas out of endoscopic reach.

In patients having had pyloroplasty or Billroth I partial gastrectomy ERCP is readily performed but after Billroth II partial gastrectomy cannulation requires intubation of the afferent loop. The papilla may be difficult to locate and cannulate. With the standard side-viewing duodenoscope, the catheter will naturally curl away from the papillary axis (Cotton & Williams 1980). Cannulation is sometimes simpler with a forward-viewing endoscope.

Diathermy ERCP and pre-cut sphincterotomy
Diathermy ERCP (Caletti et al 1980) and pre-cut sphincterotomy (Siegel 1980) are new techniques which enable the experienced endoscopist to opacify the biliary tree in cases where other techniques, including ERCP, have failed and to initiate a sphincterotomy when the papillotome cannot be introduced completely into the papilla (Cremer et al 1977). For diathermy ERCP a diathermy cutter of needle type is used (Caletti et al 1980). It is introduced through the biopsy channel of the instrument and after facing the intramural position of the common bile duct, 5–8 mm above the papilla, a small fistula 1–1.5 mm in diameter is created with the diathermy cutter. Cholangiography is then performed through the small hole. For pre-cut sphincterotomy the tip of the papillotome enters the papilla to a depth of 3–5 mm and then a pre-cut is performed which permits the passage of a cannulating catheter or which can later be enlarged to a normal sphincterotomy (Siegel 1980).

Diathermy ERCP and pre-cut sphincterotomy are applicable in cases of papillary stenosis, impacted calculi or anatomic variations, either congenital or acquired, but are not recommended by all and should only be performed by the endoscopist with experience (Siegel 1980).

Duct cytology and pancreatic juice collections
Pure bile can be collected by simple aspiration after deep cannulation of the common bile duct. Pancreatic juice for cytology should preferably be free of contrast, but this is often inevitable since it is the radiographs which provide the indication for cytology. If cancer is suspected and the pancreatic duct cannot be

cannulated, some juice may be aspirated from the orifice. Cell yields are higher from the pancreatic ducts than from bile and with direct brushing techniques. Specially designed sleeved brushes can be passed into the biliary or pancreatic ductal system. Brush cytology is most useful in the differential diagnosis of biliary strictures and in searching for small cancers within the papilla of Vater (Cotton & Williams 1980). Histological specimens can be obtained using standard biopsy forceps from some duct lesions. However, the normal forceps are too straight and too strong. Special forceps were developed (Seifert et al 1977) which are softer and more curved, and which may be guided into the biliary duct. Specimens obtained by these special forceps are, however, small and allow cytological rather than histological preparation.

Endoscopic biliary manometry

Manometry carried out by endoscopic means offers a method of evaluating pressures in the common bile duct and sphincter of Oddi (Hagenmüller et al 1977, Rösch et al 1977). Manometry is performed using two standard cannulating catheters modified by occlusion of the end-hole and creation of a 0.8 mm side-hole, 3 mm from the tip (Bar-Meir et al 1979). One catheter is passed through the channel of the duodenoscope, and is passed into the ductal system. The other catheter is attached to the side of the endoscope so as to allow simultaneous measurement of intraluminal duodenal pressure. Catheters are connected to suitable transducers and are continuously perfused with water by a pump perfusion system. All measurements are made at end-inspiration and the zero reference point is atmospheric. Baseline pressures are obtained and then a slow station pull-through from the distal common bile duct across the sphincter of Oddi is begun. Pressures are obtained at 2 mm stations, pausing for two to five minutes at each (Bar-Meir et al 1979, Cotton & Williams 1980).

In our own experience, however, endoscopic biliary manometry is unsatisfactory because the presence of a catheter may induce sphincteric contractions and delay emptying. In addition, pharmacological premedication influences the results. In most endoscopic centres manometry does not play an important role for the confirmation of diagnosis of papillary stenosis.

Complications of ERCP

All endoscopic procedures carry hazards and there are risks in ERCP. However, complications are mainly caused by inexperience and can be minimised. In large series the frequency of complications varies between 1.85% and 2.59% with a mortality rate of 0.10%–0.14% (Belohlavek et al 1977, Bilbao et al 1976, Nebel et al 1975) (Table 4.1). The serum amylase rises briskly but transiently after pancreatography, but the incidence of clinical acute pancreatitis is less than 1% (Blackwood et al 1973). Hyperamylasemia and pancreatitis following ERCP are usually short-lived and resolve within 48 hours provided a normal pancreatic system has been demonstrated. Parenchymal filling should be avoided (Demling et al 1974, Ruppin et al 1974).

ERCP is not a sterile technique and the introduction of infection into a stagnant ductal system, or especially into a pancreatic pseudocyst, should be excluded by ultrasound scanning prior to ERCP. If a pseudocyst is present, ERCP is usually

Table 4.1 Complications of ERCP

	Bilbao et al 1976	Belohlavek et al 1976	Nebel et al 1975	Author's series (unpublished)
	N = 10 435	N = 8960	N = 3884	N = 2214
Complications	270 = 2.59%	166 = 1.85%	94 = 2.42%	46 = 2.10%
Deaths	15 = 0.14%	12 = 0.13%	5 = 0.13%	2 = 0.10%

not necessary but if carried out, prophylactic antibiotics should be given and operation should follow immediately. In patients with biliary stasis due to stones or stricture the procedure may provoke cholangitis and septicaemia. In such cases antibiotic prophylaxis is advisable and the procedure should be followed by stone-removal and drainage of the biliary system either by endoscopic means or by open operation. Over-filling of the obstructed biliary system should be avoided (Keighley et al 1976, Low et al 1980, Schiller & Prout 1976). Routine antibiotic prophylaxis is considered unnecessary but indications include the obstructed biliary tree, the presence of a pancreatic pseudocyst, and immunosuppressed patients (Siegel et al 1979).

Clinical value of ERCP

The main indications for ERCP are:

1. Obstructive jaundice
2. Failure of opacification of the biliary tree or gallbladder by conventional radiology in non-jaundiced patients
3. The patient with post-cholecystectomy symptoms
4. Sensitivity to contrast material used for intravenous cholangiography

Choledocholithiasis
Calculi in the biliary system are easily diagnosed by ERCP (Anacker et al 1977, Blumgart & Salmon 1973, Wurbs & Classen 1977). Failure in the interpretation of X-ray films may occur due to inadequate filling of the biliary system or by over-filling with dense contrast. Papillary stones within the common bile duct, if not impacted, may be moved by instillation of contrast material and can be demonstrated on the screen or on X-ray. Gallbladder filling may only occur when the position of the patient is changed. Small stones within the gallbladder may only be demonstrated on late films taken 30–60 minutes after installation of contrast (Ottenjann & Classen 1979). Air bubbles inadvertently injected with the contrast material may simulate calculi but can be differentiated by changing the position of the patient (Cotton 1977). Up to one third of biliary calculi may not present with clinical symptoms and some have suggested that common bile duct stones are more dangerous when they produce minimal symptoms and remain for long periods within the ductal system (Leach 1978).

Comparison of the results of ERCP and intravenous cholangiography has demonstrated that ERCP has a significantly higher rate of correct diagnosis of biliary calculi, both in the gallbladder and common bile duct. Biliary stones may be present in patients with a normal intravenous cholangiogram and ERCP reduces the rate of diagnostic error in patients with symptoms of biliary disease (Osnes et al 1978). In the post-cholecystectomy patient intravenous cholangiography has been shown to be particularly unreliable in detecting the presence or absence of gallstones and ERPC has a much higher diagnostic yield (Blumgart et al 1977).

Complications of biliary calculi are further indications for ERCP. The Mirizzi syndrome (stone impaction in the cystic duct, cholecystitis and hepatic duct stenosis) can be clearly demonstrated by ERCP, as can the sites of perforation of stones from the gallbladder into the choledochus or adjacent viscera.

Sclerosing cholangitis

This is a rare condition which may occur primarily or be associated with inflammatory bowel disease (ulcerative colitis, Crohn's disease) (Atkinson & Caroll 1964, Brantigan & Brantigan 1973, Elias et al 1974, Halutzky & McKenzie 1964, Thorpe et al 1967). Tumours or stones in the biliary system must be excluded. This is not always easy, particularly if the stenosis is localised. There is a chronic inflammation of the bile ducts with glandular proliferation and stenosing fibrosis. Sometimes the inflammatory process is limited to the extrahepatic bile ducts (Ottenjann & Classen 1979). ERCP demonstrates irregularities of the extrahepatic biliary system with narrowing of the lumen, calibre variations and occasional areas of dilatation (Low et al 1980) (Fig. 4.1). When the intrahepatic

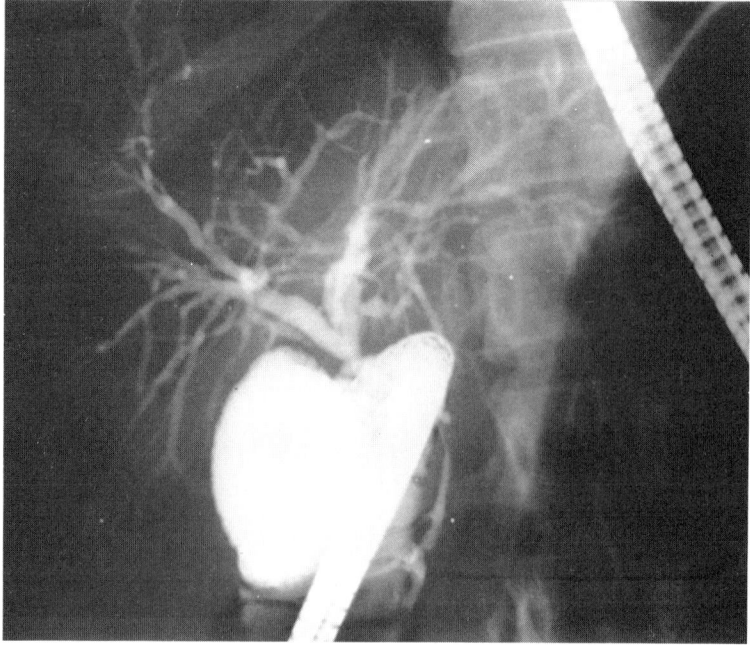

Fig. 4.1 Sclerosing cholangitis

biliary tree is involved, there are irregular areas of stenosis and dilatation and some bile ducts are totally occluded, giving an appearance of rarefaction (Geisse et al 1975, Warren et al 1966).

Tumours of the gallbladder and bile ducts

Benign tumours of the gallbladder and of the bile ducts are occasionally observed (Burhans & Myers 1971, Dowdy et al 1962). In the gallbladder they are parietal and do not change their position with movement of the patient. They must be differentiated from calculi.

Malignant tumours of the gallbladder are seldom diagnosed at ERCP. When gallbladder cancer involves the common hepatic duct it creates a stenosis close to the confluence of the hepatic ducts and simulates a primary hilar bile duct tumour. Neoplasms of the bile duct usually occur close the liver hilus or in the distal common bile duct (Seifert et al 1974, Warren et al 1972, Whelton et al 1969). ERCP reveals an irregular stenosis (Fig. 4.2). When the tumour is located in the distal common bile duct, there is usually a pre-stenotic dilatation (Seifert et al 1974). Localisation at the bifurcation produces no dilatation of the intrahepatic tree in some 20% of cases. In patients in whom the tumour is small, only minimal X-ray findings may be observed and interpretation must be cautious (Seifert et al 1974). In many cases, abrupt termination of the common bile duct is shown at ERCP (Fig. 4.3). In such cases percutaneous cholangiography is more useful in

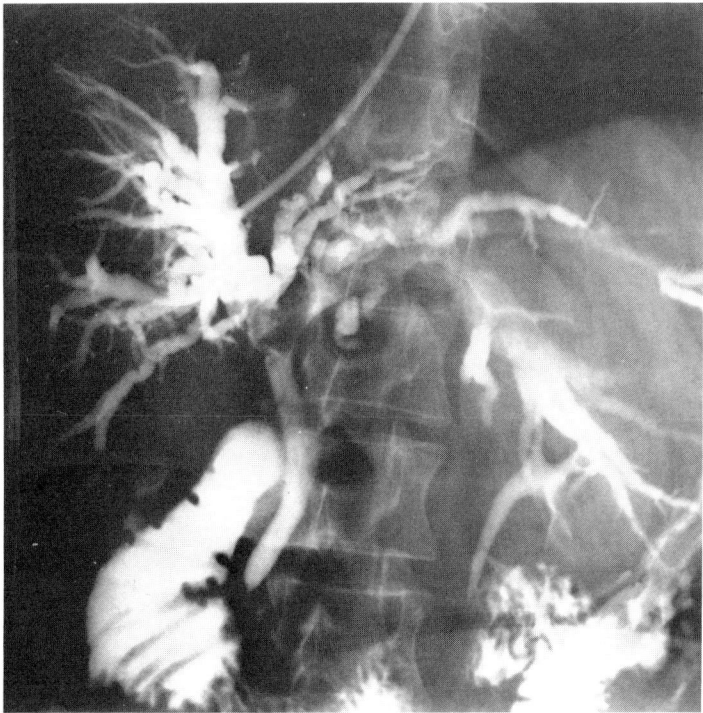

Fig. 4.2 Cancer at the common bile duct bifurcation (Tumour filling defect)

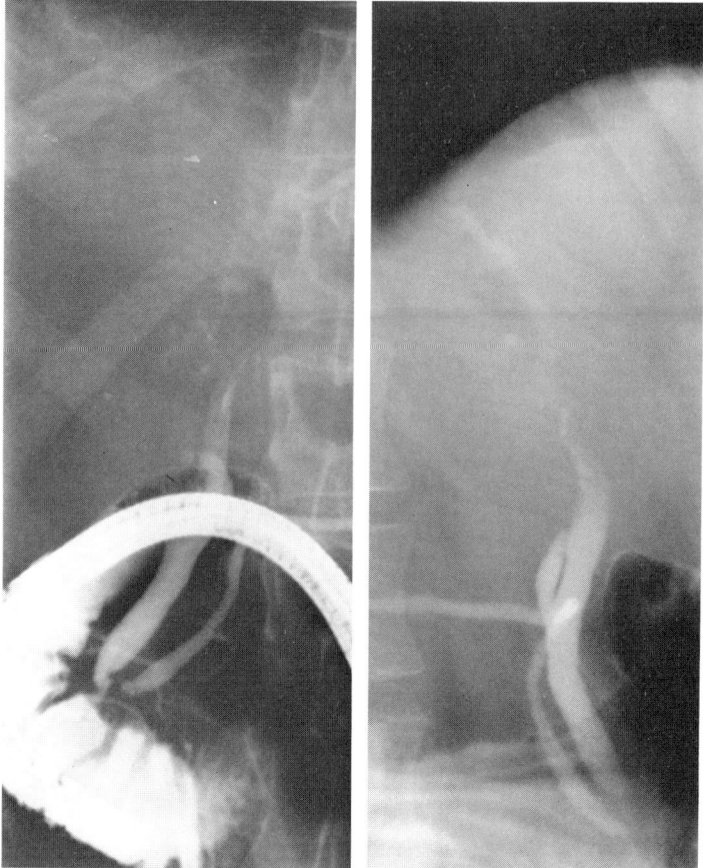

Fig. 4.3 Obstruction of common bile duct filling (cancer)

demonstrating the proximal extent of the tumour and the intrahepatic ducts (Burwood et al 1973, Classen & Demling 1973, Geisse et al 1975, Huchzermeyer et al 1975, Seifert et al 1974).

Postoperative investigation

After surgical operations, ERCP may be very valuable. Most changes observed are consequent on the creation of surgical stomata or iatrogenic error. ERCP is the most reliable diagnostic procedure in such cases, especially since it allows demonstration of the duodenal loop, visualisation of surgical stomata, and the demonstration not only of the biliary tree but also the pancreas (Blumgart et al 1970, Classen et al 1971, Ruddell et al 1980).

Most calculi found in post-cholecyestectomy patients have been overlooked at initial operation. However, some develop postoperatively and may be associated with retained sutures.

Benign iatrogenic stricture of the bile duct is seen following a variety of surgical procedures on the stomach, duodenum or pancreas, but usually follow cholecystectomy with damage to the common bile duct. Many such strictures are high in the common hepatic duct (Fig. 4.4). ERCP usually reveals a short stenosis or an abrupt termination of the common bile duct and there is no pre-stenotic dilatation of the intrahepatic ducts. PTC is generally more valuable in this situation in demonstrating the extent of the stricture and the possibilities for repair

Papillary stenosis is usually secondary to previous disease or surgery. Primary papillary stenosis in the absence of calculi and without prior surgery is extremely rare and some doubt its existence. Most papillary stenoses are found in patients with choledocholithiasis and are consequent on passage of stones through the papilla. When observed postoperatively, the diagnosis may have been missed at operation. At ERCP the common bile duct as well as the intrahepatic tree is dilated with hold-up of contrast material and delayed emptying into the duodenum. Clinical examination and laboratory tests are characteristic of cholestasis and pain may be present (Fig. 4.5). In our opinion, it is only permissible to make the diagnosis if the characteristic X-ray appearances and the clinical syndrome are present.

Sometimes fistulae from the lower common bile duct into the duodenum are found (Classen et al 1971, Hunt & Blumgart 1980). Nearly always they are observed close to the papillary orifice. Most are surgically produced and result from bouginage carried out intraoperatively in an attempt to pass a sound from the common bile duct into the duodenum. If the instrument perforates the wall of the bile duct, it is always above the papillary orifice. Similar orifices are found when surgical sphincterotomy is carried out, a false opening being made in error above the true papilla. In other cases a gallstone perforates the common bile duct at its

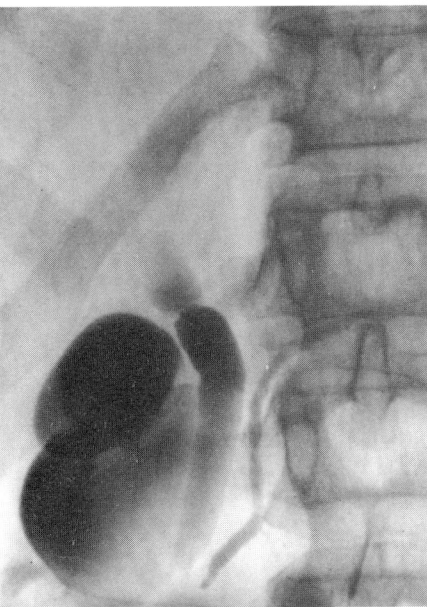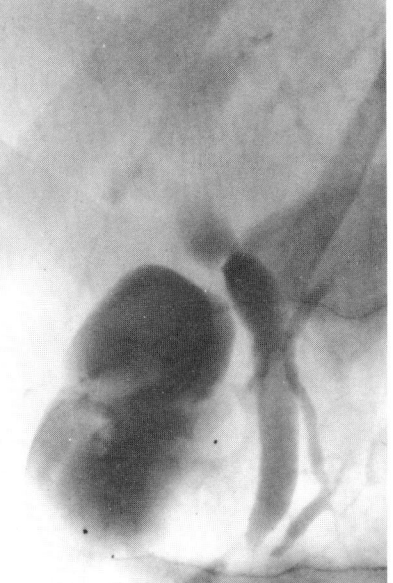

Fig. 4.4 Postoperative stricture of the common bile duct

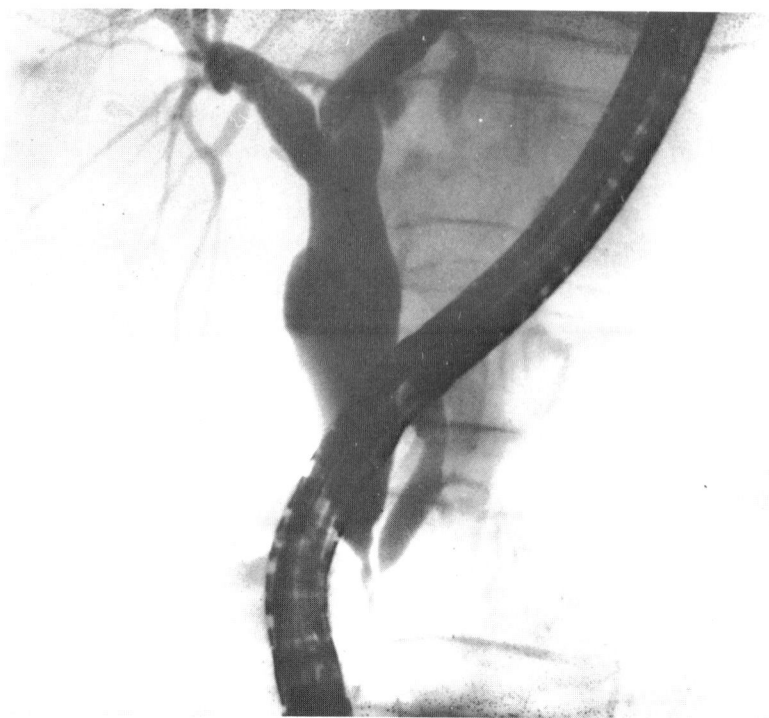

Fig. 4.5 Papillary stenosis

lowest portion and passes into the duodenum, leaving a fistulous track (Hunt & Blumgart 1980, Isch et al 1971). In such cases a second orifice exists above the papilla, and may be seen endoscopically and demonstrated radiologically after filling of the common bile duct.

Surgically performed biliary digestive anastomoses such as choledocho-duodenostomy and choledochojejunostomy may have been carried out. Chole-dochoduodenostomy can be readily inspected endoscopically and cannulated. If the choledochoduodenostomy orifice is narrow, then recurrent attacks of cholangitis may develop and this may similarly occur when a 'sump' syndrome is present with retained food or debris in the distal choledochus.

Pancreatic disease
Pancreatic diseases may compress the common bile duct. Thus carcinoma of the pancreatic head either causes stenosis at the papillary region of the common bile duct with dilatation of the prestenotic area, or results in an abrupt destruction of the choledochus above the papilla. Chronic pancreatitis usually results in a more tubular stenosis of the common bile duct (Fig. 4.6).

Other findings
Rarely, enlarged lymph nodes, especially in lymphatic system diseases, can cause compression of the biliary system. ERCP also plays a diagnostic role in the

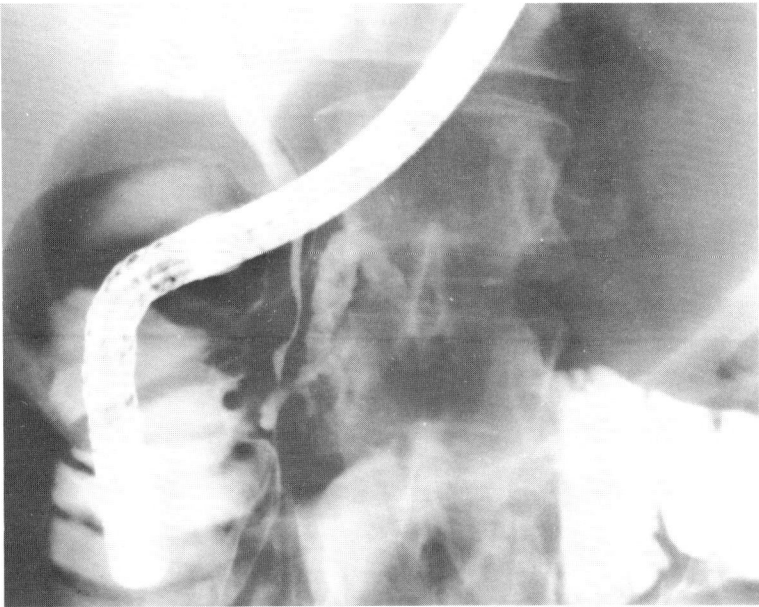

Fig. 4.6 Tabular stenosis of the common bile duct caused by chronic pancreatitis

recognition of traumatic injuries, such as haemobilia or traumatic division or rupture of the common bile duct, in a variety of liver diseases such as biliary cirrhosis, liver tumours, liver cysts, Caroli's disease, and in defining the presence of ascaris infection. Foreign bodies may also be found within the biliary system (Manegold 1981, Ottenjann & Classen 1979, Soehendra & Werner 1977).

Therapeutic procedures

Endoscopic diathermy sphincterotomy was first performed in 1973 (Classes & Demling 1974, Kawai et al 1974) and is now established as a major advance in the management of bile duct stones and is a possible therapy in a variety of other problems arising in the biliary tract (Cotton 1980, Demling & Classen 1978, Safrany 1977, 1978, Wurbs et al 1980b).

Indications
1. Presence of common bile duct stones in association with biliary tract obstruction and acute suppurative cholangitis in high risk patients (irrespective of the presence of the gallbladder)
2. Retained or recurrent common bile duct stones after cholecystectomy
3. Papillary stenosis
4. Palliative treatment of papillary tumours

Technique
After performing ERCP and confirming the presence of stones or papillary stenosis, the papillotome is inserted into the papilla of Vater. The papillotome wire

Table 4.2 Endoscopic sphincterotomy (survey from 25 centres). N = 9041

Common bile duct stones	N = 7585 = 83.90%
After cholecystectomy	N = 5347
With gallbladder in situ	N = 2238
Circumscribed papillary stenosis	N = 962 = 10.64%
Without common bile duct stones	N = 813
With common bile duct stones	N = 149
Papillary tumour	N = 187 = 2.06%
Other indications	N = 307 = 3.40%

is sheathed in a plastic tube. After insertion, the wire is bent and the roof of the papilla is cut using a high frequency current (Seifert 1977, 1978). After cutting the papilla, one may wait for spontaneous passage of the calculi or proceed to extract them immediately using a Dormia basket or Fogarty catheter, or a special loop. When calculi have not been removed and spontaneous passage has not ensued during the subsequent 8–10 days, a second procedure is necessary to remove the stones (Seifert 1978).

After endoscopic sphincterotomy duodenobiliary reflux is demonstrable in 25% of patients and aerobilia in 65%. Although a bacterobilia is almost invariable, cholangitis does not usually supervene (Burhenne 1981).

Occasionally it proves difficult to place the diathermy wire deeply into the bile duct (Seifert 1978). Some then recommend a 'pre-cut' (vide supra) in order to enlarge the papillary common channel (Cotton 1981). This allows later access to the bile duct. However, this is an uncontrolled manoeuvre and should not be undertaken by the inexperienced.

Results

We have collected the results of endoscopic sphincterotomy from 25 centres in West Germany (Table 4.2). In the period up to April 1981, 9041 procedures were performed. The main indications were common bile duct calculi in 83.9% (5347 of 7585 cases were cholecystectomised, 2238 had the gallbladder in situ). In 10.64% the indication for papillotomy was papillary stenosis with or without common bile duct stones. In 2.06% endoscopic sphincterotomy was performed because of papillary tumours, and in 3.4% because of other rare conditions. Thus choledo-cholithiasis is the main indication (Table 4.3). The success rate for endoscopic papillotomy carried out for stones was 84.06%. In 10.98% the procedure was attempted but was not successful or residual stones remained, while in 4.96% the

Table 4.3 Choledocholithiasis (N = 7585)

	N	%
Successful	6376	84.06
Not successful		
(stones remaining)	833	10.98
Not controlled	376	4.96
Op because of stones		
remaining	404	5.33

procedure was not controlled and information was incomplete. Of the 833 patients in whom the attempt at endoscopic sphincterotomy was not successful, 404 cases (5.33%) were subsequently operated upon. In this survey it was surprising that of the patients with the gallbladder in situ, only 9.83% came to cholecystectomy after endoscopic sphincterotomy.

Emergency endoscopic sphincterotomy

During recent years, emergency endoscopic papillotomy has become an important procedure. In West Germany 240 cases have been treated (table 4.4), 105 because of purulent cholangitis, 54 because of acute cholangitis and 90 with acute biliary pancreatitis (Safrany et al 1980a, Seifert 1980). Emergency endoscopic sphincterotomy may be a life-saving procedure in patients with purulent cholangitis, especially in the elderly (Seifert 1980). It is also a useful method in cases of biliary pancreatitis when an impacted calculus in the biliary tract causes obstruction of the pancreatic duct. Our experience has indicated that instillation of contrast material during an episode of acute pancreatitis does not result in clinical deterioration. Emergency endoscopic papillotomy is, in our opinion, worthy of further trial.

Table 4.4 Emergency EST (N = 241)

Purulent cholangitis	105
Acute not purulent cholangitis	44
Acute biliary pancreatitis	90
Acute bleeding after EST	2

Complications

Complications have occurred in 7.55% of cases. This is in accord with the published results of others (Table 4.5) (Cotton 1980, 1981, Ottenjann & Classen 1979, Safrany 1977, 1979, Wurbs et al 1980) and with our own data (Seifert 1977, 1978, Seifert & Wurbs 1977). However, in cases of papillary stenosis the complication rate is much higher (Gail & Seifert 1980). In patients with papillary tumours the complication rate is 5.35%.

Haemorrhage is the most common complication, followed by pancreatitis, cholangitis and perforation. Looking at the different indications for EST it can be seen that in cases of choledocholithiasis, haemorrhage occurs more often than in patients with papillary stenosis. However, perforation is more frequently encountered in patients with papillary stenosis (Gail & Seifert 1980). Cholangitis only occurs after endoscopic papillotomy carried out for common bile duct calculi (Seifert & Wurbs 1977).

Retroperitoneal perforation is usually recognised immediately or within 12 hours and contrast material may be demonstrated outside the ductal system (Seifert 1978). Haemorrhage also seems to occur immediately or within the first day, while pancreatitis and cholangitis may become manifest later and occur within 48 hours of the procedure. Acute cholecystitis subsequent to endoscopic

Table 4.5 Complications of EST

Indication		N
Choledocholithiasis	N = 7585	566 = 7.46%
Papillary stenosis (without stones)	N = 813	72 = 8.86%
Papillary tumour	N = 187	10 = 5.35%
	N = 8585	648 = 7.55%

sphincterotomy during the primary admission is usually an early complication and becomes manifest within the first 48 hours.

Treatment of complications
In our survey (Table 4.6) 451 patients developed complications after endoscopic sphincterotomy carried out for choledocholithiasis. Of these, 157 were treated surgically and 294 conservatively. In all, 17.1% died (30% of those treated surgically and 10% of those treated conservatively). Examination of the complications reveals that an attempt at conservative management is usually justifiable. Mortality rates were generally much lower for the conservative group and particularly for patients with haemorrhage, pancreatitis and cholangitis. The difference was not so marked in patients with perforation.

We would advise primary conservative treatment of the complications of endoscopic sphincterotomy and only advise operation when major bleeding is in progress and is not controlled conservatively, or in cases of perforation when signs of peritonitis are evident.

Complications developing after endoscopic sphincterotomy for papillary stenosis were particularly lethal, the overall mortality rate in this group being 25% and reaching 53% if surgical interference was attempted. Similarly, in cases of papillary tumour, the complication of bleeding was attended by a mortality rate of 10%.

Mortality of endoscopic sphincterotomy
The overall mortality of endoscopic sphincterotomy in our survey was 1.12% of 8585 treated patients (Table 4.7). This is in accord with the results published in the world literature (Cotton 1980, 1981, Ottenjann & Classen 1979, Safrany 1977, 1979, Seifert 1977, 1978, Seifert & Wurbs 1977, Wurbs et al 1980b). We did, however, demonstrate that the mortality rate was twice as high when the procedure was carried out for papillary stenosis as compared to choledocholithiasis. For papillary tumour, the mortality is low (0.53%). Although when complications did develop the mortality was high (vide supra).

Long-term results
Follow-up may be made by radiological methods or by questionnaire or clinical examination.

In 1050 patients follow-up examinations were performed by ERCP, intravenous cholangiography or PTC (Table 4.8). No stones were demonstrated in the biliary tree in 91.62% of cases. Recurrent stones were, however, demonstrated in

Table 4.6 Treatment of complications

			Surgical Deaths		Conservative Deaths
Choledocholithiasis	N = 451	157	47 = 30%	294	30 = 10%
Perforation (leakage)	N = 49	26	8 = 31%	23	6 = 26%
Haemorrhage	N = 136	44	17 = 39%	92	5 = 5%
Pancreatitis	N = 77	11	8 = 72%	66	8 = 12%
Cholangitis	N = 82	23	9 = 39%	59	10 = 17%
Cholecystitis	N = 10	4	/	6	/
Others	N = 97	49	5 = 10%	48	1 = 2%
Papillary stenosis	N = 72	19	10 = 53%	53	8 = 15%
Perforation (leakage)	N = 18	10	4 = 40%	8	5 = 63%
Haemorrhage	N = 25	3	1 = 33%	22	/
Pancreatitis	N = 28	6	5 = 83%	22	3 = 14%
Cholangitis	N = 1	/	/	1	/
Papillary tumour	N = 10	/	/	10	1 = 10%
Haemorrhage	N = 10	/	/	10	1 = 10%

Table 4.7 Mortality of EST

Indication		N
Choledocholithiasis	N = 7585	77 = 1.02%
Papillary stenosis (without stones)	N = 813	18 = 2.21%
Papillary tumour	N = 187	1 = 0.53%
	N = 8585	96 = 1.12%

Table 4.8 Long-term results of EST. Follow-up (ERCP, I.V. Cholangio etc)

		Stone-free	Recurrent stones	Stenosis
Choledocholithiasis (cholecystectomy)	N = 684	625 = 91.37%	39 = 5.70%	20 = 2.93%
Choledocholithiasis (gallbladder in situ)	N = 270†	252 = 93.33%	16 = 5.93%	2 = 0.74%
Papillary stenosis	N = 96	85 = 88.54%	/	11 = 11.46%
	N = 1050	962 = 91.62	55 = 5.77%*	33 = 3.14%

*according to all cases with choledocholithiasis
†necessary cholecystectomy N = 59 = 21.85%

Table 4.9 Long-term results of EST. Questionnaire or clinical examination (N = 1899)

		Symptom-free	Improved	Unchanged	Advanced
Choledocholithiasis (cholecystectomized)	N = 1353	888 = 65.63	392 = 28.97%	59 = 4.36%	14 = 1.04%
Choledocholithiasis (gallbladder in situ)	N = 419	384 = 91.65%		21 = 5.01%	14 = 3.34%
Papillary stenosis	N = 127	70 = 55.12%	41 = 32.28%	13 = 10.24%	3 = 2.36%
	N = 1899	1775 = 93.47%		93 = 4.90%	31 = 1.63%

5.77% but sometimes were not considered related to the patients' symptoms, jaundice, or pathological laboratory findings. When compared with surgical statistics, this number of recurrent stones is high but there is no real surgical series in which patients have been followed up in a similar way. Re-stenosis of endoscopic sphincterotomy has occurred in 3.14% and this more frequently after papillary stenosis than choledocholithiasis.

When patients were followed up by questionnaire or clinical examination, late results were available in 1889 cases (Table 4.9). Patients were found to be symptom-free or improved in 93.47% of patients.

The results were better in cases of choledocholithiasis where patients were symptom-free in 65.63% of cases as compared to only 55.12% of patients presenting with papillary stenosis. Indeed, in the group with papillary stenosis, symptoms had remained unchanged or become worse in 12.60%, this result again being not as good as that achieved for choledocholithiasis where the patient's symptoms remained unchanged or advanced in 4.4% of patients (cholecystectomised).

Special problems

The size of gallstones is a difficulty. Stones of less than 14 mm diameter will pass spontaneously with an adequate sphincterotomy but in some patients (about 30%) new stones may form, especially about retained surgical sutures, and in about 5% biliary sludge may be demonstrated (Seifert 1977, 1978). Larger stones have been removed, but the risk of bleeding and perforation increases as the sphincterotomy size is enlarged.

After removal of multiple stones, air bubbles sometimes come into the common bile duct which makes it impossible to distinguish stones from air by X-ray. In such cases it may be necessary to insert a nasobiliary tube to allow repeated radiographic control.

Endoscopic lithotripsy of stones lodged in the common bile duct has been successfully carried out (Koch et al 1977, 1980, Laurence & Cotton 1980, Demling et al 1982). For this purpose the lithotripsy probe is integrated with a Dormia basket. It is important, however, that before the stone is shattered, it should be firmly lodged in the basket. Attempts to break up stones using an ultrasound probe have also been reported.

Impaction of stones or baskets occasionally occurs and is an unavoidable complication. Should such complications occur, surgery is usually necessary.

When a T-tube is in place and retained stones are demonstrated shortly after cholecystectomy, the technique of Burhenne (Burhenne 1981) or stone-dissolution should be tried first before sphincterotomy is resorted to.

There is insufficient data to judge the efficacy and safety of using endoscopic sphincterotomy to enlarge stenosed biliary digestive anastomoses (Barkin et al 1980). We have experienced severe bleeding in an attempt to enlarge choledochoduodenostomy, and furthermore have found the procedure unsatisfactory since biliary sludge and retained food continues to accumulate despite sufficient bile outflow into the duodenum. For patients with a biliary fistula above the papilla of Vater caused by stone perforation or previous surgical instrumentation, sphincterotomy can be employed to join the main papillary orifice with the fistula.

In patients who have undergone Billroth II resection, there are major difficulties which result in a high risk and low success rate whatever methods are employed (Cremer et al 1977, Leach 1978, Safrany et al 1980b, Wurbs et al 1980a).

Special procedures
In patients with retained stones after operation and with a T-tube in situ, the papillotome can be inserted from above, down the common bile duct and then through the orifice of the papilla. Correct direction and length of incision can be controlled endoscopically. Similarly, in patients with retained biliary calculi and complicating cholangitis who cannot be treated by endoscopic papillotomy, the papillotome can be passed via the percutaneous transhepatic route (Nimura et al 1980, Urakami et al 1979). There are, however, very few indications for these procedures.

Recently the technique of nasobiliary drainage has been described whereby a catheter is left in the bile duct after sphincterotomy and brought out through the patient's nose. The tubes are well tolerated for days, or even weeks, and allow easy sequential cholangiography, bile sampling for culture, and bile duct lavage with saline or other solvents (Cotton et al 1979, Wurbs et al 1980b). A 2.5 mm tube with side-holes is passed deeply into the bile duct and preferably looped within the common hepatic ductal system. After removal of the endoscope, the tube is re-routed through the nose. A nasobiliary drainage is indicated in all cases after sphincterotomy when multiple stones have been present and complete removal is not certain, and also in cases with larger stones too dangerous to remove (Cotton et al 1979, Wurbs & Classen 1977, Wurbs et al 1980b). Suppurative cholangitis may be treated in this manner and stone solvents introduced into the biliary tree (Schenk et al 1980, Thistle et al 1980, Witzel et al 1981).

Biliary prostheses may be introduced in patients with malignant strictures of the biliary tree or papillary tumours as palliative treatment (Laurence & Cotton 1980). Endoscopic sphincterotomy is necessary before insertion of the prosthesis. Finally, peroral cholangioscopy has been carried our following endoscopic papillotomy. This allows the passage of a fine endoscope into the biliary system. The technique relies on the introduction of a smaller endoscope carried on the main instrument. At present, however, the technique is difficult and the imaging poor, and biopsy is not possible (Ariyama et al 1979, Kawai et al 1976, Sakai et al 1980, Urakami et al 1977, Urakami 1980).

The final place of these new techniques in the management of biliary disorders depends on future assessment.

References

Anacker H, Weiss H D, Kamann B 1977 Endoscopic retrograde pancreaticocholangiography (ERCP). Springer, Berlin-Heidelberg-New York

Ariyama S, Kawamura S, Guji T, Shimizu M, Azuma M, Maetani N, Harima K, Kawashima M, Nagatomi Y, Takemoto T 1979 Peroral fiber-choledochoscope — the second report Gastroent Endoscopy (Jap) 21: 1217

Atkinson A J, Caroll W 1964 Sclerosing cholangitis. Association with regional enteritis. Journal of the American Medical Association 188: 183–184

Barkin J S, Silvis S, Greenwald R 1980 Endoscopic therapy of the 'sump' syndrome. Dig Dis Sci 25: 597

Bar-Meir S, Geenen J E, Hogan W J, Dodds W J, Stewart E T, Arndorfer R C 1979 Biliary and pancreatic duct pressures measured by ERCP manometry in patients with suspected papillary stenosis. Dig Dis Sci 24: 209

Becker M, Miederer S E, Emons D, Totthauwe H W 1980 Endoskopisch-retrograde Cholangiopancreatographie im Kindesalter. Deutsche medizinische Wochenschrift 105: 1055

Belohlavek D, Koch H, Rösch W, Schaffner O, Meeder H U, Flory J, Classen M, Demling L 1976 5 years experience in endoscopic retrograde cholangio-pancreatography (ERCP). Endoscopy 8: 115

Bilbao M K, Dotter C T, Lee T G, Katon R M 1976 Complications of endoscopic retrograde cholangiopancreatography (ERCP). A study of 10 000 cases. Gastroenterology 70: 314

Blackwood W D, Vennes J A, Silvis S E 1973 Post-endoscopy pancreatitis and hyperamyluria. Gastrointestinal Endoscopy 20: 56

Blumgart L H, Salmon P R 1973 Fiberduodenoscopy and transpapillary cholangiopancreatography. In: Taylor S (ed) Recent advances in surgery. Churchill Livingstone, Edinburgh 8: 36–38

Blumgart L H, Carachi R, Imrie C W, Benjamin I S, Duncan J G 1977 Diagnosis and management of post-cholecystectomy symptoms: the place of endoscopy and retrograde choledochpancreatography. British Journal of Surgery 64: 809–816

Brantigan C O, Brantigan O C 1973 Primary sclerosing cholangitis. American Surgeon 39: 191–198

Burnhans R, Myers R T 1971 Benign neoplasms of the enterohepatic biliary ducts. American Surgeon 37: 161

Burhenne H J 1981 Radiological retrieval of bile duct stones. In: Bennett J R (ed) Therapeutic endoscopy and radiology of the gut.Chapman & Hall, London

Burmeister W, Wurbs D, Hagenmüller F, Classen M, 1980 Langzeituntersuchungen nach endoskopischer Papillotome (EPT). Zeitschrift fur Gastroenterologie 18: 527

Burwood R J, Davies G T, Lawrie B W, Blumgart L H, Salmon P R 1973 Endoscopic retrograde cholangiography. Clinical Radiology 24: 397

Caletti G. C., Verucchi G, Bolondi L, Labo G 1980 Diathermy ERCP. An alternative method for endoscopic retrograde cholangiopancreatography (ERCP). Gastrointestinal Endoscopy 26: 13

Classen M 1976 Endoscopic retrograde cholangiopancreatography. Liver symposium, Basel

Classen M 1977 Endoskopisch retrograde Cholangio-Pankreatikoskopie (ERCPS). In: Lindner H (ed) Fortschritte der gastroenterologischen Endoskopie. Witzstrock, Baden-Baden

Classen M, Demling L 1973 Retrograde Cholangiographie beim Verschlußikterus. Radiologe 13: 35

Classen M, Demling L 1974 Endoskopische Sphinkterotomie der Papilla Vateri und Steinextraktion aus dem Ductus choledochus. Deutsche Medizinische Wochenschrift 99: 496

Classen M, Frühmorgen P, Kozu T, Demling L 1971 Endoscopic radiological demonstration of biliodigestive fistulas. Endoscopy 3: 138

Cotton P B 1972 Cannulation of the papilla of Vater by endoscopy and retrograde cholangio-pancreatography (ERCP). Gut 13: 1014

Cotton P B 1977a ERCP. Gut 18: 316

Cotton P B 1977b Progress Report ERCP. Gut 18: 316–341

Cotton P B 1980 Non-operative removal of bile duct stones by duodenoscopic sphincterotomy. British Journal of Surgery 67: 1–5

Cotton P B 1981 Duodenoscopic sphincterotomy and bile-duct stone retrieval. In: Bennett J R (ed) Therapeutic endoscopy and radiology of the gut. Chapman & Hall, London

Cotton P B, Kizu M 1977 Endoscopic pancreatography and pure pancreatic juice. In: Jerzy G B (ed) Progress in Gastroenterology 3. Glass, Grune & Stratton, New York

Cotton P B, Williams C B 1980 Practical gastrointestinal endoscopy. Blackwell Scientific Publications, Oxford

Cotton P B, Burney P G J, Mason R R 1979 Transnasal bile duct catheterisation after endoscopic sphincterotomy. Gut 20: 285

Cremer M, Gulbis A, Toussaint J, de Toeuf J, Vanlaethem A, Hemanus A 1977 Technique of endoscopic papillotomy. In: Delmont J (ed) The sphincter of Oddi. Harger, Basel

Demling L 1976 5 Jahre ERCP — Pro und Contra. Deutsche medizinische Wochenschrift 20: 797

Demling L, Classen M, Frühmorgen P 1974 Atlas der Enteroskopie. Springer, Berlin-Heidelberg-New York

Demling L, Classen M (ed) 1978a Endoscopy of the small intestine with retrograde pancreatocholangiography. Thieme, Stuttgart

Demling L, Classen M 1978b Endoscopic sphincterotomy of the papilla of Vater — international workshop. Thieme, Stuttgart

Demling L, Seuberth K, Riemann J F 1982 A mechanical lithotripter. Endoscopy 14: 100

Dowdy G S, Olior W G, Stelton E L, Waldron G W 1962 Benign tumours of the extrahepatic bile ducts. Archives of Surgery 85: 503

Elias E, Summerfield J A S, Dick R, Sherlock S 1974 Endoscopic retrograde cholangiography (ERCP) in the diagnosis of jaundice associated with ulcerative colitis. Gastroenterology 67: 907

Gail K, Seifert E 1980 EPT (endoskopische Papillotomie) eine komplikationsarme Methode? In: Henning H (ed) Fortschritte der gastroenterologischen Endoskopie. Witzstrock, Baden-Baden

Geisse G, Metson G, Tedesco L, Francis J, Kelley J J, Stanley R J 1975 Stenosing lesions of the biliary tract. Evaluation with ERC and PTC. American Journal of Roentgenology Radium Therapy and Nuclear Medicine 123: 378

Hagenmüller F, Ossenberg F W, Classen M 1977 Duodenoscopic manometry of the common bile duct. In: Delmont J (ed) The sphincter of Oddi. Karger, basel

Halutzky J B, McKenzie A D 1964 Primary sclerosing cholangitis of extrahepatic bile ducts. Canadian Journal of Surgery 7: 277–283

Hess W 1973 Cholecystitis,Cholelithiasis und ihre Komplikationen. In: Demling L (ed) Klinische Gastroenterologie. Thieme, Stuttgart

Huchzermeyer H, Luska G, Otto P, Seifert E 1975 The value of the combination of antegrade and retrograde cholangiography in the diagnosis of bile duct obstruction. Endoscopy 7: 126

Hunt D R, Blumgart L H 1980 Iatrogenic choledochoduodenal fistula: an unsuspected cause of post-cholecystectomy symptoms. British Journal of Surgery 67: 10–13

Isch J H, Finneran J C, Nahrwold D L 1971 Perforation of gallbladder. American Journal of Gastroenterology 55: 451–458

Kawai K, Akasaka Y, Murakami K, Tada M, Kohli Y, Nakajima M 1974 Endoscopic sphincterotomy of the papilla of Vater. Gastrointestinal Endoscopy 20: 148

Kawai K, Nakajima M, Akasaka Y, Shimamoto K, Murakami K 1976 Eine neue endoskopische Technik: Die perorale Choledocho-Pancreatoskopie. Leber-Magen Darm 6: 121

Keighley M R B, Drysdale R B, Quoraisi A H, Burdon D W, Alexander-Williams J 1976 Antibiotics in biliary disease: the relative importance of antibiotic concentrations in the bile and serum. Gut 17: 495

Koch H, Rösch W, Walz V 1980 Endoscopic lithotripsy in the common bile duct. Gastrointestinal Endoscopy 26: 16

Koch H, Stolte M, Walz V 1977 Endoscopic lithotripsy in the common bile duct. Endoscopy 9: 95

Laurence B H, Cotton P B 1980 Endoscopic placement of palliative drainage tubes in malignant biliary obstruction. British Medical Journal: 522–526

Leach R E 1978 Endoscopic sphincterotomy. Proceedings of World Congress of Gastroenterology Madrid

Low D E, Micflikier A B, Kennedy J K, Stiver H G 1980 Infectious complications of endoscopoic retrograde cholangiopancreatography. A prospective assessment. Archives of Internal Medicine 140: 1076

Manegold B C 1981 Möglichkeiten und Grenzen der diagnostischen und therapeutischen ERCP beim Verschlußikterus. Chirurg 52: 423

Nebel O T, Silvis S E, Rogers G, Sugawa C, Mandelstam P 1975 Complications associated with endoscopic retrograde cholangiopancreatography. Gastrointestinal Endoscopy 22: 34

Nimura Y, Miyata K, Yasui K, Mukoyama N, Toyota S, Matsumoto T, Suzuki T, Hattori T, Iyomasa Y, Naito Y, Nakazawa S, Yamamoto Y 1980 Percutaneous transhepatic papillotomy. Gastroent. Endoscopy (Jap) 22: 44

Ohto M, Ono T, Tsuchiya Y, Saisho H 1978 Cholangiography and Pancreatography. Igaki Shoin

Osnes M, Larsen S, Lowe P, Gronseth K, Lotveit T, Nordshus T 1978 Comparison of endoscopic retrograde and intravenous cholangiography in diagnosis of biliary calculi. Lancet 230

Ottenjann R, Classen M 1979 Gastroenterologische Endoskopie. Lehrbuch und Atlas. Enke, Stuttgart

Rösch W, Lux G, Seuberth K 1977 A new catheter for endoscopic manometry of Oddi's sphincter. Endoscopy 9: 31

Ruddell W S J, Ashton M G, Lintott D J, Axon A T R 1980 Endoscopic retrograde cholangiography and pancreatiography in investigation of post-cholecystectomy patients. Lancet 444

Ruppin H, Ammon R, Ettl W, Classen M, Demling L 1974 Acute pancreatitis after endoscopic radiological pancreaticography (ERP). Endoscopy 6: 94

Safrany L 1977 Duodenoscopic sphincterotomy and gallstone removal. Gastroenterology 72: 238

Safrany L 1978 Endoscopic treatment of biliary tract diseases. Lancet 2: 983–985

Safrany L, Neuhaus B, Krause S, Portocarrero G, Schott B 1980a Endoskopische Papillotomie bei akuter, biliär bedingter Pankreatitis. Deutsche medizinische Wochenschrift 105: 115

Safrany L, Neuhaus B, Portocarrero G, Krause S 1980b Endoscopic sphincterotomy in patients with Billroth II gastrectomy. Endoscopy 12: 16

Sakai H, Yoshida Y, Seki H, Furusugi Y, Nogami W, Horiguchi M, Tanaka M, Ido K, Kimura K 1980 Developments of peroral fiber cholangioscope. Gastroent. Endoscopy (Jap) 22: 1221

Schenk J, Schmack B, Rösch W, Riemann J F, Koch H, Demling L 1980 Spülbehandlung von Choledochussteinen mit OCTANOAT (Capmul 8210). Deutsche medizinische Wochenschrift 105: 917

Schiller K F R, Prout B J 1976 Hazards. In: Schiller K F R, Salmon P R (eds) Modern topics in Gastrointestinal Endoscopy. Heinemann, London

Seifert E 1977 Cholelithiasis: Indikation zur Cholecystektomie, Papillotomie und Steinauflösung. Leber Magen Darm 7: 324

Seifert E 1978 Endoscopic papillotomy and removal of gallstones. American Journal of Gastroentology 69: 154

Seifert E 1980 Eitrige Cholangitis. In: Bartelheimer H, Schreiber H W, Ossenberg F W (eds) Die kranken Gallenwege. Witzstrock, Baden-Baden

Seifert E, Wurbs D 1977 Papillotomiesymposium Mai 1977. Sopron, Ungarn, unpublished

Seifert E, Safrany L, Stender H, Lesch P, Luska G, Misaki F 1974 Identification of bile duct tumors by means of endoscopic retrograde pancreato-cholangiography (ERCP). Endoscopy 6: 154

Seifert E, Urakami Y, Elster K 1977 Duodenoscopic guided biopsy of the biliary and pancreatic duct. Endoscopy 9: 154

Siegel J H 1980 Precut papillotomy: A method to improve success of ERCP and papillotomy. Endoscopy 12: 130

Siegel J H, Berger S A, Sable R A, Ho F, Rosenthal W S 1979 Low incidence of bacteremia following endoscopic retrograde cholangio-pancreatography (ERCP). American Journal of Gastroenterology 71: 465

Soehendra N, Reynders-Frederix V 1979 Palliative Gallengangsdrainage. Eine neue

Methode zur endoskopischen Einführung eines inneren Drains. Deutsche medizinische Wochenschrift 104: 206

Soehendra N, Reynders-Frederix V 1980 Palliative bile duct drainage — A new endoscopic method for introducing a transpapillary drain. Endoscopy 12: 8

Soehendra N, Werner B 1977 Zur Diagnostik der traumatischen Hämobilie und Bilhämie. Deutsche medizinische Wochenschrift 12: 428

Stewart E T, Vennes J A, Geenen J E 1977 Atlas of endoscopic retrograde cholangiopancreatography. Mosby, Saint Louis

Thistle J L, Carlson G L, Hoffman A F, Larusso N F, MacArty R L, Flynn G L, Higuchi W I, Babayan V K 1980 Monooctanoin, a dissolution agent for retained cholesterol bile duct stones: Physical properties and clinical application. Gastroenterology 78: 1016

Thorpe M E C, Scheuer P J,. Sherlock S 1967 Primary sclerosing cholangitis, the biliary tract and ulcerative colitis. Gut 8: 435

Urakami Y 1980 Peroral cholangiopancreatoscopy (PCPS) and peroral direct cholangioscopy (PDCS). Endoscopy 12: 30

Urakami Y, Nokihara M, Kishi S 1979 T-tube papillotomy under duodenoscopic control. Gastroent. Endoscopy (Jap) 21: 561

Urakami Y, Seifert E, Butke H 1977 Peroral direct cholangioscopy (PDCS) using a straight fiberscope. Endoscopy 9: 27

Warren K W, Athanassiades S, Monge J I 1966 Primary sclerosing cholangitis — a study of 42 cases. American Journal of Surgery 111: 23

Warren K W, Mountain J C, Lloyd-Jones W 1972 Malignant tumours of the bile ducts. British Journal of Surgery 59: 501

Whelton M J, Petrelli M, George P, Young W B, Sherlock S 1969 Carcinoma at the junction of the main hepatic ducts. Quarterly Journal of Medicine 28: 211

Witzel L, Wiederholt J, Wolbergs E 1981 Dissolution of retained duct stones by perfusion with monooctanoin via a teflon catheter introduced endoscopically. Gastrointestinal Endoscopy 27: 63

Wurbs D, Classen M 1976 Bedeutung der endoskopisch-retrograden Cholangio-Pankreatographie für die Differenzierung der Cholestase. Deutsche medizinische Wochenschrift 8: 291

Wurbs D, Classen M 1977 Transpapillary long standing tube for hepatobiliary drainage. Endoscopy 9: 192

Wurbs D, Hagenmüller F, Classen M 1980a Descending sphincterotomy of the papilla of Vater through a choledochoduodenostomy under endoscopic view. Another variant of endoscopic papillotomy (EPT). Endoscopy 12: 38

Wurbs D, Phillip J, Classen M 1980b Endoskopische Papillotomie mit Gallenwegsdrainage. Alternative und Ergänzung zur Chirurgie der Papillenstenose und des Gallengangssteins. Internist 21: 617

5 Interventional radiology and biliary tract disease

D. J. ALLISON and N. B. BOWLEY

Introduction

In recent years advances in radiological imaging techniques and improvements in catheter technology, together with a new and wider concept of the role of the radiologist in patient management, have contributed to the growth of a new subspeciality known as interventional radiology. Interventional techniques comprise those procedures which either achieve some direct therapeutic benefit for the patient, or, if purely diagnostic in nature, involve the use of methods that are invasive or surgical in nature compared with the techniques of conventional radiological imaging. There can be few areas of surgery in which interventional radiology has made a greater impact on patient management than the biliary system, and the various techniques now available assist in the preoperative diagnosis of biliary disorders, make the surgical procedures easier and safer, help in the management of postoperative complications, and occasionally provide either definitive or palliative treatment that obviates the necessity for any surgical procedure. Interventional techniques in the biliary system fall into three principal categories: therapeutic vascular embolization; biopsy procedures; and procedures designed to relieve or prevent biliary obstruction. These are considered in turn below.

Therapeutic vascular embolization

Therapeutic embolization is the deliberate occlusion of blood vessels by means of emboli introduced via selectively-sited vascular catheters. This technique has proved to be of great value in the management of haemobilia where it provides a safe and effective alternative to what may often be difficult and hazardous surgery.

Technique

When the clinical and endoscopic findings in a patient with gastrointestinal bleeding suggest that the source of the bleeding is the biliary tract, angiography should be performed. The vascular study is usually obtained via a femoral approach using the Seldinger technique under local anaesthesia. The likely cause or site of the haemobilia may already be suspected from the clinical history and/or the results of other less invasive imaging techniques, but the preliminary angiographic study should in any case aim to demonstrate the entire hepatic and pancreatic circulations. This is usually achieved by a pressure injection into the coeliac axis but, depending on the regional vascular anatomy, a selective superior mesenteric angiogram may also be necessary. These general studies not only show the vascular anatomy of the entire region but ensure that unsuspected or multiple lesions are not missed and, in the late phase films, give details of the portal venous circulation; an important preliminary step before any subsequent arterial embolization is undertaken. If further diagnostic detail is required of any suspicious areas, or if therapeutic embolization is to be performed directly, a super-selective angiographic study is then obtained by positioning the catheter as close as possible in the arterial tree to the vessel supplying the abnormal area. In cases of haemobilia where the source of the bleeding is unknown, the angiographic study may provide this information either by demonstrating a potential bleeding lesion such as an aneurysm or, in the case of active bleeding, by revealing the site of extravasation of contrast medium (Fig. 5.1). Most cases of haemobilia for which embolization is appropriate treatment are due to bleeding from branches of the hepatic artery, though occasionally a pancreatic lesion giving rise to haemobilia is also suitable for treatment by the technique (Fig. 5.2). The liver is a relatively safe organ in which to perform arterial embolization since normal liver tissue is able to survive on portal venous blood alone, and providing the portal circulation is intact, arterial occlusion is unlikely to lead to liver necrosis. Although arterial embolization does not usually produce major changes in hepatic function it is obviously desirable to confine the embolization (when technically feasible) to the vessels in the immediate vicinity of the abnormality; this is particularly important in the case of jaundiced patients where liver function is already compromised. A wide variety of materials can be used as embolic agents (Allison 1978), the choice of material in any particular case depending on the site and nature of the bleeding. Slow haemorrhage or haemorrhage from a small vessel may be readily controlled by the injection of sterile absorbable gelatin sponge or similar materials; in the case of massive bleeding (e.g. from trauma) the use of a rapidly setting resin such as isobutyl-2-cyanoacrylate may be more effective. Care must be taken to avoid the reflux of embolic materials into the splenic artery because of the risk of splenic infarction. Inadvertent gastroduodenal embolization is obviously undesirable, but fortunately does not usually lead to complications in practice. Following the embolization a repeat arteriogram must be performed to ensure that the bleeding has ceased and that no collateral vessels exist from which the haemorrhage could recur. Prophylactic broad spectrum antibiotics are usually given for at least six days following hepatic arterial embolization.

Indications

Embolization can be used to control haemobilia secondary to liver biopsy; liver trauma; iatrogenic damage to the hepatic arteries and biliary ducts during surgery (e.g. cholecystectomy, Fig. 5.1); and congenital or acquired vascular mal-

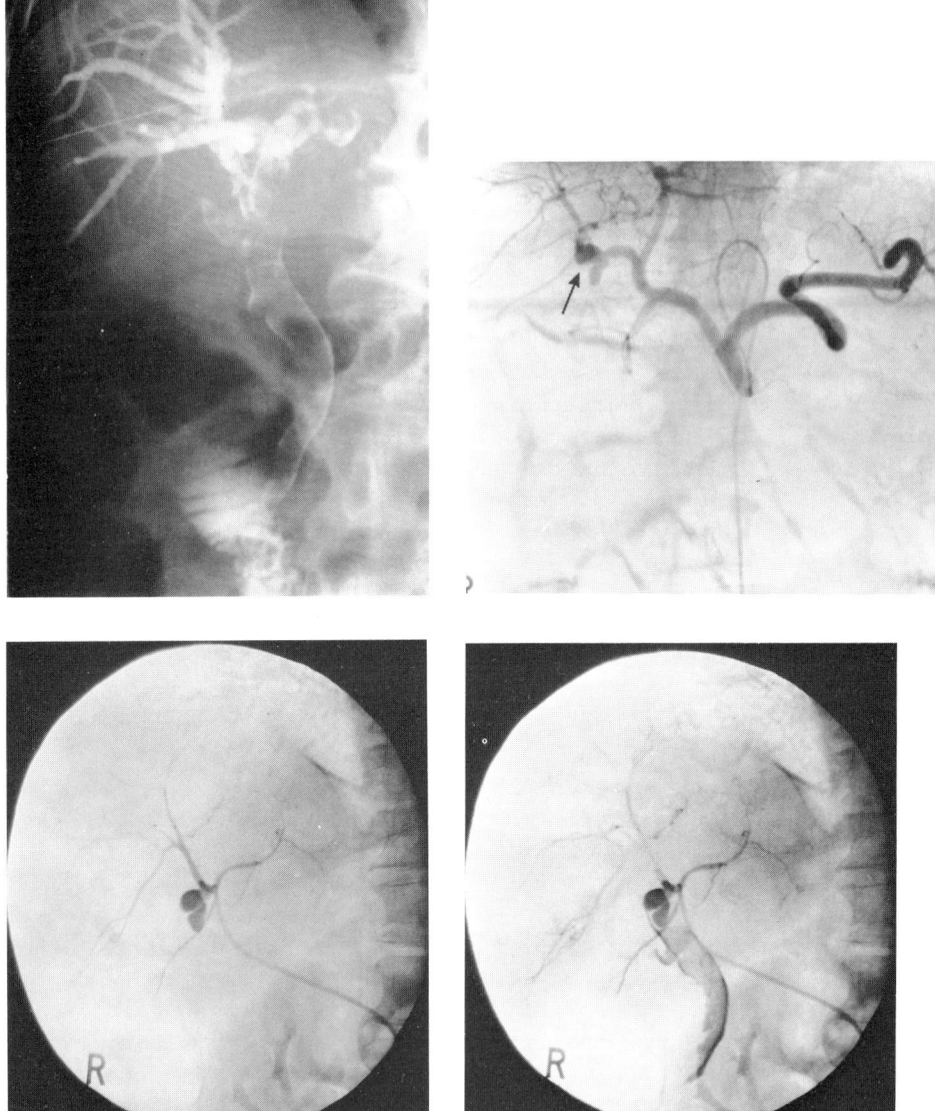

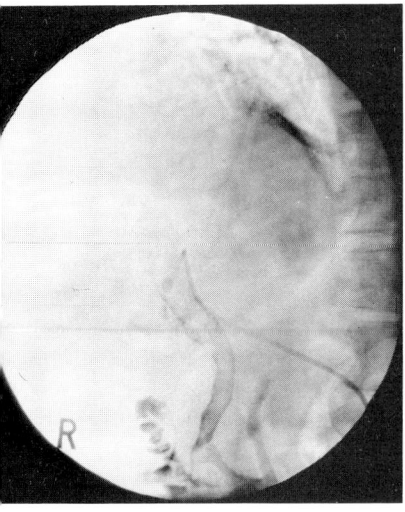
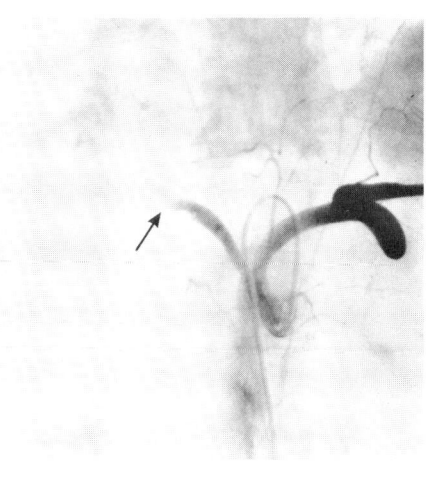

Fig. 5.1 Embolization in acute hepatic bleeding. A. Percutaneous cholangiogram in a patient with haemobilia and jaundice, showing multiple filling defects in the common bile duct due to blood clot. At cholecystectomy nine months previously, the right hepatic artery and the biliary tree had both sustained surgical damage. B. Coeliac angiogram: an iatrogenic aneurysm of the right hepatic artery is demonstrated (arrow). C. Selective hepatic angiogram showing detail of the aneurysm. D. A few seconds after the selective injection, contrast medium is seen extravasating into the common bile duct. E. The extravasated contrast medium has reached the duodenum 16 s following the arterial injection: the patient is bleeding extremely rapidly. F. The hepatic artery has been embolized with isobutyl-2-cyanoacrylate (arrow). The bleeding stopped, and the patient was discharged with no further treatment one week later.
(Reproduced by kind permission of Churchill Livingstone Ltd).

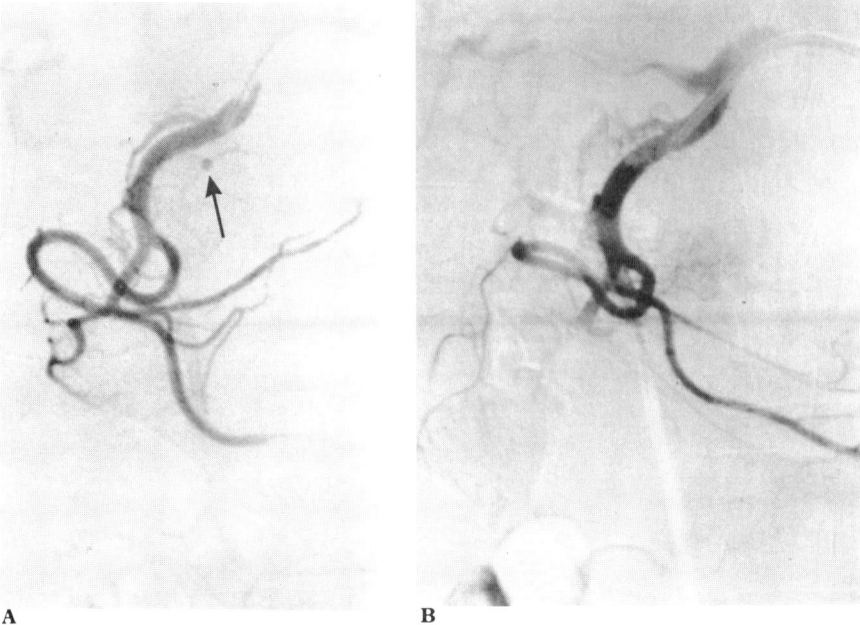

A   **B**

Fig. 5.2 Embolization in chronic haemobilia. A. Selective gastroduodenal angiogram in a man
with recurrent haemobilia. A small aneurysm is seen in the head of the pancreas (arrow).
B Repeat angiogram following emolization of the aneurysm with finely divided human dura
mater (Lyodura). The procedure successfully controlled the haemobilia.

formations and tumours. Embolization is particularly valuable in the case of
postoperative bleeding where a surgical access to the biliary tree is made difficult
and dangerous by distortion of the normal anatomy and by the presence of
adhesions. The technique is also useful in very sick patients for whom an extensive
hepatic operation under general anaesthesia would pose serious additional risks.

Contraindications and complications
Embolization of the hepatic artery should not be performed in the presence of
portal obstruction owing to the risk of massive liver necrosis, and the adequacy of
the portal circulation should always be established by preliminary indirect
splenoportography. Liver failure and extensive liver sepsis are relative contraindications to embolization, but in a case of acute biliary bleeding the risk of
embolization may still be less than the risk of surgery in such circumstances.

   Most patients experience some local discomfort or pain following liver
embolization and a transient pyrexia lasting a few days is also common. Infection is
a serious complication and may lead to death from septicaemia; prophylactic
antibiotic therapy is usually instituted to obviate this occurrence. About 10% of
patients develop a paralytic ileus following extensive hepatic embolization, but
this usually resolves within two or three days.

   Infarction of the gallbladder has been described following hepatic arterial
embolization (Jacob et al 1979, De Jode et al 1976); it has not occurred in our own
experience of over sixty procedures, however, and we believe that the small risk of

gallbladder infarction should not normally influence the decision whether or not to undertake the procedure.

Embolization versus ligation

Embolization of the hepatic artery is a preferable technique to surgical ligation of the hepatic artery in the control of haemobilia for a number of reasons. Firstly it is possible by means of arteriography at the time of the embolization to determine the exact source of the bleeding, and to ensure by a postembolization study that all the bleeding vessels and their collaterals have been occluded. This is an important consideration in the liver where anomalies of the vascular supply are common (Michels 1953, Nebesar et al 1969). Secondly even a simple surgical ligation requires an abdominal incision and (usually) general anaesthesia, both increased risk factors. Thirdly, main-stem hepatic arterial ligation is not always effective in producing vascular occlusion owing to the large number of potential collateral arterial communications to the liver (Michels 1953, Mays & Wheeler 1974, Sivula & Sipponen 1976). Embolization, by occluding peripheral hepatic vessels, reduces the risk of rebleeding from such collateral sources. Finally, surgical ligation of the hepatic artery precludes any subsequent attempt at embolization should this become necessary and makes further angiography of the liver more difficult.

Every surgeon responsible for the care of patients with liver disorders should be aware of the major contribution hepatic arterial embolization can make to the management of the difficult surgical problem of haemobilia.

Interventional biopsy procedures

A crucial step in the management of a patient presenting with a biliary lesion is to establish the nature of the disorder by histological examination. If a fragment of tissue can be obtained by one of the interventional techniques described below the need for an explanatory laparotomy or peritoneoscopy may be avoided, and the information obtained frequently has a significant influence on the subsequent management of the patient. The need for a biopsy arises most often in the case of an obstructing lesion in the biliary tree. Contrast studies of the biliary system may suggest the aetiology of an obstruction, but can be misleading and a biopsy is nearly always desirable if it can be obtained. A smooth, short stricture of the lower common bile duct may for instance be due to a carcinoma of the bile duct, ampulla or pancreas, but may also be secondary to pancreatitis, biliary duct trauma or inflammation. High biliary strictures can also result from a number of different pathological processes: differentiating a cholangiocarcinoma with secondary intrahepatic ductal fibrosis from primary sclerosing cholangitis may be difficult or impossible without the help of histology. Histological or cytological material may be obtained percutaneously (Evander et al 1978, 1980) via transhepatic drainage tubes or T-tubes (Palayew & Stein 1978, Elyaderani & Gabriele 1980, Mendez et al 1980), endoscopically (Osnes et al 1975) or transvenously (Allison 1981). The percutaneous method is usually performed from an anterior approach using a fine flexible needle (approximately 22 gauge). Fine needle aspiration biopsy (FNAB) permits diagnostic material to be obtained from deep-seated lesions without significant risk. Despite the potential complications of haemorrhage, sepsis, bowel perforation and tumour-seeding the safety record of FNAB is extremely good; there are now several large series describing the technique in liver and other abdominal organs with only negligible complication rates (Holm et al 1975, Mueller et al 1981). With pancreatic masses fluoroscopy, ultrasound or computerized axial tomography (CT) may be used for guidance (Staab et al 1979, Husband & Trott 1979). In the case of small biliary lesions the area to be biopsied may be impossible to localize by cross-sectional imaging methods, and guidance is best given by fluoroscopy after outlining the bile ducts with contrast medium (Fig. 5.3). With this method results are moderately good and in a study of all bile duct tumours Evander et al (1980) showed cytodiagnosis to be positive in 42% of cases.

Close co-operation between the cytopathology department and the radiology department is essential for the development of a successful biopsy service. The correct handling of aspirated material is critical to the outcome of the procedure and the successful development of FNAB and brush biopsy via tubes and endoscopes is due in no small part to advances in cytology (both in techniques and refinements of interpretation), that have permitted the accurate evaluation of minute quantities of aspirated material.

Transvenous liver biopsy (via the internal jugular and hepatic veins) is not applicable to small biliary lesions; it may be occasionally useful however in the

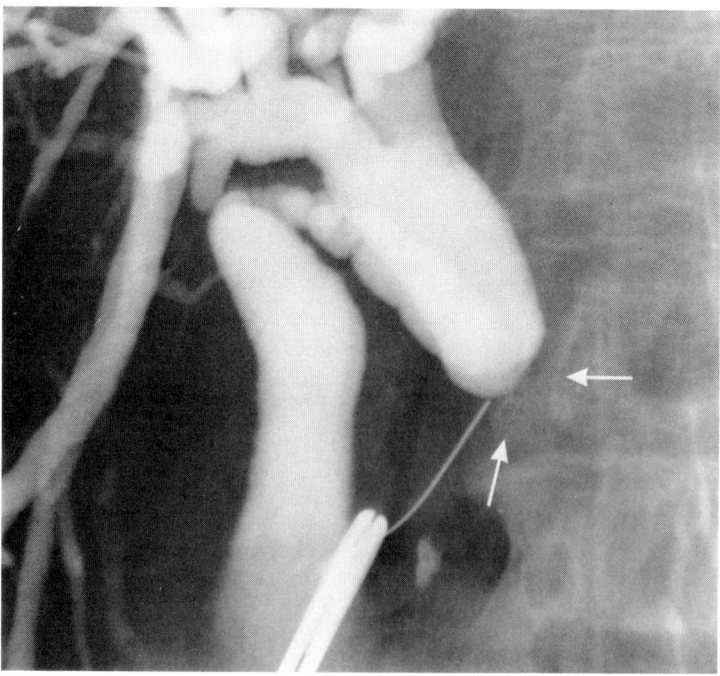

Fig. 5.3 Fine needle aspiration biopsy. An obstructing lesion was demonstrated at percutaneous cholangiography (arrows). The 22-gauge biopsy needle is foreshortened in this projection and is being held by forceps. Cytology revealed a cholangiocarcinoma.

diagnosis of diffuse biliary disorders when these are associated with disorders of blood coagulation which make conventional transperitoneal biopsy techniques hazardous (Rosch et al 1973, Gilmore et al 1978, Allison 1981).

Interventional techniques in biliary obstruction

A number of interventional radiological techniques are available for the relief or prevention of biliary tract obstruction. They include percutaneous and endoscopic drainage procedures; the insertion of radioactive seeds into biliary tumours; the percutaneous dilatation of biliary strictures; and techniques for the extraction of biliary calculi.

1. Interventional drainage techniques
Percutaneous biliary drainage originated many years ago when sheathed needles were used for diagnostic percutaneous cholangiography, and the sheath was used for drainage (Remolar et al 1956, Glenn et al 1962). In the past decade however the technique of biliary drainage as a primary therapeutic objective has developed and is now in widespread use (Molnar & Stockum 1974, Takada et al 1974, Burcharth & Nielbo 1976, Mori et al 1977, Nakayama et al 1978, Dooley et al 1979, 1981, Hellekant et al 1980, Ishikawa et al 1980, Berquist et al 1981, Irving 1981).

Technique
Percutaneous biliary drainage is usually performed under light sedation using local anaesthesia. Many centres (including our own) cover the procedure with prophylactic antibiotics, though this practice is not universal (Dooley et al 1979). The biliary system is first opacified using a fine-bore cholangiogram needle, and a catheter is then introduced using a system of guide-wires and dilators. During the procedure, bile samples are taken for culture and cytology, and a cholangiogram is performed to demonstrate the biliary anatomy and the nature, site and extent of the obstructing lesion.

Three different types of drainage procedure are possible. The simplest, which is used in the case of an impassable bile duct obstruction, is the insertion of a catheter above the stricture which drains externally only; this relieves the obstruction but the patient loses the bile unless this is replaced by some other route. More commonly, external–internal drainage is used; in this case a catheter is passed through the obstruction and sited so that drainage holes are positioned both above and below the lesion (Ring et al 1978). The tip of the catheter can lie either in the lower end of the common bile duct (in the case of a high biliary obstruction), or in the duodenum or jejunum (in the case of an ampullary lesion). If the external orifice of the catheter is clamped, bile can drain through the indwelling catheter into the alimentary tract, so obviating the problem of bile loss. This internal drainage technique is clearly preferable to the external method.

The third approach to biliary drainage is to insert an internal tube prosthesis or stent through the obstruction using a percutaneous technique. The stent has a collar at its upper end to prevent it passing into the duodenum. The catheter used to insert the stent is withdrawn completely once the internal drain is in position, leaving the patient unencumbered by any external tubes or appliances. This technique is used in the palliative treatment of inoperable biliary or pancreatic neoplasms. The techniques, pitfalls, and complications of percutaneous drainage procedures are described in detail by Bowley (1981). Percutaneous drainage kits including catheters, dilators, guide-wires and needles are now commercially available from several manufacturers. Our own preference at present is for the Ring-Lunderquist transhepatic bile duct drainage set produced by William Cook, (Europe ApS). Examples of biliary drainage procedures are shown in Figs. 5.4 and 5.5.

Indications for biliary drainage

a. Preoperative management of obstruction. Obstruction to the bile duct is associated with a deterioration in hepatic function, alterations in renal function, defective wound healing, and impairment of nutrition and blood coagulation.

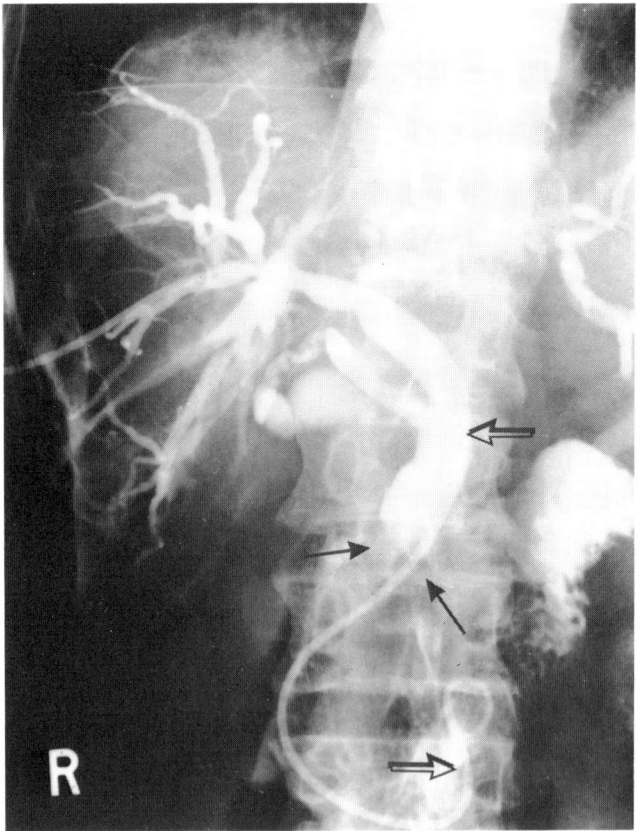

Fig. 5.4 Percutaneous biliary drainage. A catheter has been introduced percutaneously into the biliary system. The catheter passes through an obstructing tumour in the common bile duct (single arrows), through the ampulla, and into the duodenum. Sideholes in the catheter (double arrows) above and below the obstruction allow the internal drainage of bile into the gastrointestinal tract.

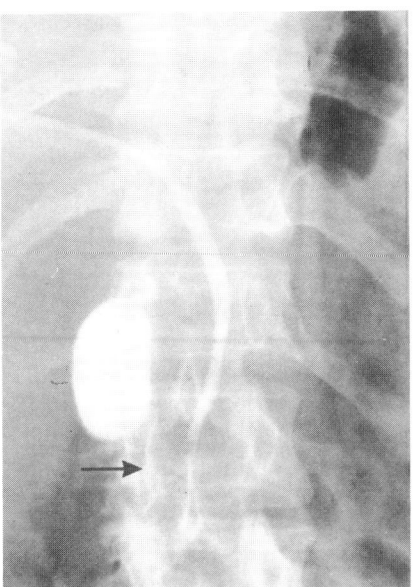 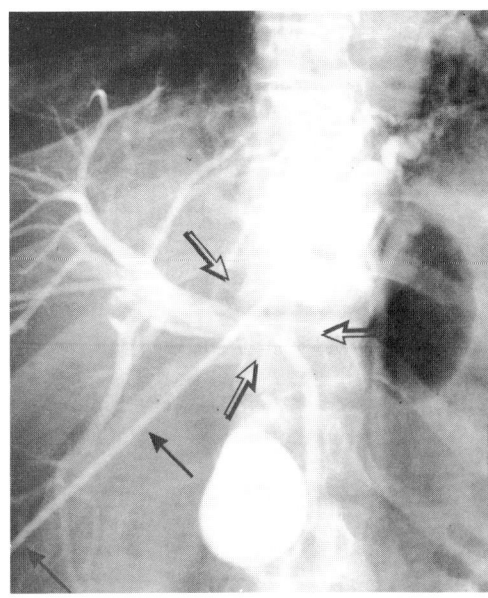

Fig. 5.5 Percutaneous biliary drainage. A. A percutaneous catheter has been passed through a hilar tumour into the common bile duct. The pig-tailed tip of the drainage catheter (arrow) lies above the ampulla. The gallbladder and cystic duct are visible. B. A second drainage catheter (single arrows) is independently decompressing the left biliary system by external percutaneous drainage. Both the right and left systems have been opacified showing the central position of the tumour (double arrows).

Because of these factors definitive surgery particularly in deep jaundice carries a high morbidity and mortality (Braasch & Gray 1977) and attempts have been made to improve the results of surgery by relieving the jaundice at a preliminary procedure. This can be done either by means of temporary surgical drainage followed later by definitive resection (Blumgart 1978), or by an initial percutaneous transhepatic approach of the type described above followed by surgery after a suitable interval of free drainage. Nakayama et al (1978) reported a reduction in mortality from 28.3% with surgery alone to 8.2% using preliminary percutaneous drainage, but many subsequent workers (including the present authors) have been unable to substantiate this improvement in mortality. Dooley et al (1979) had an operative mortality of 24% despite preliminary percutaneous drainage, and Denning et al (1981), whilst claiming a reduction in morbidity, were also unable to show any improvement in overall mortality. A number of controlled trials are at present being undertaken in the U.K., U.S.A. and South Africa in an attempt to establish the true value of preliminary drainage procedures. The criteria applied by the authors for using preliminary drainage techniques in their present management protocol are a bilirubin in excess of 300 μmol/l and/or a creatinine clearance of less than 50 ml/min. Other (relative) criteria include: the likelihood of a subsequent major resection; an albumin of less than 30 g/l; a 10% or greater recent loss of weight, and age exceeding 60 years. These criteria of course are somewhat arbitrary but attempt to take into account the known important surgical risk factors.

b. Palliative drainage. Percutaneous biliary drainage may be performed as a palliative procedure in cases of bile duct obstruction due to irresectable malignancy or sclerosing cholangitis (Pereiras et al 1978, Ring et al 1978, Dooley et al 1979, Smale et al 1981). The object of percutaneous drainage in these circumstances is to relieve the unpleasant symptoms of advanced jaundice, particularly the intolerable pruritis that commonly occurs. The technique also obviates the prolonged hospitalization that may be necessary following a palliative surgical bypass. If an external drainage catheter is used visits to hospital must be made every few months for catheter changing, but the recent introduction of the internal endoprosthesis described above means that a patient can now have the benefits of percutaneous drainage while remaining unencumbered by external tubes or appliances.

It is particularly important to ensure in those patients selected for palliative drainage that the obstructing lesion is indeed irresectable; also that every effort is made to achieve a histological or cytological diagnosis. This is because pancreatitis or lymphoma may mimic carcinoma at the lower end of the common bile duct (Oleaga & Ring 1981), leading to an incorrect assessment of the patient's prognosis.

c. Drainage in cholangitis. In patients with acute suppurative cholangitis there is increased intrabiliary pressure. This causes not only increasing jaundice but also the passage of bacteria into the bloodstream and septicaemia. Untreated, the mortality is high and early drainage is probably best achieved in these circumstances by the percutaneous technique (Dooley et al 1979) or by endoscopic sphincterotomy.

2. Iridium-192-Radiotherapy

Cholangiocarcinomas tend to remain fairly localised but are not always resectable because of vascular involvement. Conventional radiotherapy has been used but requires prolonged attendance by the patient and may have severe complications such as intractable haemorrhage, gastroduodenitis and duodenal stricture. Recently Herskovic et al (1981) have reported using 192-Ir seeds loaded 2/cm in a ribbon and inserted through the transhepatic catheter to the level of the tumour. Using single application over one or two days doses of approximately 5000 rad (50 Gy) were given. In some cases additional external beam therapy was used. Fletcher et al (1981) used 192-Ir wire loaded into a guide wire. The guide wire was introduced to the site of the tumour down either a percutaneous drain or a silastic U-tube. Doses of 4000–4800 rad (40–48 Gy) at 0.5 cm from the wire were then given over 48 hours. Results with these methods so far are promising but criteria for staging and resectability of cholangiocarcinomas have only recently begun to be defined and as with permanent drainage irradiation should not be carried out unselectively.

3. Percutaneous transhepatic transluminal choledochoplasty

It is possible to dilate benign biliary strictures with a balloon catheter (Burhenne 1974, Martin et al 1980), and this is a useful technique to facilitate the removal of biliary calculi via a T-tube track when the stones lie below a bile duct stricture (Allison & Hemingway 1982).

Dilatation of choledochoenterostomy strictures by inflating a balloon catheter across the stricture has been reported by Molnar and Stockum (1978); eight of their nine patients became asymptomatic with normal subsequent serum bilirubin values. Follow-up in all the cases was not long, but one patient who also underwent transhepatic stone removal was followed up for two years and remained well.

With continuing developments in balloon catheter technology, and the technical expertise that radiologists are acquiring using dilatation methods in the vascular system, it is possible that the procedure of percutaneous transhepatic cholangioplasty (with or without a pre existing T-tube track) may be increasingly performed in the future to the benefit of both patient and surgeon.

4. Percutaneous removal of gallstones

Despite the use of postexploratory cholangiography (Schulenberg 1969, Hall et al 1973), the choledochoscope (Finnis & Rowntree 1977) and stone extraction techniques (Fogarty et al 1968), residual biliary calculi are still a common problem following surgery in the biliary track (Larson et al 1966, Orloff 1978). They pose a serious problem since they may cause further obstruction, and surgical re-exploration in this area is a procedure carrying significant morbidity. Techniques for dissolving common duct stones have met with modified success and are only suitable for certain types of calculus. There is no doubt that if a T-tube is present, the most effective method of dealing with retained stones is to remove them through a T-tube track, using a steerable catheter and basket retrieval system (Mondet 1952, Burhenne 1973, Bean et al 1974, Mazzariello 1976).

Technique. The procedure is best done after a delay of six weeks in order to allow the track to mature. Any surgical drains placed close to the T-tube track should have been removed and their track should be closed. The technique is considerably easier to perform if a T-tube of at least 14 French has been used and the track is straight. If smaller tubes have been used it may be necessary to dilate the track and insert a larger tube for a few days prior to attempting stone extraction. For preference the tube should lead out of the lateral abdominal wall since this reduces considerably the radiation exposure to the hands of the radiologist. The procedure is performed under light sedation and if there is a history of recent cholangitis or pancreatitis antibiotic cover is provided. Following a check cholangiogram to establish that the calculi are still present and to ascertain their current position, the T-tube is removed and a steerable catheter inserted along the track. The stones are engaged in a co-axial basket system and removed. Following a final cholangiogram the track is allowed to close which it does within a few days. There may be technical problems in removing the stones but these can usually be overcome by the use of appropriate manoeuvres (Burhenne 1980). An example of stone removal is shown in Fig. 5.6.

Results. The overall success rate in the 661 patients of Burhenne's series (1980) was 95%. Others have had similar experience, Mazzariello (1976) reporting a 97.5% success. The British experience, which is somewhat younger than that of Canada, the USA and South America, has a slightly lower success of 79% in those centres treating more than 10 patients (Mason 1980). There is a morbidity of about

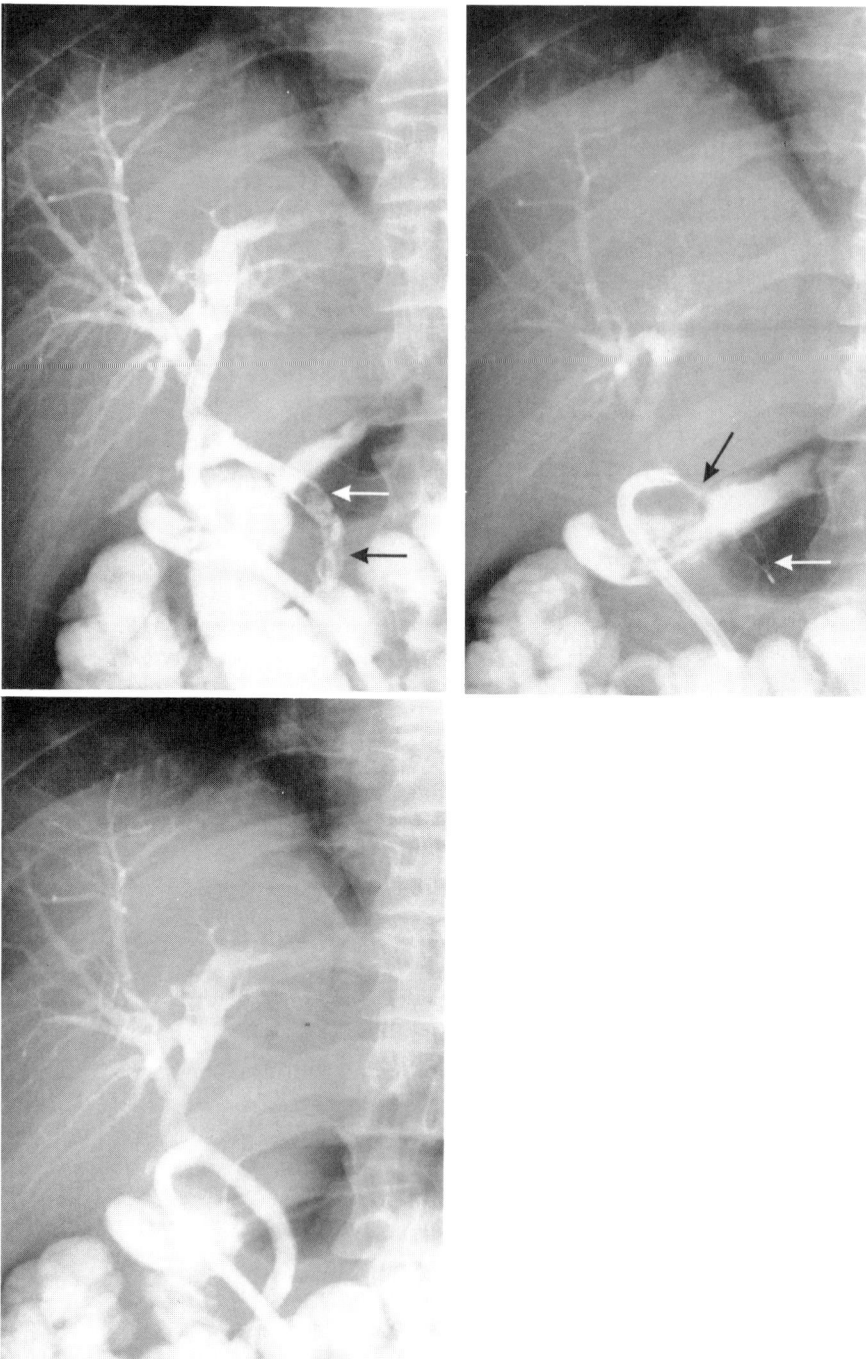

Fig. 5.6 Percutaneous removal of biliary calculi. A. A ten-day postoperative T-tube
cholangiogram shows multiple calculi in the lower common bile duct (arrows). B. The biliary
stone basket has been passed along a steerable catheter into the biliary system and has trapped
the stones (arrows). C. Post-removal study: the common bile duct is clear.

4% (Burhenne 1980). Complications include: sinus track leak, peritoneal spill, bile collections, fever and sepsis, pancreatitis and vaso vagal reactions. Perforation of the biliary tract is very unusual and deaths are exceptionally rare (Polack et al 1977, Mazzariello 1978).

Compared with the morbidity and expense of re-exploration of the biliary tree for retained calculi, the percutaneous extraction technique is outstandingly safe, economic and successful. There can be a few procedures in therapeutic radiology that are more rewarding for the patient and the radiologist, and none that has proved to be so successful in the hands of even relatively inexperienced operators.

When residual biliary calculi are present in a patient without T-tube access to the biliary tree, a more serious problem exists. It is technically feasible to extract stones with a catheter and basket using either a transhepatic puncture and dilatation method, or even a transvascular approach via the jugular and hepatic veins. These methods, however, would clearly only be attempted in the most exceptional circumstances and the usual choice to be made (if it has been elected to remove the calculi) is between surgical and endoscopic removal. Endoscopic sphincterotomy carries a failure rate of 5–22% and a mortality of 0.7–4.4%. In experienced hands surgery is successful in over 95% of cases. Although in young fit subjects the mortality is virtually nil, the overall surgical mortality is probably in the region of 1.8%, most deaths occurring in the elderly (Girard & Legros 1981). The choice between these two methods depends largely on local expertise and personal preference and is the subject of considerable controversy (Safrany 1978a, 1978b, Blumgart & Wood 1978, 1979, Cotton 1979, Motson 1979). In the elderly, patients who have already had multiple surgical attempts and those patients with cholangitis, endoscopic sphinterotomy has considerable attractions (Cotton 1980, Cotton & Vallon 1981, Mee et al 1981). On the other hand the young and otherwise healthy patient may still be best treated by the surgeon.

Conclusion

In the past decade the techniques of interventional radiology have brought about major changes in the surgical management of patients with biliary disorders. Interventional diagnostic procedures now give the surgeon important preoperative information concerning the site, nature and extent of biliary pathology; a significant contribution towards easier and less hazardous surgery. Therapeutic procedures may obviate for the patient the risks of general anaesthesia and surgery, or may allow the postponement of an operation until the increased risks imposed by infection, jaundice or haematological disturbances have been eradicated or minimized. In the post-operative patient abscesses can be drained or retained calculi extracted without recourse to further surgery, and in the incurable patient interventional techniques may assist in the palliation of unpleasant symptoms.

These benefits are significant ones and it is important for all biliary surgeons to be aware of the potential applications of interventional radiology. It is equally important for radiologists to become adept in the appropriate techniques, and to be familiar with their limitations and complications.

References

Allison D J 1978 Therapeutic embolization. British Journal of Hospital Medicine 20: 707–715

Allison D J 1981 Therapeutic aspects of radiology. Hospital Update 7: 851–871

Allison D J, Hemingway A P 1982 Removal of retained gallstones following percutaneous transluminal choledochoplasty. British Journal of Radiology 55: 304–305

Bean W J, Smith S L, Calonje M A 1974 Percutaneous removal of residual biliary tract stones. Radiology 113: 1–9

Berquist T H, May G R, Johnson C M, Adson M A, Thistle J L 1981 Percutaneous biliary decompression: Internal and external drainage in 50 patients. American Journal of Roentgenology 136: 901–906

Bowley N B 1982 The biliary tract. In: Steiner R E (ed) Recent Advances in Radiology and Medical Imaging. Churchill Livingstone, Edinburgh

Braasch J W, Gray B N 1977 Considerations that lower pancreatoduodenotomy mortality. American Journal of Surgery 133: 480–484

Blumgart L H 1978 Biliary tract obstruction: New approaches to old problems. American Journal of Surgery 135: 19–31

Blumgart L H, Wood C B 1978 Endoscopic treatment of biliary-tract diseases. Letter to the editor Lancet 2: 1249

Burcharth F, Nielbo N 1976 Percutaneous transhepatic cholangiography with selective catheterization of the common bile duct. American Journal of Roentgenology 127: 409–412

Burhenne H J 1973 Non-operative retained biliary tract stone extraction: a new roentgenologic technique. American Journal of Roentgenology 117: 388–399

Burhenne H J 1974 The technique of biliary duct stone extraction. Radiology 113: 567–572

Burhenne H J 1980 Percutaneous extraction of retained biliary tract stones: 661 patients. American Journal of Roentgenology 134: 888–898

Cotton P B 1979 Endoscopic treatment of biliary tract diseases. Lancet 1: 150

Cotton P B 1980 Non-operative removal of bile duct stones by duodenoscopic sphincterotomy. British Journal of Surgery 67: 1–5

Cotton P B, Vallon A G 1981 British experience with duodenoscopic sphincterotomy for removal of bile duct stones. British Journal of Surgery 68: 373–375

De Jode L R, Nicholls R J, Wright P L 1976 Ischaemic necrosis of the gallbladder following hepatic artery embolism. British Journal of Surgery 63: 621–623

Denning D A, Ellison E C, Carey L C 1981 Preoperative percutaneous transhepatic biliary decompression lowers operative morbidity in patients with obstructive jaundice. American Journal of Surgery 141: 61–65

Dooley J S, Dick R, Irving D, Olney J, Sherlock S 1981 Relief of bile duct obstruction by the percutaneous transhepatic insertion of an indoprosthesis. Clinical Radiology 32: 163–172

Dooley J S, Dick R, Olney J, Sherlock S 1979 Non-surgical treatment of biliary obstruction. Lancet 2: 1040–1044

Elyaderani M K, Gabriele O F 1980 Brush and forceps biopsy of biliary ducts via percutaneous transhepatic catheterisation. Radiology 135: 777–778

Evander A, Fredlund P, Hoevels J, Ihse I, Bengmark S 1980 Evaluation of aggressive surgery for carcinoma of the extrahepatic bile ducts. Annals of Surgery 191: 23–29

Evander A, Ihse I, Lunderquist A, Tylen U, Akerman M 1978 Percutaneous cytodiagnosis of carcinoma of the pancreas and bile duct. Annals of Surgery 188: 90–92

Finnis D, Rowntree T 1977 Choledochoscopy in exploration of the common bile duct. British Joural of Surgery 64: 661–664

Fletcher M S, Brinkley D, Dawson J L, Nunnerley H, Wheeler P G, Williams R 1981 Treatment of high bile duct carcinoma by internal radiotherapy with iridium-192-wire. Lancet 2: 172–175

Fogarty T J, Krippaehine W W, Dennis D L, Fletcher W S 1968 Evaluation of an improved operative technique in common duct surgery. American Journal of Surgery 116: 177–183

Gilmore I I, Bradley R D, Thompson R P H 1978 Improved method of transvenous liver biopsy. British Medical Journal 2: 249

Girard R M, Legros G 1981 Retained and recurrent bile duct stones. Surgical or non-surgical removal. Annals of Surgery 193: 150–154

Glenn F, Evans J A, Mujahed Z, Thorbjarnarson B 1962 Percutaneous transhepatic cholangiography. Annals of Surgery 156: 451–460

Hall R C, Sakiyalak P, Kim S K, Rogers L S, Webb W R 1973 Failure of operative cholangiography to prevent retained common duct stones. American Journal of Surgery 125: 51–63

Hellekant C, Jonsson K, Genell S 1980 Percutaneous internal drainage in obstructive jaundice. American Journal of Roentgenology 134: 661–664

Herskovic A, Heaston D, Engler M J, Fishburn R I, Jones R S, Noell K T 1981 Irradiation of biliary carcinoma. Radiology 139: 219–222

Holm H H, Pedersen J F, Kristensen J K, Rasmussen S N, Hanke S, Jensen F 1975 Ultrasonically guided percutaneous puncture. Radiologic Clinics of North America 13: 493–503

Husband J E, Trott P A 1980 CT guided percutaneous fine needle aspiration of intra-abdominal and pelvic masses. In: Veiga-Pires J A (ed) Intervention radiology. Excerpta Medica, Amsterdam p 340

Irving J D 1981 Relief of biliary obstruction. British Journal of Hospital Medicine 26: 329–338

Ishikawa Y, Oishi I, Miyai M, Kishimoto T, Miyamura S, Sagayama T, et al 1980 Percutaneous transhepatic drainage: experience in 100 cases. Journal of Clinical Gastroenterology 2: 305–314

Jacob E T, Shapira Z, Morag B, Rubinstein Z 1979 Hepatic infarction and gallbladder necrosis complicating arterial embolization for bleeding duodenal ulcer. Digestive Diseases and Sciences 24: 482–485

Larson R E, Hodgson J R, Priestley J T 1966 The early and long-term results of 500 consecutive explorations of the common bile duct. Surgery Gynecology and Obstetrics 122: 744–750

Martin E B, Karison K B, Fankuchen E I, Mattern R F, Casarella W J 1980 Percutaneous transhepatic dilatation of intrahepatic biliary strictures. American Journal of Roentgenology 135: 837–840

Mason R 1980 Percutaneous extraction of retained gallstones via the T-tube track — British experience of 131 cases. Clinical Radiology 31: 497–499

Mays E T, Wheeler C S 1974 Demonstration of collateral arterial flow after interruption of hepatic arteries in man. New England Journal of Medicine 290: 993–996

Mazzariello R M 1976 Residual biliary tract stones. Non-operative treatment of 570 patients. Surgical Annual 8: 113–144

Mazzariello R M 1978 A fourteen year experience with non-operative instrument extraction of retained bile duct stones. World Journal of Surgery 2: 447–455

Mee A S, Vallon A G, Croker J R, Cotton P B 1981 Non-operative removal of bile duct stones by duodenoscopic sphincterotomy in the elderly. British Medical Journal 283: 521–523

Mendez G Jr, Russell E, Levi J U, Koolpe H, Cohen M 1980 Percutaneous brush biopsy and internal drainage of biliary tree through endoprosthesis. American Journal of Roentgenology 134: 653–659

Michels N A 1953 Collateral arterial pathways to the liver after ligation of the hepatic artery and removal of the coeliac axis. Cancer 6: 708–724

Molnar W, Stockum A E 1974 Relief of obstructive jaundice through percutaneous transhepatic catheter — a new therapeutic method. American Journal of Roentgenology 122: 356–367

Molnar W, Stockum A E 1978 Transhepatic dilatation of choledochoenterostomy strictures. Radiology 129: 59–64

Mondet A 1952 Tecnica de la extracción incruenta de los calculos en la litiasis residual del coledoco. Boletines y trabajos, Sociedad de cirugía de Buenos Aires 46: 278

Mori K, Misumi A, Sugiyama M, Okabe M, Matsuoka T, Ishii J et al 1977 Percutaneous transhepatic bile drainage. Annals of Surgery 185: 111–115

Motson R W 1979 Endoscopic treatment of biliary tract diseases. Lancet 1: 377–378

Mueller P R, Wittenberg J, Ferrucci J T 1981 Fine needle aspiration biopsy of abdominal masses. Seminars in Roentgenology 16: 52–61

Nakayama T, Ikeda A, Okuda K 1978 Percutaneous transhepatic drainage of the biliary tract. Technique and results in 104 cases. Gastroenterology 74: 554–559

Nebesar R A, Kornblith P L, Pollard J J, Michaels N A 1969 Coeliac and superior mesenteric arteries. Churchill, London

Oleaga J A, Ring E J 1981 Interventional biliary radiology. Seminars in Roentgenology 16: 116–134

Orloff M J 1978 Importance of surgical technique in prevention of retained and recurrent bile duct stones. World Journal of Surgery 2: 403–410

Osnes M, Serck-Hanssen A, Myren J 1975 Endoscopic retrograde brush cytology (ERBC) of the biliary and pancreatic ducts. Scandinavian Journal of Gastroenterology 10: 829–831

Palayew M J, Stein L 1978 Postoperative biopsy of the common bile duct via the T-tube tract. American Journal of Roentgenology 13: 287–289

Pereiras R V, Rheingold O J, Hutson D, Mejia J, Viamonte M, Chiprut R O et al 1978 Relief of malignant obstructive jaundice by percutaneous insertion of a permanent prosthesis in the biliary tree. Annals of Internal Medicine 89: 589–593

Polack E P, Fainsinger M H, Bonnano S V 1977 A death following complications of roentgenologic non-operative manipulation of common bile duct calculi. Radiology 123: 585–586

Remolar J, Katz S, Rybak B, Pellizari O 1956 Percutaneous transhepatic cholangiography. Gastroenteroloy 31: 39–46

Ring E J, Oleaga J A, Freiman D B, Hustead J W, Lunderquist A 1978 Therapeutic Applications of Catheter Cholangiography Radiology 128: 333–338

Rosch J, Lakin P C, Antonovic R, Dotter C 1973 Transjugular approach to liver biopsy and transhepatic cholangiogram. New England Journal of Medicine 289: 227–231

Safrany L 1978a Transduodenal endoscopic sphincterotomy and extraction of bile duct stones. World Journal of Surgery 2: 457–464

Safrany L 1978b Endoscopic treatment of biliary-tract diseases. An international study. Lancet 2: 983–985

Schulenberg C A R 1969 Operative cholangiography: 1000 cases. Surgery 65: 723–739

Sivula A, Sipponen P 1976 The effect of hepatic dearterialization and re-dearterialization on carcinoid liver metastases. Annales chirurgiae et gynaecologiae Fennit 65: 168–175

Smale B G, Ring E J, Freiman D B, Oleaga J A, Reichman R, Mullen J L et al 1981 Successful long-term percutaneous decompression of the biliary tract. American Journal of Surgery 141: 73–76

Staab E V, Jaques P F, Partain C L 1979 Percutaneous biopsy in the management of solid intra-abdominal masses of unknwon etiology. Radiologic Clinics of North America 17: 435

Takada T, Kobayashi S, Yamada A, Uchida Y, Hanyu H 1974 Percutaneous transhepatic bile drainage by direct vision puncture. Shijutsu 28: 523

6 *Intraoperative diagnostic procedures*

LEON MORGENSTERN and GEORGE BERCI

Introduction

The intraoperative diagnostic procedures to be discussed in this chapter include operative cholangiography, cholangioscopy (choledochoscopy) and cholangiomanometry. Brief mention will also be made of operative ultrasonography and the value of liver biopsy as an adjunctive diagnostic procedure during biliary tract surgery.

The incision

Adequate exposure through a suitable incision is an essential prerequisite in carrying out any or all of the intraoperative diagnostic measures to be discussed. For cholecystectomy we prefer the right subcostal incision extending from the midline to the right anterior axillary line. The falciform ligament and ligamentum teres hepatis should be divided. In the event that exposure is inadequate with the subcostal incision alone, as may occur in obese patients or in patients with severe inflammatory reaction, conversion of the subcostal incision to the 'Kehr incision' (Fig. 6.1) is easily done by adding a vertical component at the medial extremity of the incision, ascending in the midline and to the right of the xiphisternum. This incision, with adequate retraction, opens the right upper quadrant widely and not only facilitates dissection but permits more accurate and safer performance of the diagnostic measures to be described. The addition of a vertical midline component is preferred over incision of the costal cartilages for wider retraction of the costal margin.

For re-operation on the extrahepatic biliary tract, as may be done for re-formed common duct stones or stricture, the vertical midline incision or right paramedian incision may be used. The common bile duct is a midline structure easily approached through the midline incision. Secondary operations through a new incision avoid the extensive subincisional adhesions which are usually dense in the right subhepatic area.

The essential point to be stressed is that incisions for either primary or

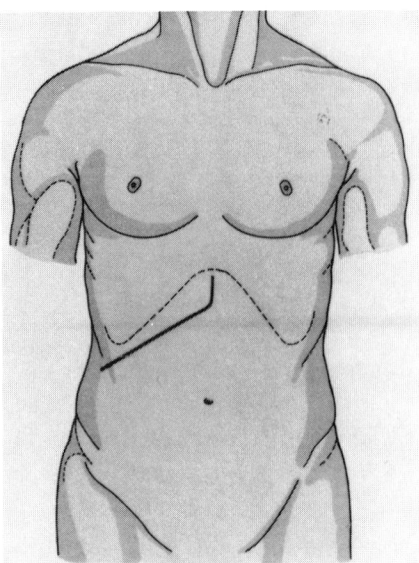

Fig. 6.1 Kehr incision, showing vertical midline extension of standard subcostal approach.

secondary biliary tract operations should be generous, affording the surgeon latitude in all directions for dissection and diagnostic manoeuvres.

Operative cholangiography

Operative cholangiography was introduced by Mirizzi in 1932 (Mirizzi 1937). Although the extent to which it should be used during routine cholecystectomy still remains controversial (Cassie & Kapadia 1981, Stark & Loughry 1980, McCarthy 1981, Berci et al 1978), there is little question that it has added greatly to our diagnostic acumen and accuracy in biliary tract surgery. We believe that its use should be routine in all cholecystectomies for the following reasons: first, in all instances, it provides accurate anatomic delineation of the biliary tree, displaying variations in cystic duct insertion as well as anomalies of importance to the surgeon; secondly, in ducts which are suspected of containing calculi, it shows the number as well as the location of the calculi; thirdly, in ducts in which stones are not suspected, it yields a discovery rate of 6–10% (Farha & Pearson 1976, Berci & Hamlin, 1981b); fourthly, in ducts in which there is some suspicion of stones, it can demonstrate that no stones are present, obviating the need for choledochotomy which is still being performed unnecessarily in 20–40% of instances if clinical indications alone are used (Schein et al 1966, Glenn 1965, Colcock & Perey 1964); finally, in conjunction with fluoroscopy, it provides useful information on the anatomy and function of the sphincteric mechanism.

Equipment for cholangiography
For optimal operative cholangiography it is necessary to equip the operating suite to a much higher degree of radiologic capability than is the custom in most

hospitals. The essentials of such equipment are a radiolucent table top with capability of side-to-side, as well as cephalocaudad movement; a mobile, overhead X-ray tube powered by an 800 mA generator; an image amplifier for placement under the operating table, with image-splitting capability so that serial 100 × 100 mm X-ray films may be coupled with fluoroscopic observation of ductal filling and emptying. Fluoroscopic imaging is displayed on television screens for viewing by both surgeon and radiologist, with the timing of fluoroscopy of film taking controlled by a double foot switch at the operating table. (Manufacturer: Siemens Co. X-ray Division, Erlangen, West Germany.)

This type of equipment permits exposures which average $\frac{1}{20}$s as compared with the required exposure of 0.5–1 s with standard portable machines. It also allows controlled filling of the ducts under direct fluoroscopic control, ensuring a complete filling of the ductal system as well as direct observation of the sphincteric mechanism. The early filling stage is one of the most important phases of the cholangiographic technique. If the duct is only partially filled (Fig. 6.2) it is easier to discover small stones within the lumen. In the average patient ten to twelve 100 mm films are made and serially mounted, giving surgeon and radiologist more information on suspicious areas and increasing diagnostic accuracy.

The patient should be positioned so that the left side is elevated. This may be achieved by folded towels, sheets or inflatable rubber pads made for this purpose. This slightly oblique position is important to avoid superimposition of the extrahepatic biliary system over the vertebral column. It is also essential to have a trained radiological technician as a member of the cholangiographic team. The technician should not only be well-versed in the technique of cholangiography but also in the traffic pattern of the operating theatre and aseptic precautions. Finally, preliminary scout films should always be taken before the operation is begun. These should be reviewed by both surgeon and radiologist so that timely corrections of any technical shortcomings can be made.

The sophisticated system just described is not available in many hospitals. With the use of portable machines it is still advisable to perform cystic duct cholangiography, rather than the customary three film completion cholangiogram after common duct exploration only. Although the advantages of fluoroscopic observation and serial aimed spot films may be lacking, *still the anatomy, integrity and function of the bile duct can and should be demonstrated before any operative manoeuvre on the common bile duct is done.*

Technique of cystic duct cholangiography

The triangle of Calot is dissected either before or after mobilization of the gallbladder from the liver bed. Dissection of the gallbladder from above downwards toward the cystic duct is done in those cases with severe inflammation where oedema and induration make identification of structures difficult. When the structures are easily identified, the cystic duct is isolated after ligation of the cystic artery. Traction applied by a clamp on Hartmann's pouch straightens the cystic duct so that its junction with the common duct can be identified. The cystic duct is singly tied or clipped at its junction with the gallbladder to prevent calculi from passing. A small incision is made in the cystic duct 1.5 cm from the junction

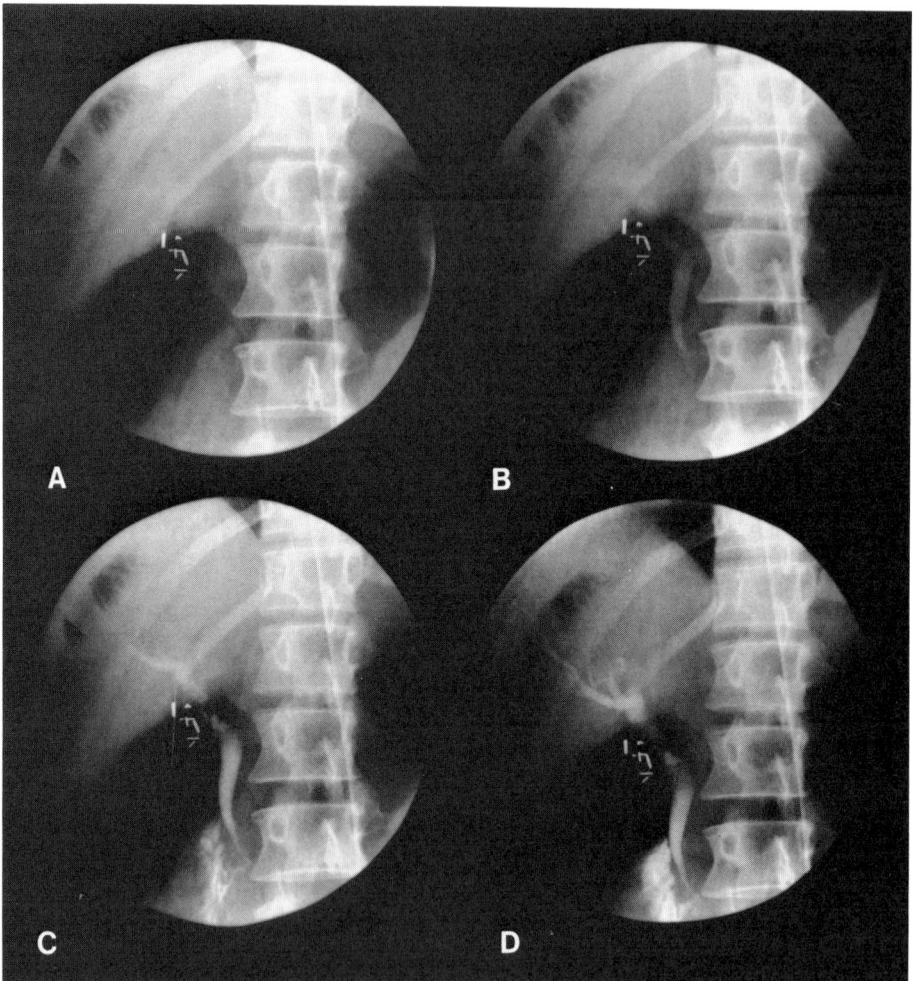

Fig. 6.2 Eight serial films (A–H) showing controlled filling of biliary ducts with small increments of contrast medium. Note changes of positions (F and G) to display all segments of the ductal system. By pressing a button electronic enlargement is achieved (E, F and G) for more structural detail. Early filling stages (B, C and D) and minute intraparenchymal hepatic ducts (H) are well seen.

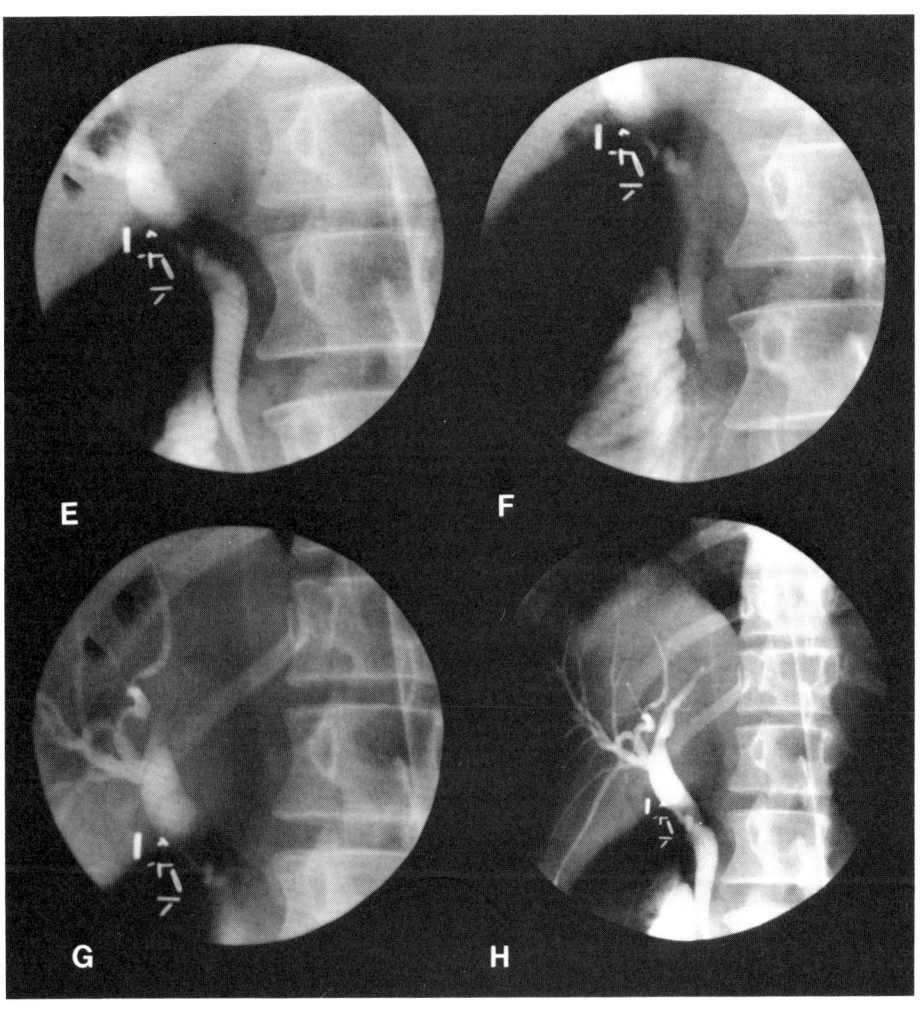

with the common duct, either with a Potts scissors or a small scalpel blade. The opening should be just wide enough to admit the cholangiography cannula. The cannula is introduced and fixed in place (Fig. 6.3A). We prefer an S-shaped metal cannula fixed in place with a modified Borge clamp (Fig. 6.3B). Other cholangiographic cannulas are available and other methods of fixation can be used. The essential points of cannula insertion are the avoidance of leakage around the cannula and the avoidance of too deep a placement, with resulting impingement on the common duct wall.

Patency and a leak-tight seal of the cannula are tested by injection of a small amount of saline. The Y-connector system of tubing for dye injection is shown in Figure 6.3B (Manufacturer: K. Storz Endoscopy Co., Tuttlingen, W. Germany). Care is taken to avoid introduction of air bubbles. If the system is working

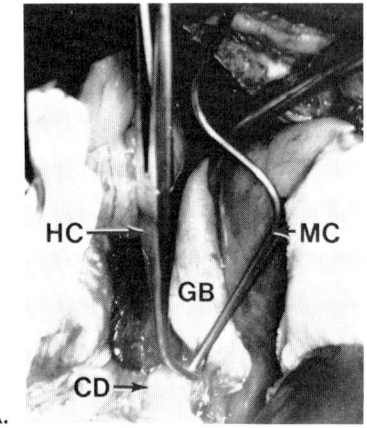

A.

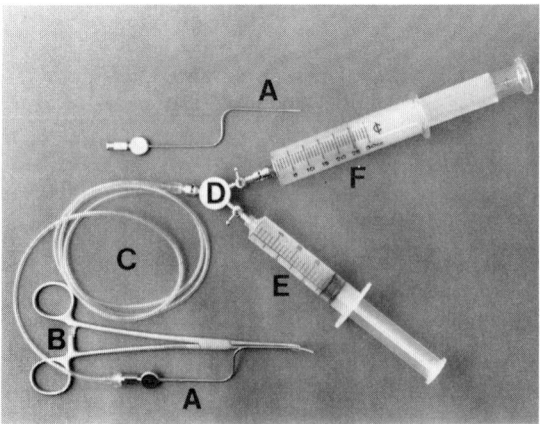

B.

Fig. 6.3 A. Metal cannula (MC) introduced into the cystic duct (CD) and fixed in position by the squeeze-lock clamp (HC). Gallbladder (GB) is in background. B. Cystic duct cannulation set. S-shaped metal cannula (A), available in two sizes (1.5 and 2.0 mm outside diameter), squeeze-lock cannula fixation clamp (B), plastic (pressure) extension tubing (C) with Luer locks, Y connector with stopcocks (D), 20 ml plastic syringe with saline (E), 30 ml glass syringe with contrast material (F).

properly, 25% Hypaque is then instilled slowly into the duct. If fluoroscopy is available, the dye is introduced in slow increments to observe the filling of the duct. Eventually the lower duct fills first and sphincteric function can be observed. If the lower duct is normal and empties well, more dye is introduced with a greater rapidity of injection to fill the common hepatic and intrahepatic ducts. *Both left and right intrahepatic ducts with their branches must be visualized.*

A two way audiovisual communication with the X-ray department is advisable. Dual observation and interpretation by both surgeon and radiologist aids greatly in diagnostic accuracy.

Cholecystocholangiography
When the cystic duct cannot be readily identified, cholangiography may be done through the gallbladder. A small catheter is introduced in the fundus of the gallbladder and fixed in place with a purse string suture of 3-0 silk. The gallbladder is emptied of its bile and 50–100 ml of 25% Hypaque introduced in the manner described above until the biliary tree is visualized.

Choledochocholangiography
When the gallbladder is absent, cholangiography is done through the common bile duct. We use a number 23 scalp vein needle with fixation of the butterfly 'wing' to the duct with a number 4-0 gastrointestinal silk or chromic suture. Since choledochotomy usually is contemplated or follows such choledochocholangio-graphy, the needle puncture is made somewhere along the site of the proposed choledochotomy, if at all possible. Cholangiography is performed as described above. As with the gallbladder, it may be necessary to first empty a tense, distended common bile duct before instillation of the dye.

T-tube cholangiography
T-tube or completion cholangiography should be done at the conclusion of all common duct explorations. We do not subscribe to primary closure of the common duct after choledochotomy.

T-tube placement should be done with the a priori assumption that intraductal manipulation may be necessary later through the T-tube tract. Since the crossbar is hemisected and tailored individually to fit the common duct, its size is of less importance than that of the stem in establishing an adequate-sized tract. The minimum size of the T-tube stem should be 18 French. We even prefer a larger tract and use up to a 22 French stem. The Whelan-Moss T-tube (Manufacturer: Davol Inc., Providence, Rhode Island, U.S.A.) is well suited for the purpose described. It incorporates a smaller sized crossbar (e.g. 18 French) with a larger sized stem (e.g. 22 French), the latter providing a good sized tract for later entry if necessary.

T-tube cholangiography should be performed as described above (under cystic duct cholangiography). Great care is necessary to avoid the introduction of air bubbles.

Following the completion cholangiogram, the T-tube is brought out *laterally* at right angles to the duct, never directly anteriorly. The lateral position of the tube allows safe and more effective postoperative intraductal manipulation should this be necessary.

Cholangiographic findings

Anomalies
The most important anomalies are those which may lead to inadvertent injury of the common duct. These include anomalous junction of the cystic duct with the right hepatic duct (Fig. 6.4) aberrant hepatic ducts and low hepatic duct bifurcation (Fig. 6.5).

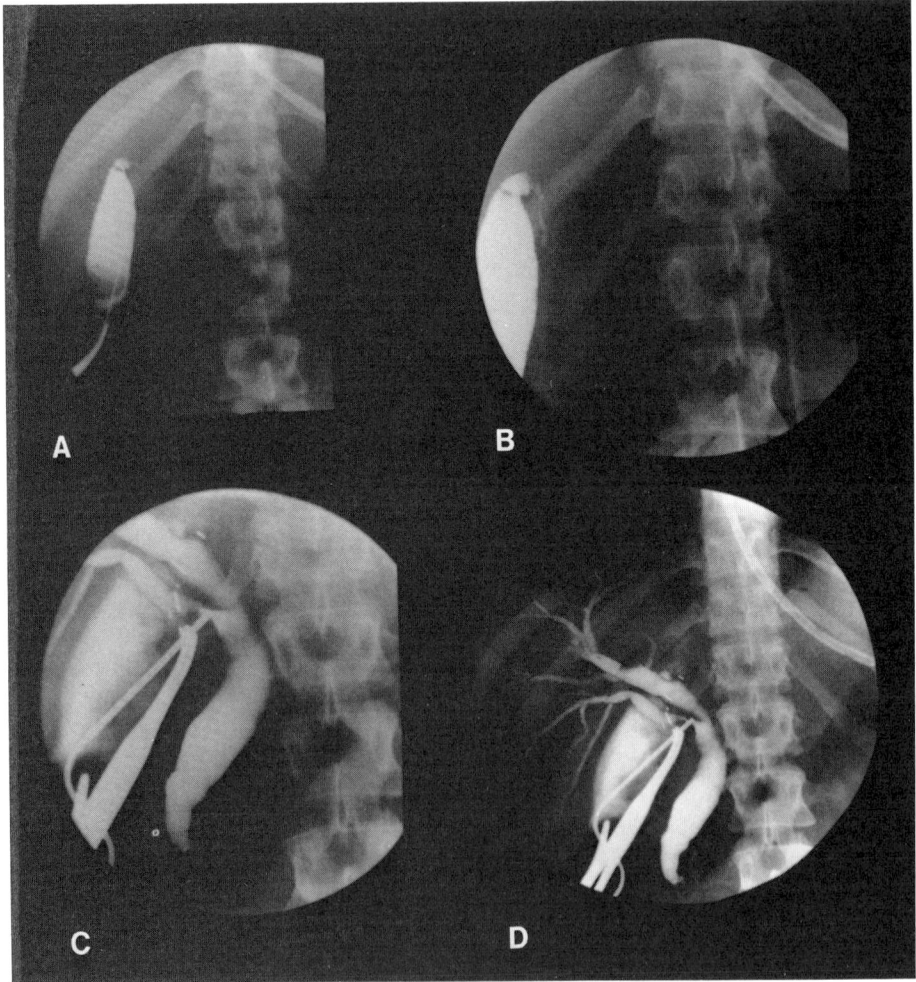

Fig. 6.4 Because of difficulties in anatomical identification of structures in the triangle of Calot, a cholecystocholangiogram was performed (A and B) showing an obstructed cystic duct (B). When the cystic duct was identified by further dissection it was seen to enter into the right hepatic duct (C and D). This anomaly was discovered before accidental injury to the right hepatic duct could occur.

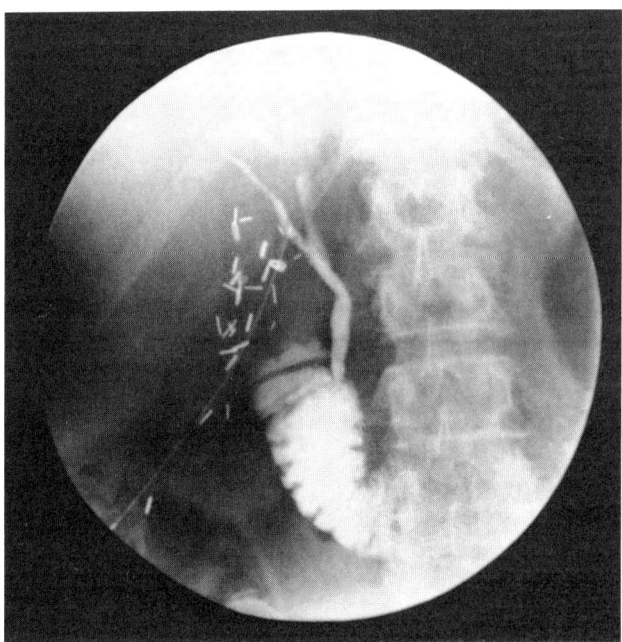

Fig. 6.5 Low junction of right and left hepatic ducts. Small cystic duct enters the right hepatic duct.

Variations in cystic duct insertion

Our studies have revealed a significant deviation from the usual concept with regard to the course and relationship of the cystic duct to the common duct. In only 17% of cases the cystic duct entered the right or lateral side of the common duct. In 41% the cystic duct entered either the anterior or posterior aspect of the common duct. In 35% of cases the cystic duct coursed in spiral fashion around the common duct (spiral duct) (Fig. 6.6). A long parallel course was seen in only 7%. In a high percentage of cases (83%), therefore, the extent of cystic duct lateral to the common bile duct is only a fraction of its total length (Hamlin 1981). The incidence of a long cystic duct remnant is much higher than previously thought. During common duct exploration, calculi have been noted to 'disappear' within a dilated spiral cystic duct (Fig. 6.7). In patients with dilated common ducts and long cystic duct stumps, we recommend concluding the exploration by gently passing a malleable probe or catheter through the stump into the common duct to detect possible calculi which may have been hidden from view during cholangioscopy.

Unsuspected stones

Unsuspected stones are present in the common duct in as many as 6–10% of cases (Farha & Pearson 1976). In our experience we have found a 5% incidence of unsuspected stones in patients undergoing routine cholecystectomy (Berci & Hamlin 1981b). If undiscovered, such unsuspected stones can lead to later complications. Spontaneous passage of stones is unpredictable.

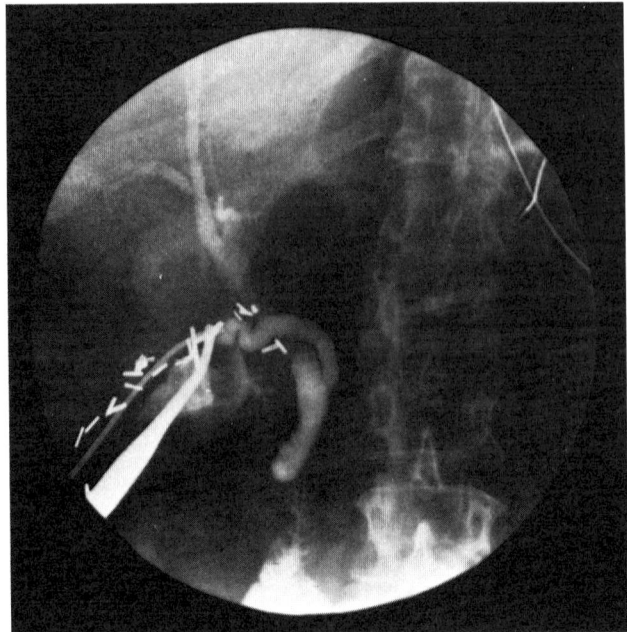

Fig. 6.6 Dilated spiral cystic duct entering the common hepatic duct.

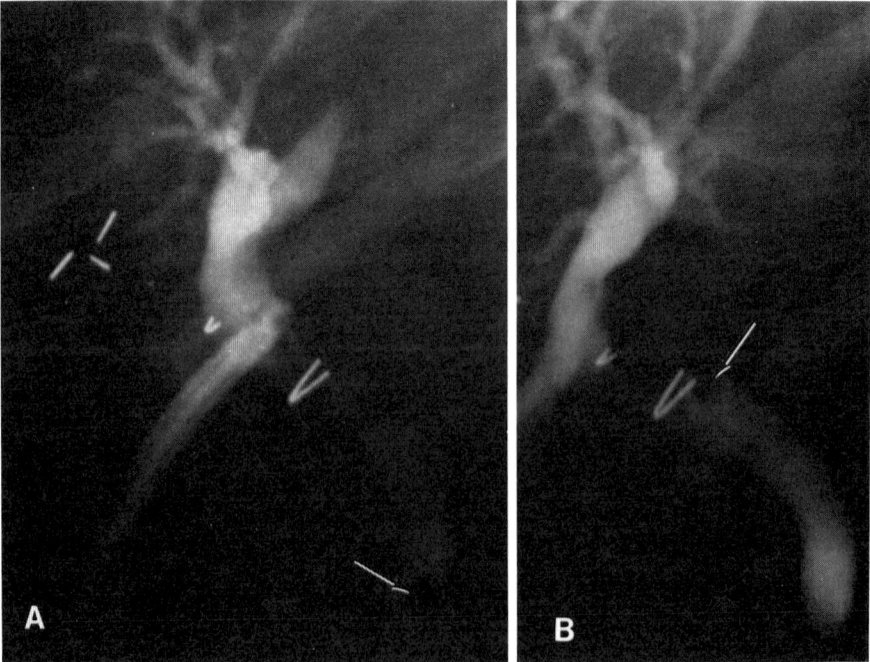

Fig. 6.7 A. T-tube cholangiogram showing stone in distal duct (arrow). B. During manipulation stone escaped into the dilated cystic duct stump (arrow) and was not visible during biliary endoscopy.

Number and location of stones
Knowledge of the number and location of stones is of great value before exploration of the common duct is undertaken. The surgeon then knows precisely where to search and to what extent the stone retrieval has been successful.

Dilated duct with stones absent
Heretofore a prior history of jaundice and the finding of ductal dilatation have been a relatively strong indication for ductal exploration. However, with good operative cholangiographic studies, unnecessary exploration of the duct can be avoided if no stones are seen and prompt emptying of the contrast is observed (Berci & Hamlin 1981c).

Sphincteric function
Serial films taken under fluoroscopic control show the cyclic opening and closing of the sphincter of Oddi. This avoids the error of misinterpretation when a pseudocalculus sign is present (Fig. 6.8). Rapidity of emptying and degree of emptying also may give a clue as to sphincteric stenosis or dysfunction. Normal sphincteric function is observed as a rhythmic opening and closure at intervals of several seconds.

Cost effectiveness of cholangiography
There have been recent reports on the cost effectiveness of operative cholangiography (Skillings et al 1979, Holmin et al 1980). These reports favour selective rather than routine operative cholangiography from the viewpoint of cost effectiveness. However, we have stressed that routine operative cholangiography is not only important for the detection of unsuspected stones and the avoidance of unnecessary exploration, but also that it is essential to demonstrate the anatomy of the ductal system. The studies on cost effectiveness do not reflect the high costs of retained stones or ductal injuries. We remain steadfast in our belief that the capital outlay for optimal equipment and the costs of its routine use are more than offset by the benefits to the patient in the reduction of operative complications.

Radiation hazard
All radiographic procedures done in the operating theatre pose a radiation hazard if adequate precautions are not observed. The surgeon in particular and operating room personnel in general are subject to varying degrees of radiation exposure during operative cholangiography. Fluoroscopy poses a greater risk than standard roentgenography, hence even greater care should be taken in limiting fluoroscopic viewing time. Fluoroscopy should be performed in short, interrupted bursts rather than by continuous observation.

The precautions to be observed are the wearing of film badges for radiation monitoring, the wearing of protective lead aprons by surgeon (gas-sterilized apron) and anesthesiologist, and all other personnel remaining in the operating theatre should place themselves behind a protective portable lead screen. The most effective way of decreasing radiation exposure to the surgeon is by increasing the distance from the operating field. A minimum of 1.2 m of plastic extension

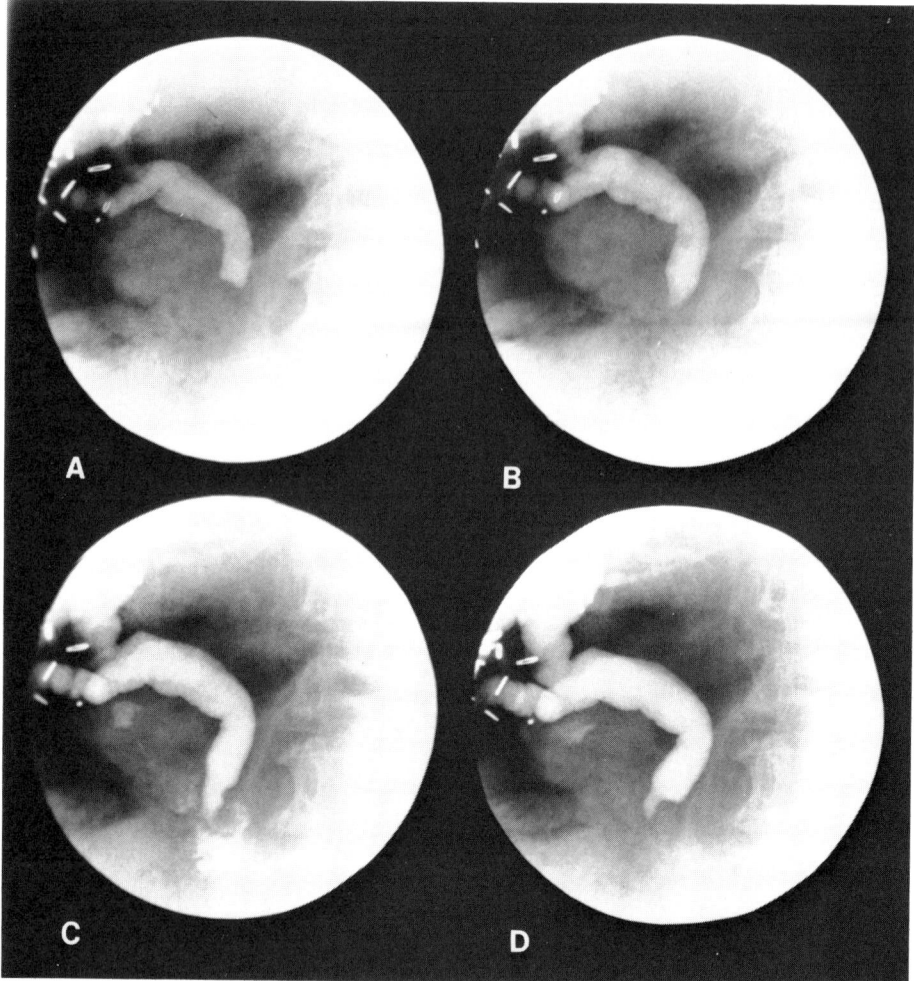

Fig. 6.8 Advantages of multiple films. Four selected X-rays from a series of eight, displaying cyclic opening and closing of sphincter. A. shows pseudocalculus sign with no dye in the duodenum, which could be interpreted as a stone in the distal duct. Fluorocholangiography can clarify this phenomenon.

tubing between the cholangiographic cannula and syringe will minimize exposure. For definitive figures regarding radiation exposure, the reader is referred to publications dealing with this subject (Linos et al 1980, Earley 1981).

Operative biliary endoscopy (cholangioscopy)

Operative biliary endoscopy does not replace cholangiography. A preliminary cystic duct cholangiogram defines the anatomy of the ductal system and serves as a guiding factor in cholangioscopy. If the distal common bile duct inserts into the second or third portion of the duodenum, or if the distal duct is long and tortuous, the Kocher manoeuvre for mobilization of the duodenum is essential. The cholangiogram also defines the number and location of intraductal stones, facilitating their identification and retrieval.

Cholangioscopy may be performed with either rigid or flexible biliary endoscopic equipment.

The rigid cholangioscope

The rigid cholangioscope (Shore et al 1971, Berci & Shore 1972) consists of a right-angled telescope with an irrigation channel and fiberoptic light carrier. The outer diameter of 5 × 3 mm permits introduction of the instrument into small as well as larger ducts. The standard 40 mm length of the horizontal limb is usually adequate for most examinations, but on occasion the duct is too long and the instrument with the 60 mm horizontal limb is needed to visualize the ampulla (Fig. 6.9 — manufacturer: K. Storz Endoscopy Co., Tuttlingen, West Germany). The Kocher manoeuvre should be used liberally to mobilize the distal duct. The latter then can be telescoped toward the end of the scope to bring the ampullary region into view (Berci & Shore 1981).

In order to provide irrigation for distention and clearing of the duct, a saline drip is placed on a stand (2 m above the floor) or enclosed within a Fenwal pressure irrigation system. The narrow irrigation channel of the scope has a high resistance and pressure is required to provide a steady flow within the ductal system. Irrigation should be applied intermittently. Illumination is provided from an external light-source by a flexible optic cable.

Operative biliary endoscopy requires training and practice before its full value can be realized. The detailed technique of cholangioscopy has been described in several previous reports (Berci & Hamlin 1981c, Nora et al 1977, Morgenstern (in

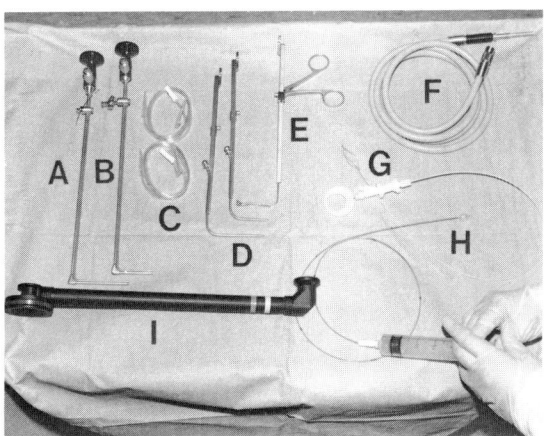

Fig. 6.9 Cholangioscopy set. A. Cholangioscope with 60 mm horizontal limb. B. Same, but with 40 mm limb. C. Venous extension tubes. D. Attachable instrument guide channels. E. Attachable stone forceps. F. Fibre-optic cable. G. Dormia stone basket. H. 4 French (arterial) balloon catheter. G and H. Accessories are introduced through instrument guide (D). I. Teaching attachment.

press), Saltzstein 1981). The endoscopist is positioned on the left of the patient for the best viewing and manoeuvrability of the instrument. The choledochotomy should preferably not be too large, so that sufficient irrigant fluid is retained for distention of the duct; the aperture can be narrowed by crossing of the two Guy sutures on either side of the choledochotomy. The room should be darkened and viewing done with the eye a short distance from the eyepiece. The scope is gently introduced into the distal duct first and advanced toward the ampulla. The rhythmic opening and closure of the ampulla should be clearly seen before this phase of the examination is deemed complete.

Examination of the proximal duct and hepatic radicles is then done by again introducing the scope in a cephalad direction. The sharp 'carina'-like area of the ductal bifurcation is a landmark denoting the confluence of right and left main hepatic ducts. Secondary branches and occasionally tertiary branches may be identified as the scope is advanced in a cephalad direction.

The lining of the biliary ducts is normally pale greyish-pink and pitted with circumferentially scattered shallow depressions. The ampullary orifice has a finely papillary appearance and varies in shape, but should always be observed as it opens and closes. The telescopic view afforded by the rigid cholangioscope displays the finely tapered diameter of the duct as it approaches the ampulla.

In the presence of cholangitis the duct lining is oedematous and often fiery red. Not only is there considerable loose fibrinopurulent exudate floating as debris within the duct, but also strands of mucopurulent and fibrinous exudate clinging to the walls of the duct. The latter are not easily dislodged by the flow of irrigation fluid, nor should the duct wall be traumatized by strenuous efforts at their removal. The cholangioscope should not be passed through the ampulla, which would only be traumatized by such a manoeuvre.

Accessories
The main accessories are depicted in Figure 6.9. A small attachable instrument channel (Fig. 6.9D) permits advancement of a Dormia basket (Fig. 6.9G) and a 4 French balloon catheter (Fig. 6.9H). These accessories are the most versatile and useful devices developed for the removal of stones under visual control.

The rigid attachable forceps (Fig. 6.9E) moves with the telescope and can be extremely useful in removing small or impacted stones from the distal duct. A biopsy forceps helps to provide tissue samples of suspicious lesions.

The invention of the Hopkins rod lens system and its application to biliary endoscopy provides a superior optical system (Shore et al 1971, Rattner & Warshaw 1981). A crisp, clear image with great depth of field is obtained. The right-angled configuration is especially suitable in patients requiring re-exploration. The rigid scope is easy to manipulate. Gas-sterilization is preferred, but in an emergency, soaking in sterilizing solution may be used. With proper maintenance, the rigid cholangioscope can be used for years without diminution in the quality of the images obtained.

Flexible fibrecholangioscope
The flexible fibrecholedochoscope was first described by Shore & Lippman in 1965. This model lacked a remote-control mechanism for the tip and required

constant refocusing. Yamakawa improved the design by adding a fixed focus and tip control in one plane (up and down) (Yamakawa et al 1976). Additional rotation is achieved by use of a twisting motion (torque). The tip movements are operated by a thumb control lever. The flexible cholangioscope is essentially a modified bronchoscope (Manufacturer: Olympus Co., Tokyo, Japan). It requires much more endoscopic skill than the rigid instrument and therefore is less useful to the general surgeon. At the present stage of fibre technology, the image quality of any flexible endoscope is far inferior to the modern rigid optical system. Surgeons who have had the opportunity to compare both systems are impressed by the superior image and the relative simplicity of the rigid cholangioscope as compared with the flexible one. As for cost considerations, the flexible scope is three or four times more expensive than the rigid one. Its delicate construction renders it more liable to damage during handling and less able to withstand repeated sterilization. These factors support our preference for the rigid system for operative biliary endoscopy. The flexible cholangioscope, however, is very useful for the removal of stones in a very long and tortuous duct or through the T-tube tract in the postoperative period (Yamakawa et al 1978, Berci & Hamlin 1981a).

Teaching cholangioscopy

The teaching attachment is an important tool in teaching endoscopic procedures. Attached to the main instrument (Fig. 6.9I) it enables the assistant to view synchronously the interior of the ducts and the technical manoeuvres within them. It avoids the necessity of awkward switching of observers to 'have a look', often with loss of position of scope and image. It facilitates training not only in the diagnostic steps of biliary endoscopy but also in the technical steps involved in stone retrieval. The attachment is gas-sterilized.

The advantages of biliary endoscopy

Detection of overlooked stones
After routine stone-retrieval techniques additional stones have been detected by endoscopy in from 10–25% of cases. In patients requiring re-exploration the incidence of error is even higher. It is therefore mandatory, in our opinion, to perform biliary endoscopy as a routine adjunctive procedure during ductal exploration.

Endoscopic removal of stones
Most stones detected by endoscopy can be removed by conventional extraction techniques. It is advisable, however, to learn and to teach the technique of endoscopic removal of stones, since this is more easily done under visual control than by blind extraction manoeuvres. The use of the Dormia basket or balloon catheter under endoscopic control expedites stone retrieval. Moreover, it avoids unnecessary damage to the sphincter of Oddi or traumatic haemobilia, both of which may occur by blind passage of instruments.

Management of impacted stones
Removal of small impacted stones in the ampullary region can sometimes be difficult. The first step should be the mobilization of the duodenum as previously mentioned. The rigid stone forceps is then attached to the instrument so that it may grasp or crush the stone. This forceps and scope move together as an ensemble. If unsuccessful efforts are too extensive or prolonged, one should consider a transduodenal removal of stones, combined with a sphincteroplasty or a choledochoduodenostomy, depending on the nature and condition of the ductal system. Stones blocking the intrahepatic orifices can be dislodged by a Dormia basket or 4 French balloon catheter advanced under visual control. Blind manipulation within hepatic branches can propel and wedge calculi more peripherally or result in perforations of the ductal system with haemobilia.

Completion T-tube cholangiogram
After choledochotomy, especially in patients with cholangitis, many artefacts can be encountered on the T-tube cholangiogram. These include air bubbles, mucoid and fibrinous debris, blood clots and pseudo-obstructive phenomena at the ampulla. Endoscopic examination can resolve many diagnostic dilemmas posed by the abnormal T-tube cholangiogram.

Diagnosis and staging of biliary tract tumours
Biopsy of biliary tract tumours for the purposes of diagnosis and staging is best done under direct visual control by endoscopy. Such tumours may be multicentric (Tompkins et al 1976) and can be most accurately staged by endoscopic methods before radical resection is undertaken.

Cholangiomanometry

Operative manometry in conjunction with cholangiography was first reported by Caroli in 1946. There have since been a number of reports using the Caroli technique and apparatus as well as modifications thereof (Mallet-Guy 1952, Daniel 1972, McCarthy 1977, Mak & Jakimowicz 1981, White & Bordley, 1978; Cushieri et al 1972; Roux & Vayre, 1976, Salomon & Roseman 1978, McCarthy 1970, White et al 1972). Nonetheless, cholangiomanometry has never achieved widespread clinical usage in biliary tract surgery, probably due to the complexity of the manometric apparatus and technique as well as the uncertainty of its significance in the diagnosis of biliary tract disorders.

Operative manometry (radiomanometry) measures the resting pressure within the common bile duct and the contrast infusion pressure required to open the sphincter of Oddi. The apparatus and technique vary in sophistication from combinations of simple glass and plastic tubing to pressure transducers and digital pressure readout systems. The essential features of all systems depend upon cannulation of the cystic duct, preferably with a metal cannula, a constant infusion of fluid through this cannula, most accurately accomplished with an infusion pump, and a means of measuring intraductal pressure at given intervals before and during the infusion, most accurately performed with a pressure transducer and an electronic recording apparatus (Fig. 6.10).

The infusion fluids reported in various studies differ, a factor which has some bearing on the pressure readings obtained. Normal saline can only be used if contrast studies are not done; in the opinion of the authors, manometric studies must be done with radiographic control to be meaningful. We recommend 25% diatrizoate sodium (Hypaque), the contrast medium used for routine cholangiography. Aimed serial spot films should be taken during the manometric measurements as with routine operative cholangiography. Sphincter function, as seen radiographically, is then correlated with the pressure measurements.

The mean resting pressure within the common bile duct is normally in the range of 15 cm of water, but considerable variation can be observed even in the normal ducts. The opening pressure, when contrast fluid is infused at a constant rate is normally approximately 2 cm greater than the resting pressure. In abnormal ducts, resting pressures are in the range of 25 cm of water and opening pressures are also correspondingly higher.

Surgeons embarking on the use of operative radiomanometry will have to choose from the diverse methods and apparatus available. Unfortunately, there is no standard method which is universally accepted or reported, a factor which has discouraged acceptance of this diagnostic manoeuvre.

We believe that cholangiomanometry is not the method of choice in the detection of common duct stones. Stones in the distal duct as well as in the intrahepatic radicles are better detected by the combined use of operative cholangiography and cholangioscopy. Cholangiomanometry appears to be the method of choice in the operative diagnosis of functional, and anatomic disorders

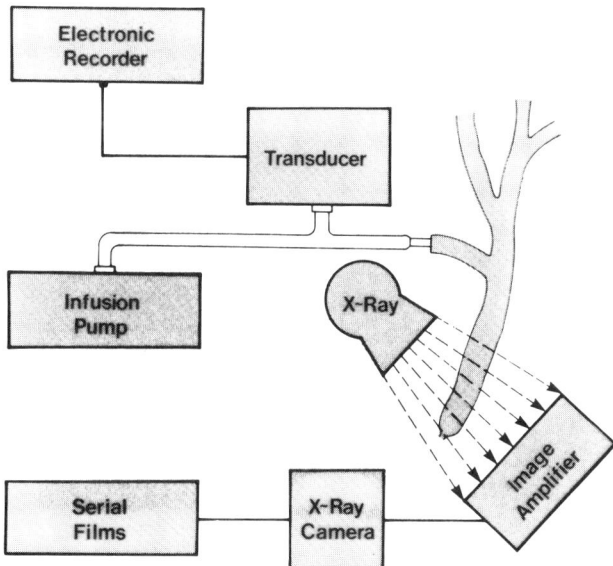

Fig. 6.10 Schematic representation of radiomanometric apparatus, showing all essential elements.

of the sphincter of Oddi. It is highly preferable to the crude method of passing a number 3 Bakes dilator through the sphincter. If high, valid resting and opening pressures are perceived by manometric methods in the absence of stones or tumour, then stenosis or spastic dysfunction of the sphincter may be inferred. Such a study may therefore give a valid, objective indication for sphincteroplasty.

In summary, operative radiomanometry (cholangiomanometry) can be a valuable adjunct in the diagnosis of biliary tract disorders. It requires, however, the use of standardized perfusion and pressure measurement equipment, standardized methodology and great care not to introduce artifactual variables. We recommend a metal cannula for cystic duct cannulation, a Harvard infusion pump for maintenance of a constant infusion rate of 25% diatrizoate sodium (Hypaque), a disposable pressure transducer, and an electronic digital readout recording apparatus. Less sophisticated systems may be used if the surgeon is aware of the advantages as well as the shortcomings of each system.

Intraoperative ultrasound

Intraoperative ultrasonography has been described by Sigel et al in 1981 for the diagnosis of biliary and pancreatic disease. It requires a portable real-time B-mode ultrasound apparatus which can be brought to the operating room. The transducer probe is either gas-sterilized or covered by a sterile plastic envelope so that it can be hand-held and directed by the operating surgeon. The

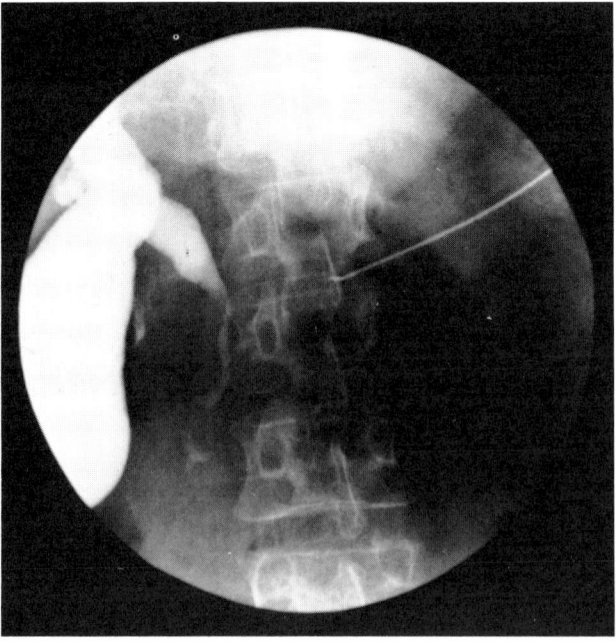

Fig. 6.11 Operative cholangiogram in patient with known pancreatitis, showing narrowing of distal common duct due to oedematous pancreatic head.

probe is held directly over the structure to be examined (gallbladder, common bile duct, pancreas) and then moved vertically or horizontally over the structure to obtain meaningful images. The images obtained at the operating table with the abdomen open are superior to those obtained by routine preoperative ultrasonic imaging.

We feel that this operative diagnostic manoeuvre has limited applicability in operations on the biliary tract. It may be useful in locating an obscured, dilated common duct in re-operative procedures on the biliary tract. It is doubtful that it can approach the accuracy and specificity of cholangiography for the detection and location of calculi.

Ultrasonic imaging at this time appears to hold the most promise in the diagnosis of pancreatic pathology in the vicinity of the distal common duct. Shown in Figure 6.11 is the operative cholangiogram in a patient with known pancreatitis. Preoperative ultrasonography had shown only a 2 cm pseudocyst in the pancreatic head. Operative imaging ultrasonography clearly showed multiple pseudocysts in an enlarged pancreatic head and was successful in delineating the dilated pancreatic duct (Fig. 6.12).

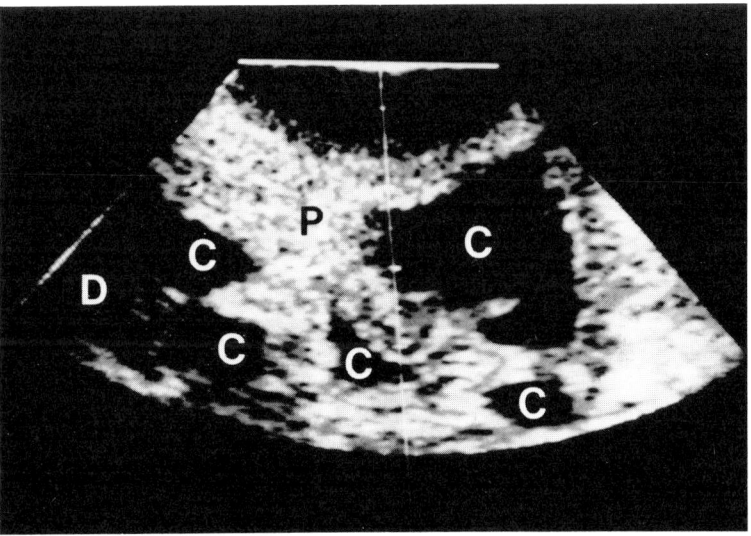

Fig. 6.12 Operative ultrasonogram showing multiple pseudocysts (C) within pancreatic parenchyma (P) and adjacent duodenum (D). Preoperative sonogram had shown only one cyst.

Liver biopsy

Liver biopsy has limited usefulness as an intraoperative diagnostic manoeuvre during biliary tract surgery. However, it can provide valuable information which may be of use in the postoperative period. We have reported a surprisingly high incidence of abnormal findings in hepatic histology when liver biopsy is performed routinely during biliary tract operations (Michel et al 1977). Among the findings which may be of use to surgeons in the postoperative period are fatty infiltration (indicating nutritional depletion or alcohol abuse), cholangitis and triaditis, unsuspected hepatitis, hemochromatosis, and abnormal pigment deposition (hemosiderosis, Dubin-Johnson syndrome). In long-standing biliary tract disease with recurrent jaundice, liver biopsy helps to substantiate the degree of hepatic damage. In patients with jaundice in whom no obstructive calculi are found in the common bile duct, the existence of cholangitis or focal necrosis may help explain jaundice and enzyme abnormalities. Early portal fibrosis, not visible grossly, may also be detected on liver biopsy.

Biopsy may be performed either by needle (Menghini) or by excising a small wedge from the edge of right or left lobes. In wedge biopsies, it is essential to obtain a biopsy deep enough to avoid capsular artifacts.

In view of our findings and those of others (Lygidakis 1981), we recommend the judicious use of liver biopsy as an adjunctive intraoperative diagnostic procedure.

Summary

Operative cholangiography is a simple, effective means of detecting anomalies, calculi and functional abnormalities during operations on the biliary tract. The information it provides is indispensable, and it should be used routinely in all biliary tract operations. When combined with fluoroscopy, its value is enhanced and more functional information is obtained. The accuracy of cholangiography in the detection of ductal calculi should be in the range of 95%.

Choledochoscopy should be performed in all cases which require choledochotomy, the rare exception being the small thin-walled common duct, too fragile to accept the choledochoscope (Reitsma 1981). The rigid choledochoscope with the Hopkins rod-lens system provides the best optical system for intraductal examination. Flexible choledochoscopes are more expensive, have a shorter life and provide less resolution than the rigid choledochoscope. However, they can be useful in examination and stone retrieval in long, tortuous ducts.

The overall diagnostic accuracy for the combined procedures of cholangiography and choledochoscopy should be 98–99%. Moreover, the two methods, used adjunctively, eliminate blind intraductal manipulation and instrumentation. The scraping of the delicate linings of the duct with scoops, probes, forceps and other instruments does unwarranted damage. Similarly, the blind passage of the Fogarty catheter into the proximal ductal system is fraught with the danger of ductal rupture and hemorrhage. Cholangiographic and endoscopic visualization of the sphincter of Oddi is vastly preferable to blind probing and 'dilatation' with Bakes dilators. We mention sphincteric dilatation for purposes of condemnation only; passage of the 3 mm dilator may be an acceptable intraoperative manoeuvre with the Bakes dilators for the assessment of sphincteric stenosis but is rarely necessary given the availability of cholangiography and choledochoscopy.

Cholangiomanometry is as yet not well established universally as an intraoperative diagnostic measure. Many techniques as well as instrumentation have been described. With the newer cholangiographic cannulas, transducers and recording devices, it is possible that this too can become a routine intraoperative procedure. It appears to be most useful in the diagnosis of disorders of the sphincter of Oddi.

Real-time ultrasonic imaging performed during operation can be of value in disorders of the (intrapancreatic) distal common duct and head of the pancreas. The apparatus is as yet cumbersome and interpretation difficult.

Operative liver biopsy, judiciously used, may yield useful information for the postoperative management of selected patients.

Acknowledgments

The authors gratefully acknowlege the invaluable assistance of the following individuals in the preparation of this chapter: Dr J. A. Hamlin for cholangiographic interpretation; Ms Pamela Amodeo and Ms Deena Bailey for preparation of the manuscript; Ms Margaret Paz-Partlow and Ms Maureen DeBose for illustrations; and Ms Judi Lippe for bibliographic research.

References

Berci G, Hamlin J A 1981a A combined fluoroscopic and endoscopic approach for retrieval of retained stones through the T-tube tract. Surgery, Gynecology and Obstetrics 153: 237–240

Berci G, Hamlin J A 1981b Unsuspected stone(s). In: Operative biliary radiology. Williams & Wilkins, Baltimore, ch 9, p 137

Berci G, Hamlin J A 1981c Critical analysis. In: Operative biliary radiology. Williams & Wilkins, Baltimore, ch 17, p 203

Berci G, Shore J M 1972 Advances in cholangioscopy. Endoscopy 4: 29–31

Berci G, Shore J M 1981 Operative biliary endoscopy (cholangioscopy). In: Berci G, Hamlin J A (eds) Operative biliary radiology. Williams & Wilkins, Baltimore, ch 14, p 169

Berci G, Shore J M, Morgenstern L, Hamlin J A 1978 Choledochoscopy and operative fluorocholangiography in the prevention of retained bile duct stones. World Journal of Surgery 2: 411–427

Caroli J 1946 La radiomanometrie biliaire. La Semaine des Hôpitaux de Paris 22: 1985–2000

Cassie G F, Kapadia C R 1981 Operative cholangiography or extra-ductal palpation: an analysis of 418 cholecystectomies. British Journal of Surgery 68: 516–517

Colcock B P, Perey B 1964 Exploration of the common bile duct. Surgery, Gynecology and Obstetrics 118: 20–24

Cushieri A, Hughes J H, Cohen M 1972 Biliary-pressure studies during cholecystectomy. British Journal of Surgery 59: 267–273

Daniel O 1972 The value of radiomanometry in bile duct surgery. Annals of the Royal College of Surgeons of England 51: 357–372

Earley D 1981 Radiation hazard. In: Berci G, Hamlin J A (eds) Operative biliary radiology. Williams & Wilkins, Baltimore, ch 4, p 27

Farha G J, Pearson R N 1976 Transcystic duct operative cholangiography: personal experience with 500 consecutive cases. American Journal of Surgery 131: 228–231

Glenn F 1965 Chronic and acute cholecystitis and common duct stone. American Journal of Gastroenterology 44: 232–244

Hamlin J A 1981 Biliary ductal anomalies. In: Berci G, Hamlin J A (eds) Operative biliary radiology. Williams & Wilkins, Baltimore, ch 8, p 109

Holmin T et al 1980 Selective or routine intraoperative cholangiography: a cost-effectiveness analysis. World Journal of Surgery 4: 315–322

Linos D A, Gray J E, McIlrath D C 1980 Radiation hazard to operating room personnel during operative cholangiography. Archives of Surgery 115: 1431–1433

Lygidakis N J 1981 Histologic changes and intrahepatic biliary abnormalities in extrahepatic biliary tract obstruction. Surgery, Gynecology and Obstetrics 153: 532–536

McCarthy J D 1970 Radiomanometry during biliary operations. Archives of Surgery 100: 424–429

McCarthy J D 1977 Radiomanometric guides to common bile duct exploration. American Journal of Surgery 134: 697–701

McCarthy J D 1981 Surgical pros and cons (editorial). Surgery, Gynecology and Obstetrics 153: 249

Mak B, Jakimowicz J J 1981 Technique and preliminary results of peroperative electronic manometry in the bile ducts. The Netherlands Journal of Surgery 33: 46–49

Mallet-Guy P 1952 Value of peroperative manometric and roentgenographic examination in the diagnosis of pathologic changes and functional disturbances of the biliary tract. Surgery, Gynecology and Obstetrics 94: 385–393

Michel S L, Lipsky R, Morgenstern L 1977 'Routine' liver biopsy in upper abdominal surgery. Archives of Surgery 112: 959–961

Mirizzi P L 1932 La colangiografia durante las operaciones de las vías biliares. Boletines y Trabajos, Sociedad de cirugia de Buenos Aires 16: 1133–1161

Mirizzi P L 1937 Operative cholangiography. Surgery, Gynecology and Obstetrics 65: 702–710

Morgenstern L (In Press) Exploration of the common bile duct for stones (including operative cholangiography and choledochoscopy). In: Way L M, Dunphy J E (eds) Surgery of the gallbladder and bile ducts. W B Saunders, Philadelphia

Nora P F et al 1977 Operative choledochoscopy: results of a prospective study in several institutions. American Journal of Surgery 133: 105–110

Rattner D W, Warshaw A L 1981 Impact of choledochoscopy on the management of choledocholithiasis: experience with 499 common duct explorations at the Massachusetts General Hospital. Annals of Surgery 194: 76–79

Reitsma B J 1981 Common duct stones — a reappraisal of aetiology and surgical management with special emphasis on operative biliary endoscopy. Akademisch Proefschrift, Maastricht, Holland

Roux M, Vayre P 1976 Morphological and functional study of the common bile duct in biliary surgery (value of intraoperative radiomanorheometry: an assessment of 25 years' experience) Chirurgia Gastroenterologia 10: 71–81

Salomon J, Roseman D L 1978 Intraoperative measurement of common duct resistance. Archives of Surgery 113: 650–653

Saltzstein E C 1981 Operative choledochoscopy and the retained common duct stone (editorial). Current Surgery 38: 371–373

Schein C T, Stern W Z, Jacobson H G 1966 The common duct. Operative cholangiography, biliary endoscopy and choledocholithotomy. Thomas, Springfield Mass

Shore J M, Lippman H N 1965 A flexible choledochoscope. Lancet 1: 1200–1201

Shore J M, Morgenstern L, Berci G 1971 An improved rigid choledochoscope. American Journal of Surgery 123: 567–568

Sigel B, Coelho J C U, Spigos D G, Donahue P E, Wood D K, Nyhus L M 1981 Ultrasonic imaging during biliary and pancreatic surgery. American Journal of Surgery 141: 84–89

Skillings J C, Williams J S, Hinshaw J R 1979 Cost-effectiveness of operative cholangiography. American Journal of Surgery 137: 26–31

Stark M E, Loughry C W 1980 Routine operative cholangiography with cholecystectomy. Surgery, Gynecology and Obstetrics 151: 657–658

Tompkins R K, Johnson J, Storm F K, Longmire W P 1976 Operative endoscopy in the management of biliary tract neoplasms. American Journal of Surgery 132: 174–182

White T T, Bordley J 1978 One percent incidence of recurrent gallstones six to eight years after manometric cholangiography. Annals of Surgery 188: 562–569

White T T, Waisman H, Hopton D, Kavlie H 1972 Radiomanometry, flow rates, and cholangiography in the evaluation of common bile disease: a study of 220 cases. American Journal of Surgery 123: 73–79

Yamakawa T, Komaki F, Shikata J 1978 Experience with routine postoperative choledochoscopy via the T-tube sinus tract. World Journal of Surgery 2: 379–385

Yamakawa T, Mieno K, Nogucki T, Shikata J 1976 An improved choledochofiberscope and non-surgical removal of retained biliary calculi under direct visual control. Gastrointestinal Endoscopy 22: 160–164

7 *Cholecystitis*

ROGER W. MOTSON and
LAWRENCE W. WAY

Introduction

Gallstone disease is extremely common, affecting approximately 10% of the adult population. In the USA alone more than 15 million people are affected. Each year 800 000 new cases present and 400 000 cholecystectomies are performed. Although symptomless gallstones are sometimes demonstrated during the investigation of another illness, the majority of patients present with symptoms of acute or chronic cholecystitis.

Chronic cholecystitis

The term chronic cholecystitis is used to describe both patients with continuous low-grade symptoms and patients with recurrent acute attacks of colic. The symptoms are produced by inflammation of the wall of the stone-containing gallbladder or obstruction of the cystic duct by stone resulting in biliary colic. The pain is of visceral origin and poorly localized, increases over 15–60 minutes, remains constant for minutes to hours, and then gradually fades. Although frequently described as right hypochondrial pain, biliary colic may be felt in the epigastrium or even the left hypochondrium. Referred pain felt in the back or right scapula occurs in one third of patients and is occasionally the only symptom. The attacks of pain may occur in almost any pattern. In some subjects they are years apart, whereas in others symptoms are experienced almost every day. Nausea and vomiting occasionally accompany the pain.

The other principal symptoms of chronic cholecystitis are dyspepsia and heartburn. Although most patients have pain, these may be the only symptoms in some. Prospective studies have shown that only about half the patients seeking medical help for flatulent dyspepsia have gallstones. Although this suggests that there may be no direct connection between cholecystitis and dyspepsia, it has been found that cholecystectomy eliminates dyspepsia in 80% of patients (Johnson 1975, Kingston & Windson 1975).

In chronic cholecystitis the physical examination usually adds little to the history. There may be mild tenderness in the right hypochondrium and the gallbladder is rarely palpable.

Diagnosis

Oral cholecystography remains the most widely used investigation. Approximately 10% of patients have opaque stones visible on plain abdominal X-ray, but it is essential that a cholecystogram be performed to confirm that the stones are within the gallbladder. In approximately 25% of patients the gallbladder does not opacify, and in these cases a further dose of contrast should be given. This will opacify the gallbladder in 60% of patients whose initial study was unsuccessful. Failure to opacify the gallbladder after a double dose of contrast indicates more than a 95% chance of gallbladder disease. Oral cholecystography yields few false negatives (perhaps 1 or 2% of gallbladders that contain stones), and the radiographs are easy to interpret.

Ultrasound scanning can also demonstrate gallstones and other abnormalities of the gallbladder and is now being more widely used in the diagnosis of cholelithiasis (Lee et al 1980). With increasing experience and improvement in scanning equipment diagnostic accuracy has steadily increased. Using a real-time scanner Cooperberg and Burhenne failed to detect gallstones in only five out of 261 patients, a sensitivity of 98%; quite comparable to oral cholecystography. In 43 patients subsequently confirmed not to have gallstones the scan correctly demonstrated their absence in all except one, a specificity of 98% (Cooperberg & Burhenne 1980). In another recent series the sensitivity was 92% and specificity 91% (Lee et al 1980). Ultrasound scanning does not rely on concentration or opacification by a dye, is unaffected by liver disease, and does not expose the patient to radiation. However, it may be difficult to obtain a good scan in obese patients, and intestinal gas overlying the gallbladder may make it impossible to obtain a satisfactory study. Furthermore the images are more difficult to interpret than are X-rays.

In chronic cholecystitis the two techniques are complementary, with oral cholecystography being preferred for the uncomplicated non-urgent case. Ultrasonography is of greatest value in patients suffering from liver disease, those who are pregnant, or those who have had an unsuccessful oral cholecystogram. Intravenous cholangiography is not recommended to diagnose stones in the gallbladder. The gallbladder is often opacified, though poorly, but stones are not well demonstrated, and there are many false negative studies. Furthermore the infusion of contrast produces unpleasant side effects in many patients and occasionally a serious sensitivity reaction.

Differential diagnosis in chronic cholecystitis includes peptic ulcer disease, hiatus hernia, reflux oesophagitis, chronic pancreatitis, angina pectoris, irritable bowel syndrome, carcinoma of the right colon and functional disorders. Barium meal, endoscopy, pancreatography, electrocardiogram and barium enema will be necessary in some cases.

Acalculous chonic cholecystitis

The management of patients with symptoms of cholecystitis who are shown to have gallstones on oral cholecystography or ultrasound scan is straightforward.

However, a substantial number of patients with similar symptoms are found to have a normal cholecystogram. Indiscriminate cholecystectomy in these patients is likely to result in a high frequency of post-cholecystectomy pain. Nevertheless, there are some patients with acalculous cholecystitis whose symptoms will be relieved by cholecystectomy. Can they be identified?

It is obviously important to exclude other causes of right hypochondrial or epigastric pain, and barium studies or endoscopy will be necessary in many cases. The cholecystogram should be repeated to confirm that it is normal.

In patients with symptoms typical of gallbladder disease whose oral cholecystogram and ultrasound scan is normal an ERCP should be performed. Occasionally, gallstones that have eluded detection by these other tests are first demonstrated in this way.

If the ERCP is also normal and there is still a strong suspicion that the gallbladder could be the source of the patient's complaints, the duodenum should be intubated and a sample of duodenal bile examined for the presence of cholesterol crystals or bilirubinate granules. Empirically, there is a strong correlation between abnormalities on this study and the presence of gallbladder disease. Furthermore, Sedaghat & Grundy (1980) have shown that irrespective of the absolute value of the cholesterol saturation index of the bile, cholesterol crystals only form in the bile of subjects with gallstone disease. In other words, subjects with supersaturated bile but no gallstone disease have no crystals in their bile.

A large series of 62 patients with acalculous cholecystitis were treated surgically by Keddie et al (1976). Adenomatosis (48%) and chronic inflammation (39%) were the principal pathologic findings. Cholesterosis (10%) and acute inflammation (3%) accounted for the remainder. In this series 90% of patients were completely relieved of their symptoms, a higher success rate than most have achieved (Gunn et al 1973, Anderson et al 1971).

Treatment

In the majority of patients with symptomatic chronic cholecystitis there is little difficulty in recommending cholecystectomy. The results are likely to be excellent in terms of symptom relief, and operative morbidity and mortality are very low. More difficult are patients with minimal symptoms, those without symptoms whose stones have been found fortuitously, and patients with other medical problems for whom the risk of surgery is greater.

We feel there is little urgency in performing cholecystectomy in patients with minimal symptoms or no symptoms. Follow-up studies of subjects without symptoms show about a 2% per year risk of symptoms (i.e. colic) appearing and a very low risk of complications (Gracie & Ranschoff 1981). It is also true, however, that the risk of cholecystectomy in asymptomatic individuals is low. In essence, the decision may be difficult, but it is not very weighty — the risk of either treating or not treating the patient is very low. On the other hand, we would definitely recommend prophylactic cholecystectomy for patients with diabetes mellitus or those with a non-opacifying gallbladder on oral cholecystography, because even if asymptomatic they are more likely to encounter complications of their disease.

Chenodeoxycholate (CDC) and ursodeoxycholate are capable in some patients of dissolving cholesterol gallstones. About $1-1\frac{1}{2}$ years of continuous therapy is required before dissolution becomes complete, and the highest success rate in carefully selected patients is about 30%. Complete dissolution was seen in only 15% of the group receiving 'high dose' (750 mg/d) CDC in the randomized controlled trial conducted in the USA (Schoenfield et al 1981). The effects of dissolution on the patient's symptoms and the natural history of the disease has not been adequately documented; no effect was observed in the American trial. Following dissolution and interruption of therapy, the rate of gallstone recurrence inexorably increases as time passes. In one study the recurrence rate was 50% after a median period of observation of 23 months (Ruppin & Dowling 1982). The relatively low efficacy and temporary nature of the benefits make it difficult to judge whether dissolution therapy has any well-defined role at present. It would seem that elderly patients with coexisting cardiopulmonary disease and no contraindications to dissolution (i.e. their gallstones are radiolucent and small, and the gallbladder opacifies on oral cholecystogram) might better be treated with drugs than by surgery. In most other kinds of patients, however, surgery remains preferable to dissolution.

Acute cholecystitis

In most cases acute cholecystitis is the result of obstruction of the cystic duct by stone. Acute inflammation develops in the gallbladder initially due to the irritant action of bile salts (i.e. it is a chemical inflammation). Proliferation of bacteria, almost always present once stones have formed, usually begins only after the acute cholecystitis is established, but suppuration does not develop in the average uncomplicated case. An attack is terminated either by the stone passing into the common duct or falling back into the gallbladder. The natural course of the disease is to resolve spontaneously within one week, but in a minority of patients the disease progresses and empyema may form or the gallbladder may perforate.

Diagnosis

Oral cholecystography in the acute attack fails to opacify the obstructed gallbladder and cannot therefore provide direct evidence of gallbladder disease. Intravenous cholangiography can be used for diagnosis, but it has now been largely superseded by radionuclide excretion studies. With either a radionuclide study or an IVC, imaging of the common duct with no imaging of the gallbladder strongly supports the diagnosis of acute cholecystitis. The radionuclide test is performed by hepatobiliary scanning with a gamma camera after intravenous injection of technetium 99m-labelled HIDA (Hall et al 1981, O'Callaghan et al 1980, Ram et al 1981, Weissmann et al 1981). A clear image of the biliary ducts and gallbladder is obtained, followed by recognizable entry of the radionuclide into the duodenum. Rare false negative studies may occur in patients with acute acalculous cholecystitis whose cystic duct is patent. False positive studies are occasionally seen with chronic cholecystitis (in the absence of acute inflammation) and with acute pancreatitis. There is a high correlation between the result of the HIDA scan and the presence or absence of acute cholecystitis, but the facilities to perform this investigation are not available in all hospitals.

Treatment

The treatment of acute cholecystitis is more controversial than that of chronic cholecystitis, with arguments advanced both for early surgery and for conservative treatment of the acute attack followed by elective cholecystectomy six to eight weeks later.

The basis of the conservative argument is that most cases of cholecystitis will settle on expectant management, that early surgery may spread localized infection into the general peritoneal cavity, that operation may be more difficult since inflammation around the bile ducts obscures the anatomy, and that exploration of the common duct cannot be so readily performed. The advocates of early surgery argue that the complications of failed conservative treatment — empyema and perforation — are avoided, that in the early stages the inflammation is confined to the gallbladder, and that difficulties in exploring the common bile duct are not insurmountable. In addition the patient spends less time in hospital (i.e. costs of medical care and lost income are less), suffers less pain and may be spared further acute attacks or chronic symptoms while awaiting elective surgery (Fowkes & Gunn 1980).

We subscribe to the latter view providing that the diagnosis can be confirmed by one of the methods described above and the patient's general health is suitable for early surgery. To answer specifically the arguments for conservative management, it is certainly true that about two-thirds of cases settle spontaneously. However, the remainder do not, and emergency surgery later in the attack in an unfit patient may well turn out to be more hazardous and difficult than is planned early surgery. Spreading of infection into the peritoneal cavity might occur if an inflammatory mass is disturbed, but in practice this does not seem to be a major problem. In this respect, acute cholecystectomy may be regarded as analogous to acute appendectomy. Because the infection is confined to the gallbladder the cystic duct and common bile duct are normal, only affected by secondary oedema. Dissection of the ducts and cystic artery therefore usually presents little additional difficulty, and operative cholangiography, common duct exploration and choledochoscopy can all be performed with no greater morbidity than in an elective case (van der Linden & Edland 1981). Furthermore, elective cholecystectomy after a six to eight week interval is not always straightforward. A thickened, shrunken gallbladder adherent to the bile ducts is not infrequently encountered, and it is often true that the dissection would have been simpler during the acute attack.

We therefore recommend that a patient presenting with acute cholecystitis should have the diagnosis confirmed by ultrasound or Tc99 HIDA scanning and undergo early cholecystectomy. If the patient's general condition renders him a poor risk for early surgery (because of ancillary conditions, such as cardiac or pulmonary disease) a conservative policy is favored, followed by confirmation of the diagnosis by oral cholecystography four weeks later and elective cholecystectomy six to eight weeks after the acute attack. If a patient treated conservatively fails to settle or deteriorates, then emergency operation should be performed.

Table 7.1 Controlled trials comparing early and delayed (interval) cholecystectomy for
acute cholecystitis

Author	Timing of Cholecystectomy (No. of Patients)	
	Early	Delayed
van der Linden (1970)	70	58
McArthur et al (1975)	15	15
Lahtinen et al (1978)	49	44
Jarvinen et al (1980)	80	75
Total	214	192

Cholecystostomy is indicated only rarely. The decision to perform cholecystostomy is usually based on preoperative findings, and the most common
situation is a desperately ill patient from suppurative cholecystitis who is a poor
risk for a general anaesthetic and anything but the briefest operation.

The results of four controlled trials all support the more aggressive surgical
management of uncomplicated acute cholecystitis. These trials and the numbers
of patients randomly treated by early or late cholecystectomy are listed in Table
7.1; the results are summarized in Table 7.2. It is obvious that surgical mishaps are
not more common during cholecystectomy performed during the acute attack, and
that the benefits of this approach have been verified. The evidence suggests that
early surgery decreases mortality by obviating the need for urgent laparotomy in
the occasional patient whose condition deteriorates during expectant management
(van der Linden & Edlund 1981).

Table 7.2 Consolidated results of the four controlled trials listed in Table 7.1 comparing early
and delayed cholecystectomy for acute cholecystitis. 'Failure of regimen' means cholecystectomy
was not performed as planned.

Timing of cholecystectomy	Patients	Deaths	Duct injuries	Total mean Hospital stay	Failure of regimen
Early	214	0	0	10.9	0%
Delayed	192	5	0	20.1	19%

Conclusion

Chronic cholecystitis continues to be the most frequent
presentation of cholesterol gallstone disease. With the safety of modern surgical
treatment cholecystectomy should be recommended in the great majority of cases.
This should decrease the incidence of complications of gallstone disease, such as
common duct obstruction, cholangitis, empyema of the gallbladder, perforation of
the gallbladder and gallstone ileus. Acute cholecystitis can now be diagnosed
accurately early in the course of an attack in most cases. Early surgery reduces the
duration of the patient's illness, is not associated with any additional hazard, may
reduce the incidence of difficult cholecystectomy in elective cases, and reduces
hospital costs.

References

Anderson A, Bergdahl L, Boquist L 1971 Acalculous cholecystitis. American Journal of Surgery 122: 3

Cooperberg P C, Burhenne H J 1980 Real time ultrasonography. Diagnostic technique of choice in calculous gallbladder disease. New England Journal of Medicine 302: 1277

Fowkes F G R, Gunn A A 1980 The management of acute cholecystitis and its hospital cost. British Journal of Surgery 67: 613

Gracie W A, Ransohoff D F 1981 The natural history of silent gallstones. Gastroenterology 80: 1161

Gunn A, Keddie N C, Fox M 1973 Acalculous gallbladder disease. British Journal of Surgery 60: 213

Hall A W, Wisbey M L, Hutchinson F, Wood R A B, Cushieri A 1981 The place of hepatobiliary scanning in the diagnosis of gallbladder disease. British Journal of Surgery 68: 85

Jarvinen H J, Hastbacka J 1980 Early cholecystectomy for acute cholecystitis. A prospective randomised study. Annals of Surgery 191: 501

Johnson A G 1975 Cholecystectomy and gallstone dyspepsia. Clinical and physiological study of a symptom complex. Annals of the Royal College of Surgeons of England 59: 69

Keddie N C, Gough A L, Galland R B 1976 Acalculous gallbladder disease: a prospective study. British Journal of Surgery 63: 797

Kingston R D, Windson C W O 1975 Flatulent dyspepsia in patients undergoing cholecystectomy. British Journal of Surgery 62: 231

Lahtinen J, Alhava E M, Aukee S 1978 Acute cholecystitis treated by early and delayed surgery. A controlled clinical trial. Scandinavian Journal of Gastroenterology 13: 673

Lee J K T, Melson G L, Koehler R E, Stanley R J 1980 Cholecystosonography: Accuracy, pitfalls and unusual findings. American Journal of Surgery 139: 223

van der Linden W, Edlund G 1981 Early versus delayed cholecystectomy: the effect of a change in management. British Journal of Surgery 68: 753

van der Linden W, Sunzel H 1970 Early versus delayed operation for acute cholecystitis. A controlled clinical trial. American Journal of Surgery 120: 7

McArthur P, Cuschieri A, Sells R A, Shields R 1975 Controlled clinical trial comparing early with interval cholecystectomy for acute cholecystitis. British Journal of Surgery 62: 805

O'Callaghan J D, Verow P W, Hopton D, Craven J L 1980 The diagnosis of acute gallbladder disease by technetium-99m-labelled HIDA hepatobiliary scanning. British Journal of Surgery 67: 805

Ram M D, Hagihara P F, Kim E E, Coupal J, Griffen W O 1981 Evaluation of biliary disease by scintigraphy. American Journal of Surgery 141: 77

Ruppin D C, Dowling R H 1982 Is recurrence inevitable after gallstone dissolution by bile-acid treatment? Lancet, January: 181

Schoenfield L J, Lachin J M et al 1981 Chenodiol (chenodeoxycholic acid) for dissolution of gallstones: The national cooperative gallstone study. A controlled trial of efficacy and safety. Annals of Internal Medicine 95: 257

Sedaghat A, Grundy S M 1980 Cholesterol crystals and the formation of cholesterol gallstones. New England Journal of Medicine 302: 1274

Weissmann H S, Rosenblatt R, Sugarman L A, Freeman L M 1981 An update in radionuclide imaging in the diagnosis of cholecystitis. Journal of the American Medical Association 246: 1354

8

Cholecystectomy and common duct explorations

C. K. McSHERRY

Little change in the incidence of calculous biliary tract disease is anticipated during the next several decades. The population of the United States in 1981 was 226 million, 80% of whom were adults. Based on postmortem studies and clinical reports, approximately 12%, or 22 million people, have or have had gallstones. There is much to suggest that these statistics are applicable to most other developed nations. In the absence of preventive measures and safe, effective cholelitholytic agents, cholecystectomy will continue to be the primary treatment for cholelithiasis and its sequelae.

The recent report of the National Cooperative Gallstone Study (1981) on the effectiveness and safety of chenodeoxycholic acid (chenodiol) to dissolve cholesterol gallstones was a disappointment. Of the 611 patients treated with chenodiol, only 50 (8%) had complete dissolution of their stones by cholecystographic criteria after two years of treatment. In addition, the incidence of undesirable side-effects was much higher than anticipated. There were 98 patients who dropped out or withdrew from the study; major elevations of serum aminotransferase were experienced by 39 patients, some of whom required liver biopsy for further evaluation; and significant elevations of serum cholesterol occurred in 29 patients. McSherry (1981) estimated the morbidity of chenodiol therapy to be 27%. It is unlikely that chenodiol therapy will displace cholecystectomy as the primary treatment of cholelithiasis. Further research, however, is anticipated to yield more effective gallstone dissolving agents in the not too distant future.

Although there is agreement that cholecystectomy is the treatment of choice in patients with recurrent attacks of biliary colic, the management of patients with asymptomatic or 'silent' gallstones is still controversial. Cholelithiasis is a common disease, but knowledge of its natural history untreated is scant. Surgeons, convinced that the morbidity and mortality rates of cholecystectomy are significantly higher in the older age group and in those patients with acute cholecystitis and common duct obstruction, recommend early cholecystectomy. Other physicians interpret the same data and conclude that in many patients with asymptomatic stones, operation will never prove necessary.

Until recently, published reports indicated that in many patients asymptomatic gallstones do not remain 'silent' indefinitely. Lund (1960) reported on 526 patients with cholelithiasis observed for from 5 to 20 years. Of this group, 50% of the women and 30% of the men had symptoms of biliary calculous disease, usually within five years of the diagnosis. Acute cholecystitis and/or common duct obstruction occurred in 25% of the patients. Wenckert & Robertson (1966) reported the development of symptoms in 51% of 781 patients and Comfort et al (1948), 46% of 112 patients followed for up to 20 years. In 1981, Gracie & Ransohoff reported a group of 123 faculty members at the University of Michigan with asymptomatic gallstones that were followed for 10–15 years and noted that only 13% became symptomatic and 2.4% had serious sequelae. This experience, which is quite different from that reported in the older literature, is difficult to explain on grounds other than the select nature of this patient population. There is an obvious need for comparable studies of larger numbers of patients more representative of the population at risk. Clinical practice at the present time is to evaluate the relative risks and benefits for each patient and to individualize the appropriate course of action.

Cholecystectomy performed in accordance with accepted indications is very effective. It interrupts the progression of the disease process and prevents recurrence of calculi. The technical aspects of the operation require careful attention to detail in order to minimize the risks of the procedure. These include partial or complete interruption of the common bile duct or its main tributaries, the right and left hepatic ducts; impairment of the blood supply to the liver; and transection of unobserved anomalous ductal and vascular channels between the liver and gallbladder or cystic duct. The ability to recognize anomalies of the ductal system and its blood supply and to deal with unexpected hemorrhage is the cornerstone of the skills required.

In most patients, a right subcostal incision provides the optimum exposure. In patients with narrow costal arch, a paramedian incision may be preferred. More important than the type of incision is its length; abdominal incisions should be of sufficient extent to afford adequate exposure without undue retraction.

After the peritoneal cavity is entered and the falciform ligament divided, a complete exploration of the abdomen is carried out. The viscera that occupy the right hypochondrium adjacent to the liver are retracted to expose the gallbladder and inferior surface of the liver. The structures in the hepatoduodenal ligament are placed on tension by retraction of the stomach and duodenum inferiorly. With additional retractors elevating the costal margin and inferior surface of the liver, the contents of the gallbladder can be palpated and any variation from the normal of the course of the bile ducts noted. With a finger in the foramen of Winslow, the distal duct can be palpated for stones. The duodenum, especially the area of the ampulla of Vater, and the head of the pancreas should also be palpated in search of calculi or tumour.

The dissection to remove the gallbladder is begun by incising the peritoneum overlying the triangle of Calot. The base of this anatomic triangle is the cystic artery and the junction of the cystic and common hepatic ducts, the apex. The cystic duct and cystic artery are exposed by blunt dissection. A silk ligature is then placed around each of these structures and secured with a single knot (Fig. 8.1). This is done to minimize blood loss and impede the dislodgement of small calculi into the common bile duct during the dissection of the gallbladder from its

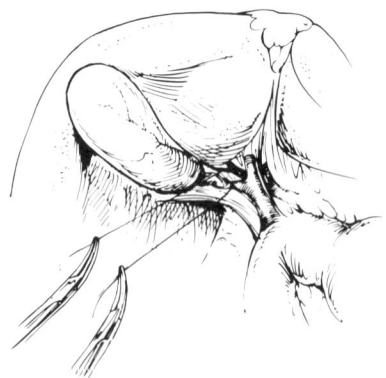

Fig. 8.1 Silk ligatures are placed around the cystic duct and cystic artery for the purposes of identification and traction on these structures.

capsule. The peritoneum surrounding the gallbladder is incised at a distance of 1–1.5 cm from the liver. The gallbladder is then separated from its peritoneal attachment to the liver by a combination of both blunt and sharp dissection beginning at the fundus and proceeding to the ampulla, the so-called 'antegrade' technique (Fig. 8.2). The entrance of the cystic artery on to the anterior wall of the gallbladder is identified, and the vessel is secured between two clamps and then divided. The stump of the cystic artery is ligated with non-absorbable suture. A lymph node is often encountered along the course of the cystic vessels that is variable in size dependent on the extent of present and prior inflammation. Occasionally sufficient scarring is encountered, and separation of the cystic artery and cystic duct requires careful technique. When the gallbladder has been dissected completely from its capsule and the cystic artery divided, the cystic duct is traced to its true junction with the common hepatic duct. Anomalies are frequent in this area and the length of the cystic duct variable. If an operative cholangiogram is to be performed, a suture-ligature is placed in the wall of the cystic duct approximately 1 cm proximal to its junction with the common bile duct (Fig. 8.3). A small incision is made in the cystic duct, and the plastic cholangiography catheter is inserted into it and secured by the previously placed suture-ligature. Care is taken to avoid the introduction of air bubbles into the ductal system. Radiopaque contrast solution, usually 8–12 ml, is instilled slowly into the ductal system. If ciné radiography is available, over distension of the ductal system can be avoided and radiographs obtained after the contrast agent has entered the duodenum. The availability of ciné radiography facilitates operative cholangiography by reducing the need for multiple injections and repeat radiographs. If the operative cholangiogram is normal and there are no findings to prompt exploration of the common bile duct, the cholangiography catheter is removed and the cystic duct is divided 5–8 mm from its junction with the common hepatic duct. The cystic duct is divided between clamps as illustrated in Fig. 8.4 and its stump secured with a ligature and a transfixion suture of non-absorbable material.

An alternative technique is to remove the gallbladder by initiating the dissection

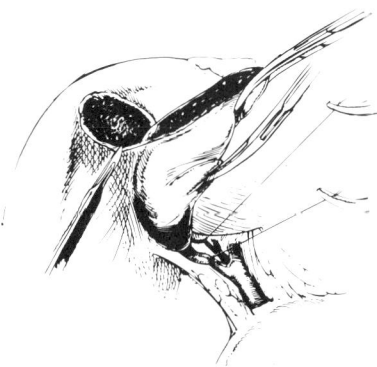

Fig. 8.2 The peritoneal attachments of the gallbladder to the liver are severed proceeding from the fundus to the ampulla, the 'antegrade' technique of cholecystectomy.

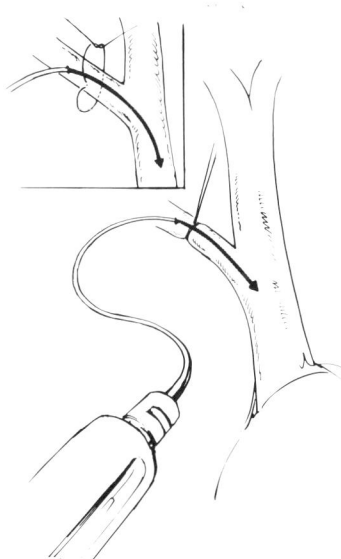

Fig. 8.3 A cholangiography catheter is secured in the cystic duct in preparation for introducing contrast agent into the ductal system during the performance of operative cholangiography

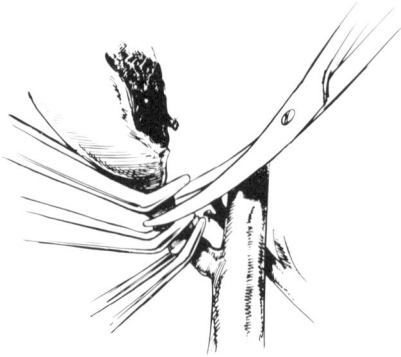

Fig. 8.4 The stump of the cystic duct is secured with both a ligature and a suture of non-absorbable material.

in the region of the ampulla and proceeding to the fundus, the 'retrograde' method. As illustrated in Fig. 8.5, an incision is made in the peritoneal fold of the hepatoduodenal ligament at the level of the presumed junction of the cystic and common hepatic ducts. The cystic duct is dissected free from the surrounding tissue, and a silk ligature is passed about it. As traction is made on the cystic duct by the ligature, the peritoneum is incised superiorly toward the cystic artery where it enters the wall of the gallbladder. Following division of the cystic artery, the remainder of the cystic duct is more easily exposed to complete its dissection and division as previously described. With traction on the divided cystic duct, the peritoneum overlying the gallbladder is incised 1–2 cm from the liver capsule. The dissection of the gallbladder is then accomplished in retrograde fashion, beginning at the ampulla and proceeding to the fundus.

If there are clinical or radiologic indications to explore the common bile duct for additional stones, two fixation sutures are placed one to two centimeters distal to the junction of the cystic and common ducts. An incision is then made through the anterior wall equal in length to the diameter of the duct as depicted in Fig. 8.6. After sufficient bile has been obtained for microbiologic studies, the lumen of the duct is searched for additional stones. There are several acceptable methods for ductal exploration. My own preference is to explore the duct firstly in the direction of the ampulla and then in the direction of the liver using successively stone (Randall) forceps (Fig. 8.7), small pituitary spoons, Fogarty catheters and then irrigating catheters (Figs. 8.8 and 8.9). If necessary, the descending segment of the duodenum should be mobilized by incising its lateral peritoneal reflection (Kocher manoeuvre). This permits digital manipulation of the retropancreatic segment of the common bile duct and may facilitate dislodgement of stones (Fig. 8.10). In a small proportion of patients with common duct stones, efforts to remove calculi from the ampullary segment of the duct via the choledochotomy incision are unsuccessful. In these patients, it is necessary to approach the lower end of the common bile duct through the duodenum. A lateral longitudinal duodenotomy is made opposite the ampulla (Fig. 8.11), and the duct is explored retrograde. Division of the sphincter of Oddi is often necessary to remove

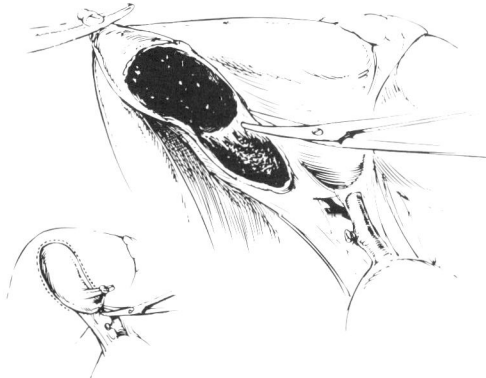

Fig. 8.5 The 'retrograde' method of cholecystectomy.

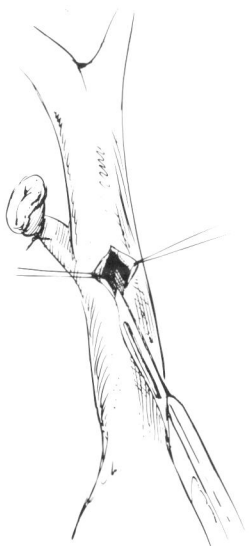

Fig. 8.6 The common bile duct is incised distal to the junction of the cystic and common hepatic ducts to permit exploration for stones.

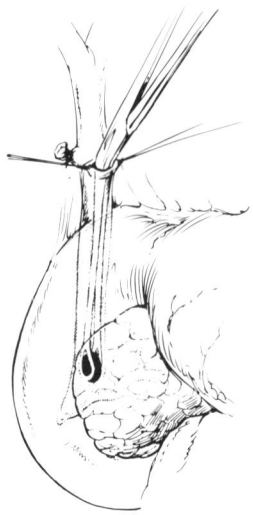

Fig. 8.7 Stone-grasping forceps are used to extract calculi from the common bile duct.

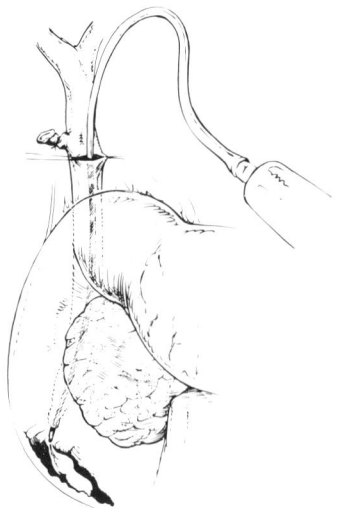

Fig. 8.8 Soft, flexible catheters are used to irrigate the ductal system to flush small stones and debris.

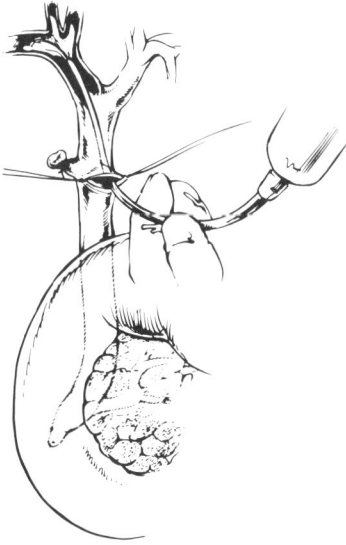

Fig. 8.9 Saline irrigation of the intrahepatic ducts and the use of balloon-tipped catheters are often preferred techniques for removing calculi from the right and left hepatic ducts.

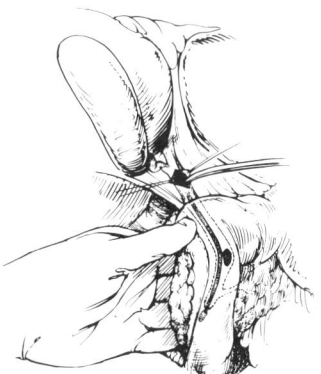

Fig. 8.10 Mobilization of the second portion of the duodenum by the Kocher manoeuvre facilitates exploration of the lower end of the duct.

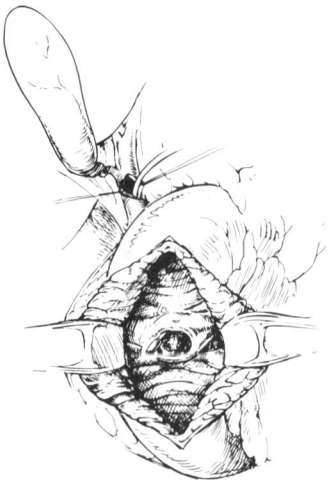

Fig. 8.11 Longitudinal duodenotomy to expose a stone impacted at the ampulla of Vater. The probe in the ampulla is helpful in selecting the appropriate site for duodenotomy.

impacted calculi. This is best accomplished by dividing the sphincter at the 11 o'clock position (Fig. 8.12) and then suturing the duodenal mucosa to the mucosa of the common bile duct with absorbable catgut (Fig. 8.13). Upon completion of the procedure, the duodenotomy is closed transversely.

Choledochoscopy is performed in the course of common duct exploration to identify stones or other lesions and to minimize or reduce the incidence of retained or overlooked calculi (Fig. 8.14). In ducts of small diameter, this technique is not feasible and may indeed result in needless trauma. Both flexible and rigid choledochoscopes are available, and each has its proponents. My own preference at the present time is for the rigid instrument.

Upon completion of choledochoscopy, a T-tube is placed in the common bile duct and the choledochotomy closed with chromic catgut (Fig. 8.15). Our preference is to employ the Whelan-Moss modified T-tube because the limb exiting from the abdomen has a larger diameter than that which remains in the bile duct. This facilitates the extraction of retained common duct stones through the T-tube tract if such becomes necessary. After the T-tube has been secured in place, an operative cholangiogram is obtained and carefully examined for evidence of residual stones. It is most advantageous to have these cholangiograms also interpreted by an experienced radiologist. In any event, the abdomen should not be closed until the surgeon has satisfied himself that the ductal system is free of calculi.

With respect to operative technique, debate continues on the routine use of drains and operative cholangiography. The majority of surgeons continue to drain the subhepatic space in all patients who undergo cholecystectomy. The rationale for the use of drains is to prevent the accumulation of bile and blood which, if infected, would result in a subhepatic abscess. Other authors (Kambouris et al 1973) have been more selective in the use of drains and report fewer postoperative complications and a shortened hospital stay.

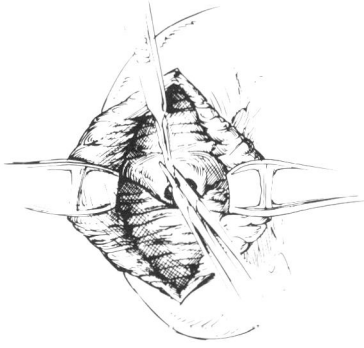

Fig. 8.12 If necessary, the sphincter of Oddi is divided to facilitate extraction of calculi. The incision through the sphincter should be at the 11 o'clock position to avoid injury to the pancreatic duct.

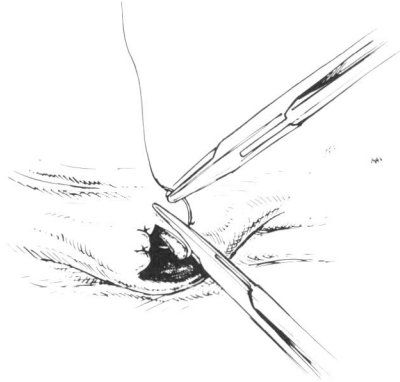

Fig. 8.13 Sphincteroplasty is accomplished by approximating the mucosa of the duodenum and common bile duct with absorbable suture.

Operative cholangiography is an essential element of successful biliary tract surgery. It reduces the frequency of unnecessary exploration of the common bile duct and is the principal means of reducing the incidence of residual and overlooked common duct stones. Saltzstein et al (1973) have reported their experience with cystic duct operative cholangiography in 423 of 506 consecutive patients undergoing cholecystectomy. In 79 patients with clinical indications for common duct exploration, operative cholangiograms were normal in 39 (50%) and therefore obviated the need for choledochotomy in these patients. Unsuspected common duct stones were demonstrated in 8 (1.8%) of 427 patients without clinical indications for common duct exploration. There is general agreement that as the frequency of operative cholangiography has increased, the number of common bile duct explorations has decreased, but the proportion of patients with stones recovered from the ductal system at exploration has increased. Therefore, operative cholangiograms should be performed in most patients subjected to

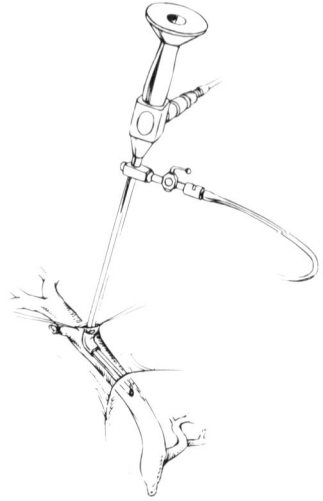

Fig. 8.14 The choledochoscope is used in search of calculi in the biliary ductal system.

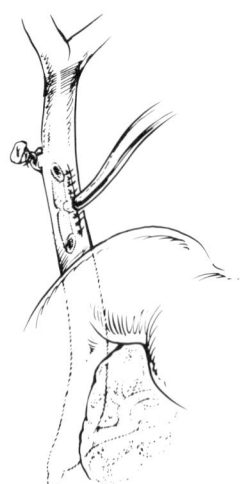

Fig. 8.15 A T-tube has been placed in the common bile duct and the choledochotomy closed with interrupted suture.

Table 8.1 Surgical treatment for non-acute biliary tract disease

	Patients	Deaths	Mortality Rate
A. Cholecystectomy	7956	38	0.5%
B. Cholecystostomy	115	10	8.7%
A or B plus choledochotomy	1533	53	3.5%
Choledochotomy (secondary in search of calculi)	353	7	1.98%
Procedures for strictures and miscellaneous conditions	259	20	7.7%
Total operations	10216	128	1.3%

cholecystectomy. Patients with a solitary large cholesterol stone and those with very small calibre cystic ducts are examples of patients in whom operative cholangiography may be omitted.

Statistics accumulated by Dr Frank Glenn at The New York Hospital–Cornell Medical Center over a period of almost five decades suggest that approximately 80% of patients operated upon for calculous biliary tract disease have chronic cholecystitis and cholelithiasis. From 1932 through 1980 12 693 patients had operative therapy for non-malignant biliary tract disease at that institution. Of this group of patients 10 216 were considered to have 'nonacute' biliary tract disease and 2477 'acute' disease.

The operations employed in the group of patients considered to have nonacute biliary tract disease and their associated mortality rates are listed in Table 8.1. Comparable data for patients with acute cholecystitis are listed in Table 8.2. Age and the occurrence of acute cholecystitis were the major determinants of operative risk in patients with calculous biliary tract disease. In this group of 12 693 patients, there were 5679 less than 50 years of age, and there were 19 deaths, a mortality rate of 0.3%. Of 4288 patients aged 50 to 64 years, there were 71 deaths, a mortality rate of 1.6%; and of the 2726 patients 65 years and older, there were 134 fatalities (4.9%). The mortality rate following cholecystectomy for chronic cholecystitis and cholelithiasis was 0.5% amongst 8052 patients. In contrast, it was 1.3% of 1707 patients that underwent cholecystectomy for acute cholecystitis.

A major and as yet unsolved problem in the field of biliary tract surgery is the problem of the retained common duct stone. In the above described group of 12 693 patients operated upon for nonmalignant biliary tract disease, 12 434 had a primary operation for biliary calculi, viz., cholecystectomy or cholecystostomy alone or combined with common duct exploration. Indeed common duct

Table 8.2 Surgical treatment for acute cholecystitis

	Patients	Deaths	Mortality Rate
A. Cholecystectomy	1707	22	1.3
B. Cholecystostomy	381	41	10.8
A or B plus choledochotomy	389	33	8.5
Total operations	2477	96	3.9

explorations were performed in 2275 patients (18.3%), and stones were recovered from the common duct in 1434 (63%). There were 74 patients with retained stones in the entire group of 12 693, an incidence of 0.6%. Considered only in the context of the number of patients that underwent common duct exploration, the incidence of retained common duct stones was 3.3%.

The principal techniques available to minimize and reduce the incidence of retained common duct stones are choledochoscopy and operative cholangiography. These techniques are complementary and not mutually exclusive of each other. Operative cholangiography, because it can be employed in all patients without regard to the diameter of the ductal system, is used with greater frequency than choledochoscopy.

The effectiveness of operative cholangiography is enhanced by ciné radiography (Berci et al 1978). This technique permits the surgeon to visualize the distribution of contrast agent in the ductal system as it is injected. Thus overdistension of the ducts, the use of an excessive amount of contrast agent and improper positioning of the X-ray equipment are avoided. In addition, the ability to secure radiographs as contrast enters the duodenum eliminates the need for repeated injections of contrast to demonstrate patency of the ampullary segment of the duct. The use of glucagon to differentiate spasm of the sphincter of Oddi from an impacted stone at the distal end of the duct has been a useful adjunct to the technique of operative cholangiography (Bordley & Olsen 1979). In most patients, the inability to demonstrate the passage of contrast material from the common bile duct into the duodenum is an indication for duodenotomy and retrograde exploration of the duct via the ampulla of Vater.

In their effort to avoid the problem of retained common duct stones, some surgeons advocate the frequent use of sphincteroplasty or, more commonly, a biliary-intestinal anastomosis in patients with common duct calculi. These procedures are presumed to mitigate the consequences of residual stones and improve bile flow. Residual common duct stones are presumed to be of no clinical consequence because the biliary-intestinal anastomosis permits decompression of the extrahepatic ductal system in the presence of distal obstruction. The procedure employed most frequently has been the lateral or side-to-side choledochoduodenostomy. Proponents of this operation cite its ease of performance as an alternative to the difficulty of extracting stones from the hepatic ducts and the intramural, transduodenal segment of the common bile duct. Indeed Schein et al (1978) advocate choledochoduodenostomy in all patients with calculous biliary tract disease and a common bile duct of 1.4 cm or larger in diameter.

Sphincteroplasty has not enjoyed the same degree of acceptance as choledochoduodenostomy, perhaps because it is technically more difficult to perform and is associated with a higher morbidity rate. Proponents of sphincteroplasty assume that many patients with soft, friable 'stasis' stones have a functional or anatomic derangement of the sphincter of Oddi that results in impaired bile flow and stone formation. Unfortunately there is lack of agreement as to what constitutes stenosis of the ampulla of Vater and the Oddi sphincter.

McSherry & Fischer (1981) have recently reported a small group of patients who continued to experience symptoms attributed to residual common bile duct stones after surgery that included a biliary-intestinal anastomosis. In some patients, symptoms appeared to be related to stricture of this anastomosis and in others, occurred despite a widely patent anastomosis. In some patients, symptoms were attributed to ductal obstruction and cholangitis and, less frequently, pancreatitis. The authors suggested that if the patient's condition permitted, every effort should be made to remove all calculi from the common bile duct at operation and to confirm this by operative cholangiography and/or choledochochoscopy. Choledochoduodenostomy was recommended only for poor risk patients and those individuals with objective evidence of stricture and obstruction of the distal common bile duct.

When confronted with a patient who has a residual common bile duct stone as evidenced by postoperative T-tube cholangiography, removal of this stone by non-operative measures should be attempted with anticipation of a high degree of success. Our initial approach is to attempt chemical dissolution by the continuous administration of monoctanoin through the T-tube as described by Mack et al (1981). In our hands, this technique has proved successful in approximately 50% of patients, and the success rate appears to be inversely proportional to the size of the retained stone(s). If chemical dissolution is unsuccessful, the patient is discharged from the hospital with the T-tube in situ to allow maturation of a well-defined T-tube track. This usually is accomplished after four to six weeks, and the patient is then re-admitted for extraction of the stones by the Burhenne technique (Burhenne 1980) through the T-tube track. Our experience with this technique in 25 patients indicates a success rate of over 90% and is comparable to others (Mason 1980). In the very rare instance when the above measures have been unsuccessful, the patients are evaluated for endoscopic papillotomy. This technique has been particularly useful in patients with stones less than 2 cm in diameter. It is most unusual that patients with retained common bile duct stones require reoperation if they have a T-tube in place.

Our ability to deal effectively with biliary tract calculi in the vast majority of patients is one of the major accomplishments of modern surgery. Safe and effective operative techniques are available to deal with the protean clinical manifestations of biliary calculous disease. Further developments in this field await the development of more effective and safe cholelitholytic agents.

References

Berci G, Shore J M, Hamlin J A, Morgenstern L 1978 Operative fluoroscopy and cholangiography. American Journal of Surgery 135: 32

Bordley J IV, Olson J E 1979 The use of glucagon in operative cholangiography. Surgery, Gynecology and Obstetrics 149: 583

Burhenne H J 1980 Percutaneous extraction of retained biliary tract stones: 661 patients. American Journal of Roentgenology 134: 889

Comfort N W, Gray H K, Wilson J M 1948 The silent gallstone: a 10–20 year follow-up study of 112 cases. Annals of Surgery 128: 931

Gracie W A, Ransohoff D F 1981 The natural history of silent gallstones: the innocent gallstone is not a myth (Abstract). Gastroenterology 80 (2): 1161

Kambouris A A, Carpenter W S, Allahen R D 1973 Cholecystectomy without drainage. Surgery, Gynecology and Obstetrics 137: 613

Lund J 1960 Surgical indications in cholelithiasis: prophylactic cholecystectomy elucidated on the basis of long-term follow-up on 526 nonoperated cases. Annals of Surgery 151: 153

Mack E, Patzer E M, Crummy A B, Hofmann A F, Babayan V K 1981 Retained biliary tract stones. Archives of Surgery 116: 341

McSherry C K 1981 The National Cooperative Gallstone Study report: A surgeon's perspective (editorial). Annals of Internal Medicine 95: 379

McSherry C K, Fischer M G 1981 Common bile duct stones and biliary-intestinal anastomoses. Surgery, Gynecology and Obstetrics 153: 669

Mason R 1980 Percutaneous extraction of retained gallstones via the T-tube track — British experience of 131 cases. Clinical Radiology 31: 657

Saltzstein E C, Evani S V, Mann R W 1973 Routine operative cholangiography. Archives of Surgery 107: 289

Schein C J, Shapiro N, Gliedman M L 1978 Choledochoduodenostomy as an adjunct to choledocholithotomy. Surgery, Gynecology and Obstetrics 146: 25

Schoenfield L J, Lachin J M 1981 The Steering Committee: The National Cooperative Gallstone Study Group. Chenodiol (chenodeoxycholic acid) for dissolution of gallstones: a controlled trial of efficacy and safety. Annals of Internal Medicine 95: 257

Wenckert A, Robertson B 1966 The natural course of gallstone disease. Eleven-year review of 781 nonoperated cases. Gastroenterology 50: 376

9 *The post-cholecystectomy patient*

L. H. BLUMGART and N. J. LYGIDAKIS

The majority of patients with biliary calculi are cured following cholecystectomy and where necessary choledocholithotomy (Burnett & Shields 1958, Le Quesne et al 1959, Schofield & MacLeod 1966, Le Quesne 1974). Indeed, of all patients submitted to cholecystectomy for gallstones it is likely that only 5% have significant persistent or recurrent symptoms (Bodvall 1973).

Post-cholecystectomy problems

There is no such entity as a specific post-cholecystectomy syndrome (Schofield & MacLeod 1966). Although symptoms may arise as a result of abnormality within the biliary tree or pancreas, they may also be the result of associated disease such as peptic ulceration, hiatus hernia or diverticular disease of the colon. Furthermore, neuromuscular disorders associated with bile reflux into the stomach may occur in some patients with gallstones and this may account for persistent flatulent dyspepsia (Johnson 1972, 1975). A recent study has shown a close correlation between late gastritis and previous cholecystectomy (Kalima & Sjöberg 1980). In addition, in the absence of precise diagnosis it has been proposed that many of these patients have a psychosomatic origin for their symptoms, and indeed psychological stress acting through the autonomic nervous system may be a factor in some cases (Johnson 1975, Valberg et al 1971). It is thus most important in the diagnosis of post-cholecystectomy symptoms to differentiate disorders arising in the biliary tree from associated diseases and in particular to try to ensure that the symptoms complained of are related to demonstrable abnormalities.

The symptom complex in the post-cholecystectomy patient usually comprises dyspepsia or biliary pain, although the more severe clamant presentation associated with jaundice, cholangitis or pancreatitis is not infrequent. Symptoms may appear immediately after cholecystectomy and this is especially likely if there has been iatrogenic damage to the biliary ductal system. However, some patients only develop symptoms many months or even years after operation. In a study carried out in our clinic patients were classified on admission according to their predominant symptom (Blumgart et al 1977). It was found that 21 of 52 patients suffered from upper abdominal pain. 18 from persistent or recurrent attacks of jaundice, 5 from recurrent attacks of cholangitis and 8 from recurring attacks of biochemically proven pancreatitis. Many patients, of course, had a combination of these symptoms. The complexity of these cases is emphasised by the fact that no fewer than 10 had already been submitted to at least one further laparotomy and in 5 of these a further operative procedure had been carried out. Despite this all remained symptomatic. In a further study we assessed 157 patients, symptomatic after cholecystectomy (Hunt & Blumgart 1982). The predominant problem leading to referral was recurrence of pain similar to that present before cholecystectomy in 57, development of a new pain considered on clinical grounds to be of biliary origin in 26, development or recurrence of pain with raised amylase levels in 14 and jaundice in 57. One patient had rigors as a sole problem and in two the postoperative T-tube cholangiogram was equivocal.

In patients presenting with biliary colic or dyspepsia, especially when this is similar in nature to symptoms before cholecystectomy, there is less frequently a demonstrable abnormality than in patients presenting with jaundice, with cholangitis or with pancreatitis, where we have found abnormality on ERCP in every case. Coincidental upper gastrointestinal pathology is particularly likely in the dyspeptic group and duodenal ulcer not uncommon even in the presence of a previous normal barium meal series (Blumgart et al 1977). It is important in such patients that the biliary tract and pancreas are shown to be normal and not also involved (Ruddell et al 1980, Blumgart et al 1975).

Despite the importance of recognising associated disease, the majority of patients have abnormalities within the biliary or pancreatic ductal apparatus. Frequently, but by no means always, the symptoms arise as a result of residual common bile duct stones or are consequent on disease of the biliary tract. However, unsuspected pancreatic disease may be present at the time of the original cholecystectomy and pass unnoticed (Ruddell et al 1980) or indeed a tumour may be present at the time post-cholecystectomy symptoms appear. We have found the persistence of jaundice after cholecystectomy and exploration of the common bile duct particularly sinister in this respect (McCloy et al 1982). Indeed, in a total series of 218 patients symptomatic after cholecystectomy, we have found 9 cases of carcinoma of the papilla, common bile duct, or pancreas.

In other cases, symptoms result from complications of additional operative procedures carried out at the time of cholecystectomy. This applies particularly to transduodenal exploration of the common bile duct and interference with the papilla of Vater or is associated with traumatic passage of metal dilators into the duodenum during exploration of the common bile duct from above (McCloy et al 1982, Hunt & Blumgart 1980).

Diagnosis

Diagnosis may be extremely difficult and the need for further laparotomy not clear. In addition while laparotomy dictated by symptoms may result in operative diagnosis, this may frequently not be the case. Adhesions hinder exploration and operative cholangiography poses a special problem in a patient previously submitted to surgery. Abnormalities at the site of previously constructed surgical stomata are not readily diagnosed at laparotomy. For these reasons re-operation without the benefit of preoperative diagnosis frequently results in frustration for the surgeon and continued symptoms for the patient (Blumgart et al 1977). It is clear that the need for precise preoperative information in biliary tract surgery is nowhere more evident than in this group of patients.

In the past intravenous cholangiography has been a mainstay in the diagnosis of patients symptomatic after cholecystectomy, and indeed gives positive information in a proportion of cases. However, it has been shown to be valueless in the presence of jaundice and inaccurate and imprecise in many non-jaundiced patients (Blumgart et al 1977). Indeed, even when ductal anatomy is outlined by means of intravenous cholangiography, a definite diagnosis may not be possible and stones may be present in a common bile duct thought to be of normal calibre (Fig. 9.1) or absent from a clearly dilated ductal system.

The past decade has seen extraordinary innovations in the imaging techniques

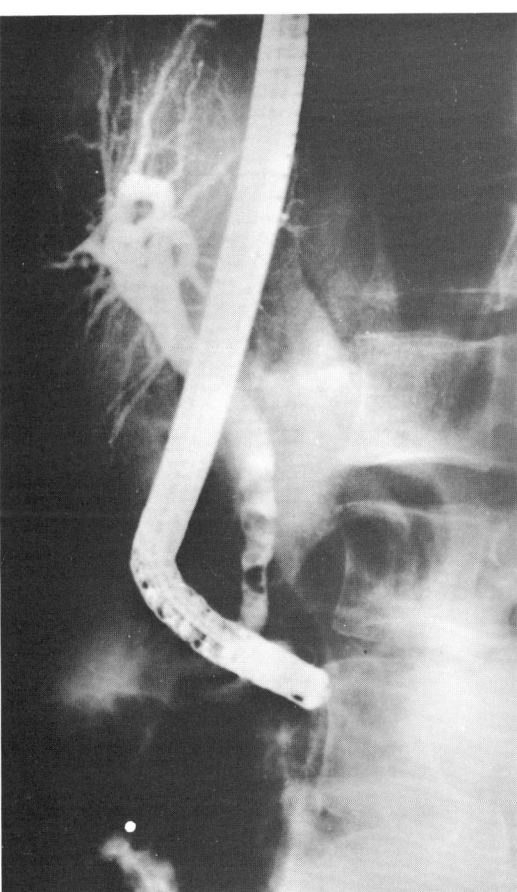

Fig. 9.1 Endoscopic retrograde cholangiography in a woman referred with intermittent attacks of pain and jaundice following cholecystectomy. Intravenous cholangiography revealed a normal calibre common bile duct and failed to confirm the presence of gall stones. Note that the biliary ductal system is not grossly dilated. There are multiple stones in the low common bile duct.

available for diagnosis of biliary tract disorders. These developments have provided hitherto unforeseen possibilities in allowing exact information on which to base therapy and have resulted in the formation of new diagnostic approaches especially in jaundiced patients. Such approaches to diagnosis have attempted to define the timing and place of the various procedures available (Elias et al 1976, Blumgart 1978). In our clinic an integrated approach to the diagnosis of biliary tract obstruction has been established (Benjamin et al 1978, Benjamin & Blumgart 1978). This relies on the initial use of ultrasonography and fine needle percutaneous transhepatic cholangiography (PTC). Endoscopic retrograde cholangiopancreatography (ERCP) is reserved for those patients in whom ductal anatomy is not outlined by fine needle PTC. This approach is not adhered to in the post-cholecystectomy patient where it is frequently important to obtain not only cholangiography but pancreatography (Blumgart et al 1977), cytology and biopsy, and where inspection of the papilla of Vater or surgically created stomata are often essential for full diagnostic information (Blumgart et al 1977, Ruddell et al 1980, Blumgart et al 1975, Hunt & Blumgart 1980).

Patients referred to our Department with post-cholecystectomy symptoms have usually already undergone extensive investigation and multiple radiological studies. Previous X-rays including operative cholangiograms, T-tube cholangiograms and intravenous cholangiograms are studied and this may reveal an unsuspected diagnosis. However, even if the biliary ductal system has been completely visualised and considered normal, ERCP is proceeded with provided there is clinical or biochemical evidence suggestive of upper gastrointestinal pathology, biliary obstruction or pancreatitis. Endoscopy and ERCP are carried out in the X-ray Department. The endoscopic and radiological techniques have been previously described (Burwood et al 1973, Blumgart & Salmon 1973). In all patients an attempt is made to outline both the biliary and pancreatic ductal system, although if a clear abnormality is demonstrated in either the biliary or pancreatic duct and the diagnosis is evident, prolonged attempts to cannulate the remaining duct are not always pursued. During the examination the duodenal cap and stomach are examined for associated pathology such as duodenal or gastric ulceration. Following examination, the patients are kept in hospital overnight, serum amylase being measured within three hours of the procedure and again 15 hours later if pain or nausea are present. Complications are recorded.

In a recent group of 75 patients symptomatic after cholecystectomy, submitted to endoscopy and ERCP at Hammersmith Hospital, we have been able to define the diagnosis in 70 (93%) with only 3 (4%) failed cannulations and 2 (3%) complications (Blumgart & McCloy 1981).

Specific problems which might arise after cholecystectomy are considered below and the value of endoscopy and ERCP evaluated. In addition, recently developed techniques (Classen & Safrany 1975, Cotton et al 1976) allowing endoscopic papillotomy and removal of gallstones from the common bile duct are critically assessed.

Stones

In Western countries, most stones in the common bile duct come from the gallbladder, although occasionally they may arise primarily within the common bile duct on the basis of biliary stasis and infection (Lygidakis 1981). Careful and precise pre-operative diagnosis helps to eliminate associated lesions and reduce error arising as the result of double pathology. For instance, periampullary or bile duct carcinoma may coexist with common bile duct stones, the presence of the tumour being missed at initial exploration and the final diagnosis being made at endoscopy. In jaundiced patients we now usually recommend simple duodeno-scopy before operation, even if gallstones are known to be present. Similarly, common bile duct stones may be responsible for intermittent bouts of jaundice and yet be associated with co-existent hepatocellular disease such as primary biliary cirrhosis or chronic active hepatitis. Such patients may remain jaundiced after choledocholithotomy.

The routine use of operative cholangiography during cholecystectomy, and in particular post-exploratory cholangiography and/or choledochoscopy, has markedly reduced but not abolished the incidence of residual bile duct stones (Faris et al 1975, Hicken & McAllister 1964, Schulenberg 1969, Le Quesne 1980, Berci & Hamlin 1980). Thus, in a recent series of 127 patients submitted to chole-cystectomy, we have noted only one retained stone. In addition, information gleaned at operative cholangiography provides anatomical information which is useful in dissection and may prevent operative trauma. Common bile duct stones may not only remain after exploration of the duct and be detected during post-operative T-tube cholangiography, but in a proportion of patients the common bile duct has never been explored and operative cholangiography never carried out. The presence of stones at operation has thus never been recognised.

There is a high rate of complication associated with residual common bile duct stones (Faris et al 1975) and since many of these are of a potentially serious nature, the detection of the stones and their removal is usually advisable. Indeed, of 31 patients we treated who presented with jaundice, cholangitis or recurrent pancreatitis after cholecystectomy, common bile duct stones or biliary mud were present and demonstrated at ERCP in 16 (Fig. 9.2). Even in the absence of major complications, we found low grade ill-health and vague upper abdominal pain in 3 further cases who had no history of jaundice and in 2 in whom there was no abnormality of the liver function tests (Blumgart et al 1977).

Jaundice
While jaundice after cholecystectomy is frequently the result of a residual common bile duct stone or biliary ductal stricture, there are occasions where this is not so. Sometimes the patient is referred for consideration with a T-tube in situ draining freely despite the fact that the patient is still jaundiced. In others there is no T-tube and here again endoscopic retrograde choledochopancreatography is invaluable since it may demonstrate retained stones, a normal biliary tree or a residual carcinoma missed at initial laparotomy.

Perhaps the important point is that no patient jaundiced after cholecystectomy and particularly after exploration of the common bile duct should be submitted to surgery without precise pre-operative cholangiography.

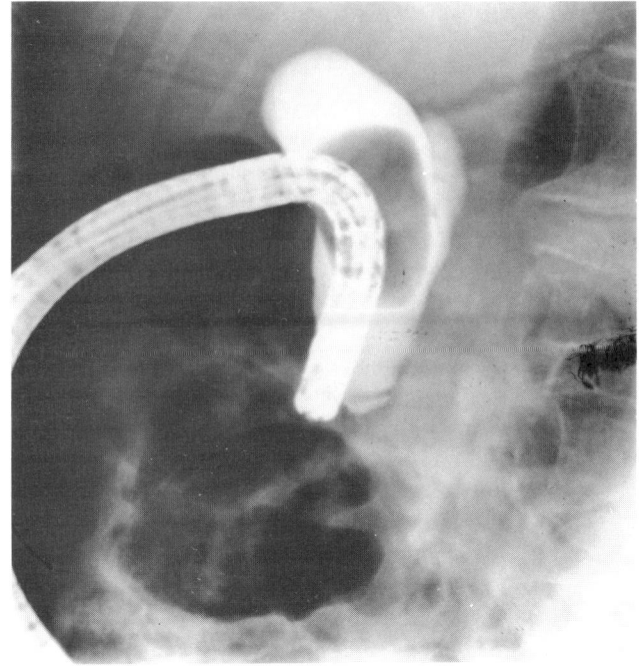

Fig. 9.2 Huge common bile duct stone demonstrated in a grossly dilated duct. Patient suffered from recurrent attacks of pain, fever and jaundice.

Pancreatic disease

In a significant proportion of patients found symptomatic after cholecystectomy, there is associated disease of the pancreas (Blumgart et al 1977, Ruddell et al 1980). In some cases there is recurrent acute pancreatitis consequent upon residual common bile duct stones and such attacks always abate after removal of the offending calculi. In others. a previous attack of acute pancreatitis has left damage resulting in a pancreatic ductal stricture or pancreatic cyst. Such a stricture may result in the development of chronic pancreatitis presenting in due course with increasing pain. It is important to recognise that a patient may be submitted to cholecystectomy for proven gallstones on the grounds of upper abdominal pain, and the presence of demonstrable chronic pancreatic damage missed. We have seen several such patients presenting with continued pain in the postoperative period.

The advent of endoscopic retrograde pancreatography has emphasised the latter point and indeed it has now been demonstrated that chronic pancreatitis with gross ductal abnormality associated with biliary disease (but not necessarily caused by it) may be revealed at ERCP even in asymptomatic patients. Such changes are not very different to those described by Nardi (1973) and thought to be associated with papillary stenosis. Operation in such cases should not be dictated by the presence of abnormal findings on pancreatography but by persistent symptoms and only then if there has been a period of abstinence from alcohol. In other words, the endoscopist and the surgeon must not be misled by radiological abnormalities of the pancreatic duct no matter how gross.

Complications of surgery
Persistent symptoms may occur as a result of complications of operative procedures performed at the times of primary cholecystectomy and choledocholithotomy. Such complications arise as a result of damage to the common bile duct, stenosis of surgically created stomata or surgical errors occurring in the region of the papilla of Vater.

Over 80% of stenoses or strictures of the common bile duct are consequent upon operative trauma and the majority follow cholecystectomy which the surgeon regarded as being simple and without incident. The majority present soon after surgery with jaundice or biliary fistula and there is often a history of prolonged biliary drainage or a septic course following surgery. There may, however, be a delayed presentation with late onset of jaundice and cholangitis. Precise documentation of such lesions is usually possible with percutaneous cholangiography sometimes combined with ERCP.

Supra-duodenal choledochotomy would seem to be the preferred method of exploring the common bile duct at primary operation. The procedure is simple in most instances and there is only a small increase in the morbidity and mortality associated with cholecystectomy. It should be noted, however, that there should not be any attempt to traverse or dilate the papilla of Vater by the passage of metallic dilators from above. This is unnecessary and particularly if operative cholangiography has demonstrated free flow of contrast medium into the duodenum. Such attempts at dilatation may be associated with post-operative secondary acute pancreatitis (Fig. 9.3) or the development of late secondary papillary stenosis (Tondelli et al 1979). In addition, the instrument may readily perforate the biliary tree proximal to the true papilla, thus producing a choledochoduodenal fistula (Fig. 9.4) and this may be associated with late symptoms (Blumgart 1978, Hunt & Blumgart 1980). We have now seen 12 such fistulae in patients referred with recurrent symptoms after cholecystectomy. Our practice is to refrain from instrumentation of the papilla unless operative cholangiography shows failure of passage of contrast into the duodenum. In such cases, a fine gum elastic bougie or a Fogarty biliary catheter can be gently passed into the duodenum and palpated in the common bile duct behind the mobilised head of the pancreas.

Some advocate the use of transduodenal sphincterotomy or sphincteroplasty for primary exploration of the common bile duct (Wright 1960, Hardy & Davenport 1969, Hunter 1972, Carter 1973, Peel et al 1974, Jones 1973), but there seems no strong argument for this unless there is an additional indication for deliberate augmentation of biliary drainage. While the procedure is safe in some hands and particularly where widely practised (Partington 1977, Aubrey & Edwards 1978), the mortality rate is generally higher than for supraduodenal exploration of the common bile duct (Braasch & McCann 1967, Colcock & Perry 1964, Mahoner & Browne 1955, Shieber 1962, Rottwell-Jackson 1968, Stuart & Hoerr 1972). Quite apart from peri-operative mortality and complications, the late morbidity of sphincterotomy or sphincteroplasty is not inconsiderable. Restenosis may occur in

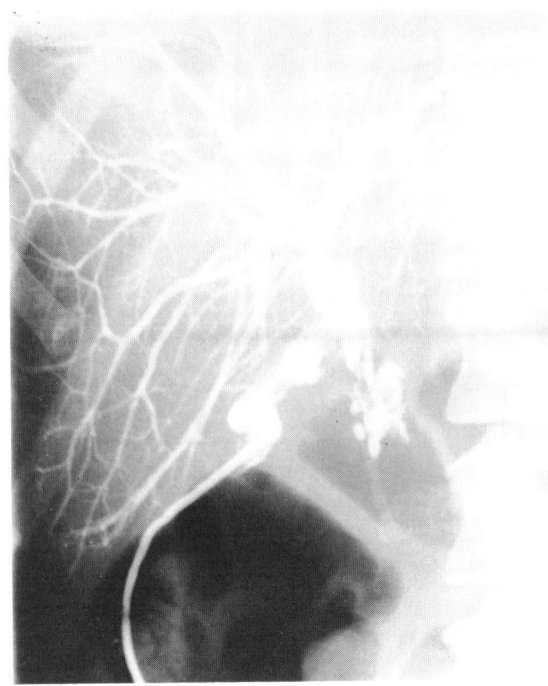

Fig. 9.3 T-tube cholangiogram obtained after cholecystectomy and exploration of the common bile duct. The postoperative course was complicated by postoperative acute pancreatitis. The operative note referred to forcible dilatation of the lower end of the common bile duct. The lower end of the T-tube lies within the pancreatic substance; there is no flow into the duodenum and there is filling of irregular cavities within the pancreatic head. This patient developed a low bile duct stricture for which choledochojejunostomy Roux-en-Y was necessary.

a proportion of patients and there may be associated damage to the orifice of the pancreatic duct with resultant late pancreatitis. Even in the presence of a patent sphincteroplasty orifice, there may be rigidity of the margins of the stoma with peristomal inflammation and proximal hold-up of debris within a dilated ductal system (Blumgart 1978). In addition, some surgeons, when performing sphincteroplasty and particularly if there is difficulty in identifying the papilla of Vater at operation, carry out a supra-duodenal choledochotomy, a probe being passed down into the papilla from above. This does not always readily pass (Aubrey & Edwards 1978) and in any event the method has disadvantages since a false passage may be produced (McCloy et al 1982, Blumgart 1978), the probe or dilator being forced into the pancreatic tissue (Fig. 9.3) through the duodenal wall proximal to the papilla and a 'sphincteroplasty' created in error at this point. In our experience the common clinical presentation of such a fistula may be vague upper abdominal pain and ill-health, or the more severe symptoms of jaundice, cholangitis or recurrent acute pancreatitis (Hunt & Blumgart 1980) (Fig. 9.4). Only endoscopy allows precise diagnosis in this situation.

It should be noted that on the grounds of the high incidence of recurrent or residual stones, some authors recommend drainage of the common bile duct at

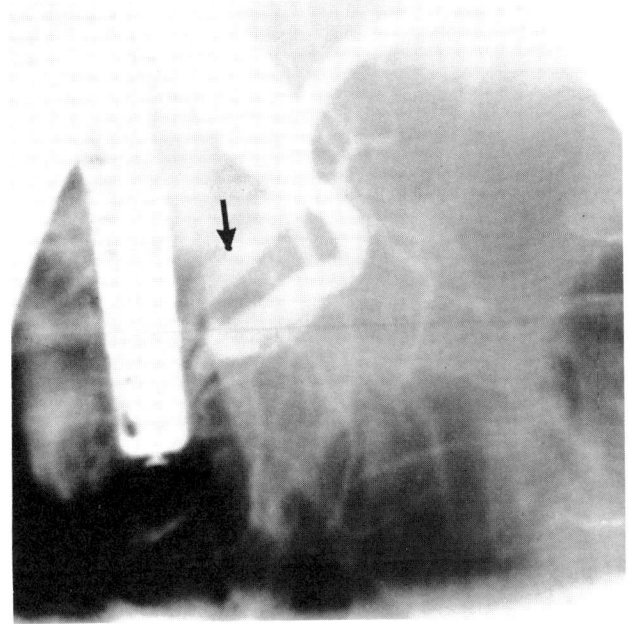

Fig. 9.4 ERCP in a patient with choledochoduodenal fistula. The original operative note stated that cholecystectomy had been performed. At endoscopy there was a normal papilla but above it a false passage has been created. Both were cannulated individually. Cannulation of the fistula outlined a track (arrow) running into the common bile duct. Cannulation of the papilla revealed the low common bile duct in its supra-papillary portion and the pancreatic duct. This woman also had a cyst in the region of the tail of the pancreas, demonstrated both at ultrasound and at ERCP and required cyst gastrostomy.

primary operation (Rutledge 1976, Aldrete 1977, Saharia et al 1977). Such deliberate choledochal incontinence has been advocated as a valuable adjunct to choledocholithotomy and prophylactic against recurrent stones (Schein 1977). Those who oppose the use of such routine drainage procedures do so on the grounds of increased late morbidity from biliary sepsis consequent upon reflux of duodenal contents into the bile duct or upon the 'sump syndrome' caused by debris remaining or accumulating within the intrapancreatic portion of the bile duct after choledochoduodenostomy. We have carried out side-to-side chole-dochoduodenostomy for benign conditions using similar indications and techniques to those advocated by Madden (1973) and Stuart & Hoerr (1972), and provided the anastomosis is created to a ductal incision 2 cm in length in a common bile duct no smaller than 15 mm diameter, we have never encountered a case of ascending cholangitis (Lygidakis 1981). Similar results are reported by Madden (1973) and Schein (1981). Nevertheless, there is no doubt that complications can occur, especially where choledochoduodenostomy has been carried out on dubious grounds to a bile duct of normal calibre perhaps producing a small stoma. The stomal orifice can be readily visualised at endoscopy and the surgical stoma and papilla individually catheterised. These patients suffer from low-grade chronic cholangitis and we have noted infected inspissated bile aggregates in the

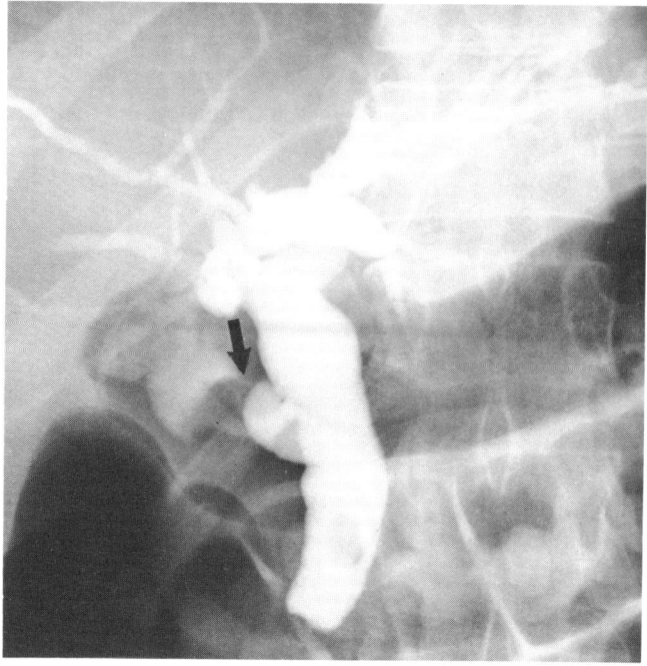

Fig. 9.5 Endoscopic retrograde cholangiography in a woman submitted to cholecystectomy exploration of the common bile duct and choledochoduodenostomy. In the post-operative period she experienced recurrent attacks of cholangitis and pain. Endoscopy revealed a normal papilla and a tiny orifice in the apex of the duodenal cap. The papilla and this orifice were cannulated independently. The common bile duct was dilated and contained a residual stone. There was a cystic duct remnant and the cystic duct had been anastomosed to the duodenum, there now being only a narrow communication between the two (arrow). Choledochoduodenostomy had in fact never been performed but the anastomosis had been made to the cystic duct.

common bile duct after ill-considered operation (Blumgart et al 1977). We have on record one case in which a choledochoduodenostomy had been recorded but in which the anastomosis had been made to an enlarged cystic duct (Fig. 9.5).

Endoscopic papillotomy and removal of gallstones

The advent of endoscopic papillotomy allows successful removal of residual common bile duct stones in a high proportion of patients. Thus, in a recent series Cotton (1980) reports 134 patients referred for attempted removal of retained stones. Residual stones (or failure in the attempt) occurred in 11% of patients; a figure similar to that reported by Safrany (1978). Complications occurred in 10 patients, three required emergency surgery and there was one death. In particular, it is worth noting that when the stones were 2 cm or more in size, the failure rate rose to 38%, being worse than any surgical series in which there is judicious use of some form of biliary enteric bypass at open surgical operation (Lygidakis 1981, Stuart & Hoerr 1972, Schein & Gliedman 1981). Not all results for endoscopic sphincteroplasty are so successful. Indeed, another series in the United Kingdom (Sloof et al 1980) shows a bed occupancy of 9.5 +/– 5 days for the procedure with a clear duct in only 70% of patients and a complication rate of 30%. One patient of 37 died as a result of the procedure and another within a year, whose death the authors feel could have been prevented by initial surgery.

A recently published survey of British Centres employing endoscopic sphincterotomy for removal of common bile duct stones (Cotton & Vallon 1981) reveals overall success in 76% of patients. Seven deaths (1%) were recorded in a total of 679 attempts of which 590 were successful with an overall morbidity rate of 8.5%. When complications arise, the majority are related to haemorrhage, pancreatitis or cholangitis, and it is in this group that the mortality is highest. Indeed, of 58 patients with complications, 11 required an operation within hours or a few days and seven died. The precise nature and extent of the operation required to achieve control is not detailed. The authors acknowledge, as do others experienced in this field, that the long-term result remains to be assessed. The results of this series and most other series describing endoscopic papillotomy for residual stones are compared favourably with surgical series showing a higher mortality and morbidity rate. Indeed, of the 14 centres contributing to the survey (Cotton & Vallon 1981), 7 were of the opinion that they would always advise endoscopic sphincterotomy, even in low-risk post-cholecystectomy cases. However, as pointed out by Girard & Legros (1981) the surgical mortality for re-operation on the common bile duct should be less than 2%. Indeed, in an analysis of 6 recent series of re-operations for retained or recurrent bile duct stones, they found a mortality rate of 1.8% in 498 operations, most of this being in the elderly. In another series (McSherry & Glenn 1980) 341 patients were reported in whom choledocholithotomy was carried out for retained or recurrent calculi. Of these patients 2.1% died, but if patients with cholangitis and pancreatitis were excluded, only four patients (1.2%) died after secondary choledocholithotomy. Thus, the acceptance of endoscopic sphincterotomy on the basis of a lower mortality and morbidity rate in comparison to surgical therapy may well be unjustified.

There is no question that endoscopic sphincterotomy is ingenious and reasonably safe and can remove retained stones. There seems good evidence that this may well be the preferred approach in the elderly and in high risk patients who should perhaps not be offered surgery. On the other hand, there is no doubt that endoscopic techniques are operative and have real risks. There seems little justification for the use of the technique in the young or fit patient, or in patients with large stones (Fig. 9.2) or a very large common bile duct, where the method would seem to be associated with an unacceptable failure rate, and where choledochoduodenostomy appears to offer an alternative approach with a mortality rate of 0–3% and good long-term results (Lygidakis 1981, Stuart & Hoerr 1972, Schein & Gliedman 1981). There is no doubt, however, that the operative mortality for surgical interference at the sphincter of Oddi is higher (Nardi 1973, Braasch & McCann 1967, Colcock & Perry 1964). The majority of the deaths are consequent on secondary acute pancreatitis (Imrie et al 1978). In addition to mortality, there is a morbidity associated with sphincterotomy or sphincteroplasty (Blumgart et al 1977, Hunt & Blumgart 1980, 1982). These facts can be used as arguments against surgical interference with the papilla of Vater as compared to supra-duodenal methods for exploration of the common bile duct (see above) but are not a justification for the preferential use of endoscopic methods as suggested by Demling (1977).

Finally, experience of surgical interference with the sphincter of Oddi leads one to expect that endoscopic papillotomy may well have a higher incidence of long term effects and late stenosis than has yet been reported.

Perhaps the most important of the facts, emphasised as a result of the development of endoscopic papillotomy, is the high incidence of retained or recurrent bile duct stones after exploration of the common bile duct. This represents a fearful indictment of surgical approaches to the biliary tree and, in particular, a major criticism of primary operation for gallstones. These problems are almost certainly associated with failure to perform pre- and post-exploratory cholangiography (Le Quesne 1980) or choledochoscopy, and a lack of a clear understanding of the indictions for biliary enteric bypass procedures (Lygidakis 1981, Schein & Gliedman 1981).

References

Aldrete J 1977 In discussion of Saharia et al. Annals of Surgery 185: 598

Aubrey D A, Edwards J L 1978 The selective use of combined supraduodenal and transduodenal exploration of the common bile duct. British Journal of Surgery 65: 246

Benjamin I S, Blumgart L H 1978 Biliary bypass and reconstructive surgery. In: Wright R, Alberti G, Karran S R, Sadler H M (eds) Liver and biliary disease: a pathophysiological approach. W B Saunders, London

Benjamin I S, Allison M E M, Moule B, Blumgart L H 1978 The early use of fine needle percutaneous transhepatic cholangiography in an approach to the diagnosis of jaundice in a surgical unit. British Journal of Surgery 65: 92

Berci G, Hamlin J A 1980 Operative biliary radiology. Williams and Wilkins, Baltimore

Blumgart L H 1978 Biliary tract obstruction — new approaches to old problems. American Journal of Surgery 135: 19

Blumgart L H, McCloy R 1981 Endoscopic techniques after cholecystectomy. In: Way L (ed) Surgery of the gallbladder and bile ducts. San Francisco

Blumgart L H, Salmon P R 1973 Fiberduodenoscopy and transpapillary cholangiopancreatography. In: Taylor S (ed) Recent advances in surgery. Churchill Livingstone, Edinburgh

Blumgart L H, Sokhi G S, Duncan J G 1975 Endoscopy and retrograde choledochopancreatography in the diagnosis of post-cholecystectomy symptoms. Bulletin de la Société internationale de chirurgie 6: 587

Blumgart L H, Carachi R, Imrie C W, Benjamin I S, Duncan J G 1977 Diagnosis and management of post-cholecystectomy symptoms: the place of endoscopy and retrograde choledochopancreatography. British Journal of Surgery 64: 809

Bodvall B 1973 The post-cholecystectomy syndrome. Clinical Gastroenterology 2: 103

Braasch J W, McCann J C Jr 1967 Observations on single section of the sphincter of Oddi. Surgery, Gynecology and Obstetrics 125: 355

Burnett W, Shields R 1958 Symptoms after cholecystectomy. Lancet 1: 923

Burwood R J, Davies G T, Lawrie B W 1973 Endoscopic retrograde choledocho pancreatography. A review with a report of a collaborative series. Clinical Radiology 24: 397

Carter A E 1973 Kocher's perampullary approach for common bile duct calculi. British Journal of Surgery 60: 117

Classen M, Safrany L 1975 Endoscopic papillotomy and removal of gallstones. British Medical Journal 4: 371

Colcock B P, Perry B 1964 Exploration of the common bile duct. Surgery Gynecology and Obstetrics 118: 20

Cotton P B 1980 Non-operative removal of bile duct stones by duodenoscopic sphincterotomy. British Journal of Surgery 67: 1

Cotton P B, Vallon A G 1981 British experience with duodenoscopic sphincterotomy for removal of bile duct stones. British Journal of Surgery 68: 373

Cotton P B, Chapman M, Whiteside C G, Le Quesne L P 1976 Duodenoscopic papillotomy and gall stone removal. British Journal of Surgery 63: 709

Demling L 1977 Endoscopic papillotomy and removal of gall stones. Journal of the Royal College of Surgeons of Edinburgh 22: 385

Elias E, Hamlyn A N, Jain S, Long R G, Summerfield J A, Dick R, Sherlock S 1976 Randomised trial of percutaneous transhepatic cholangiography with the Chiba needle versus endoscopic retrograde cholangiography for bile duct visualisation in jaundice. Gastroenterology 71: 439

Faris I, Thompson J P S, Grundy D J, Le Quesne L P 1975 Operative cholangiography. A re-appraisal based on a review of 400 cholangiograms. British Journal of Surgery 62: 966

Girard R M, Legros G 1981 Retained and recurrent bile duct stones. Surgical or non-surgical removal? Annals of Surgery 193: 150

Hardy E G, Davenport T J 1969 The transduodenal approach to the common bile duct. British Journal of Surgery 56: 667

Hicken N E, McAllister A J 1964 Operative cholangiography as an aid in reducing the incidence of 'overlooked' common bile duct stones: a study of 1293 choledocholithotomies. Surgery 55: 753

Hunt D R, Blumgart L H 1980 Iatrogenic choledochoduodenal fistula: an unsuspected cause of post-cholecystectomy symptoms. British Journal of Surgery 67: 10–13

Hunt D R, Blumgart L H 1982 Endoscopic abnormalities in patients presenting with post-cholecystectomy problems (in preparation)

Hunter R R 1972 Choledochotomy and transduodenal sphincterotomy. Annals of the Royal College of Surgeons of England 51: 250

Imrie C W, McKay A J, Benjamin I S, Blumgart L H 1978 Secondary acute pancreatitis: aetiology, prevention, diagnosis and management. British Journal of Surgery 65: 399

Johnson A G 1972 Pyloric function and gallstone dyspepsia. British Journal of Surgery 59: 449

Johnson A G 1975 Cholecystectomy and gallstone dyspepsia. Annals of the Royal College of Surgeons of England 56: 69

Jones S A 1973 Sphincteroplasty (not sphinterotomy) in treatment of biliary tract disease. Surgical Clinics of North America 53: 1123

Kalima T V, Sjöberg J 1980 Bile reflux gastritis after cholecystectomy. Scandinavian Journal of Gastroenterology 15: 903

Lygidakis N J 1981 Choledochoduodenostomy in biliary calculous diseases. British Journal of Surgery 68: 762

McCloy R F, Jaffe V, Blumgart L H 1982 Endoscopy and postcholecystectomy problems. In: Salmon P (ed) Proceedings of Growing Points in Endoscopy. Associate Book Publishers (Andover) Ltd

McSherry C K, Glenn F 1980 The incidence and cause of death following surgery for non-malignant biliary tract disease. Annals of Surgery 191: 271

Madden J L 1973 Common duct stones: their origin and surgical management. Symposium on Surgery of the Biliary Tree. Surgical Clinics of North America 53: 961

Mahorner H, Browne E R 1955 Results following transduodenal choledochoampulotomy. Annals of Surgery 141: 607

Nardi G L 1973 Papillitis and stenosis of the sphincter of Oddi. Surgical Clinics of North America 53: 1147

Partington P F 1977 Twenty-three years of experience with sphincterotomy and sphincteroplasty for stenosis of the sphincter of Oddi. Surgery, Gynecology and Obstetrics 145: 161

Peel A L G, Hermon-Taylor J, Ritchie H D 1974 Technique of transduodenal exploration of the common bile duct. Annals of the Royal College of Surgeons of England 55: 237

Le Quesne L P 1974 In: Maingot R (ed) Abdominal Operations, 6th edn. Appleton-Century-Crofts, New York,

Le Quesne L P 1980 In: Maingot R (ed) Abdominal Operations, 7th edn. Appleton-Century-Crofts, New York

Le Quesne L P, Whiteside T G, Hand B 1959 The common bile duct after cholecystectomy. British Medical Journal 1: 329

Rothwell-Jackson R L 1968 Sphincteroplasty in the treatment of biliary and pancreatic disease. British Journal of Surgery 55: 616

Ruddell W S J, Ashton M G, Lintott D J, Axon A T R 1980 Endoscopic retrograde cholangiography and pancreatography in investigation of post-cholecystectomy patients. 1: 444

Rutledge R H 1976 Sphincteroplasty and choledochoduodenostomy for benign biliary obstructions. Annals of Surgery 183: 476

Safrany L 1978 Endoscopic treatment of biliary tract diseases. Lancet 2: 983

Saharia P C, Zuidema G D, Cameron J L 1977 Primary common duct stones. Annals of Surgery 185: 598

Schein C J 1977 Choledochal incontinence as a purposeful adjunct to choledocholithotomy. Surgery, Gynecology and Obstetrics 144: 571

Schein C J, Gliedman M L 1981 Choledochoduodenostomy as an adjunct to choledocholithotomy. Surgery, Gynecology and Obstetrics 152: 797

Schofield G E, MacLeod R G 1966 Sequelae of cholecystectomy. British Journal of Surgery 53: 1042

Schulenburg C A R 1969 Operative cholangiography: 1000 cases. Surgery 65: 723

Shieber W 1962 Duodenotomy with common duct exploration. Archives of Surgery 85: 944

Sloof M, Baker R, Lavelle M I, Lendrum R, Venables C W 1980 What is involved in endoscopic sphincterotomy for gallstones? British Journal of Surgery 67: 18

Stuart M, Hoerr S 1972 Late results of side-to-side choledochoduodenostomy and of transduodenal sphincterotomy for benign disorders. A twenty year comparative study. American Journal of Surgery 123: 66

Tondelli P, Gyr K, Stalder G A, Allgower M 1979 The biliary tract. Clinical Gastroenterology 8(2): 487

Valberg L S, Jabbari M, Kerr J W, Curtis A C, Ramchand S, Prentice R S A 1971 Biliary pain in young women in the absence of gall stones. Gastroenterology 60: 1020

Wright A D 1960 Surgery of the biliary tract. Annals of the Royal College of Surgeons of England 27: 373

10 *The obstructed biliary tract*

IRVING S. BENJAMIN

Definition

The term biliary tract obstruction requires precise definition. It is clearly inadequate to equate biliary tract obstruction with jaundice. Similarly, obstruction and dilatation of the biliary tree are not synonymous, and the classical biochemical changes associated with complete obstruction may be absent or unreliable in many cases. It is necessary for the clinician to recognise at least four categories of biliary tract obstruction:

(i) *Complete obstruction* producing jaundice.

(ii) *Intermittent obstruction* which produces symptoms and typical biochemical changes, but may or may not be associated with attacks of clinical jaundice.

(iii) *Chronic incomplete obstruction* with or without classical symptoms or the observation of biochemical changes, but producing pathological changes in the bile ducts or liver.

(iv) *Segmental obstruction*, in which one or more isolated segments of the intrahepatic biliary tree are obstructed. This obstruction may take the form of complete, intermittent, or chronic incomplete obstruction, as defined above.

It is important to recognise these nuances of biliary obstruction, since they may produce subtle clinical syndromes whose true nature may pass unrecognised. In particular, the entity of segmental biliary obstruction has been poorly recognised and described in the past, but may now be diagnosed confidently as a result of advances in radiological imaging techniques, particularly percutaneous transhepatic cholangiography. The biochemical evidence of segmental obstruction may be masked by the available mass of adequately functioning non-obstructed liver. It may nevertheless produce important symptoms, and have serious sequelae, including infection in an obstructed segment.

Any table of the potential causes of biliary tract obstruction is necessarily incomplete, but Table 10.1 provides a general framework and illustrates the way in which a variety of pathological entities may fall into each of the above four categories. This chapter will consider firstly the effects of biliary obstruction, physiological, pathological, biochemical and functional. The clinical syndromes and approaches to diagnosis and treatment will then be considered, with emphasis

157

Table 10.1 Lesions commonly associated with biliary tract obstruction

I Complete obstruction
    Tumours, especially of the pancreatic head
    Ligation of the common bile duct
    Cholangiocarcinoma
    Parenchymal liver tumours, primary or secondary

II Intermittent obstruction
    Choledocholithiasis
    Periampullary tumours
    Duodenal diverticula
    Papillomas of the bile duct
    Choledochus cyst
    Polycystic liver disease
    Intrahiliary parasites
    Haemobilia

III Chronic incomplete obstruction
    Strictures of the common bile duct:
        congenital
        traumatic (iatrogenic)
        sclerosing cholangitis
        post-radiotherapy
    Stenosed biliary-enteric anastomoses
    Stenosis of the sphincter of Oddi
    Chronic pancreatitis
    Cystic fibrosis
    ?Dyskinesia

IV Segmental obstruction
    Traumatic (including iatrogenic)
    Hepatodocholithiasis
    Sclerosing cholangitis
    Cholangiocarcinoma

on the current state of our knowledge of the pathophysiology of the drained biliary tree.

The effects of biliary tract obstruction

Physical and pathological effects

Back pressure

The normal secretory pressure of bile is 120–250 mm H_2O (11.8–24.5 kPa) (Lynn 1969). When the intrabiliary pressure is raised to more than 300 mm H_2O (29.4 kPa) there is total inhibition of hepatic bile secretion. The effects on secretion of bile salts, cholesterol and phospholipids are unequal (Strasburg et al 1971), and the return of these secretory functions following relief of bile duct obstruction may be asynchronous. Proximal dilatation of the biliary tree above an obstruction is the rule, and this is seen in its most marked form in acute complete obstruction of a previously normal biliary tract. However, there is an extremely variable relationship between obstruction and dilatation. The degree of dilatation depends on the nature and the duration of the obstruction, but also on the pliability of the extrahepatic bile ducts and of the supporting skeleton of the intrahepatic bile ducts. Since prolonged biliary obstruction leads to inflammation and fibrosis of the biliary tract (vide infra), even long-standing obstruction may occur without significant proximal dilatation. Such lack of dilatation of the intrahepatic biliary tree in the presence of an organic stricture is not only a radiological pitfall, but may also be a grave prognostic sign indicating possible impaired hepatocellular function, and raising the suspicion of portal hypertension. In addition, this type of fibrotic non-dilated duct poses a technical problem for the surgical reconstruction of the obstructed biliary tree.

The changes of ductal dilatation are readily reversible after decompression of the biliary tree in a liver which has not undergone significant secondary damage. Such prompt collapse of the bile ducts may be seen quite dramatically following percutaneous transhepatic catheter drainage.

Effect on blood flow

It is reasonable to assume that obstruction of the large bile ducts, by raising the intrahepatic hydrostatic pressure, will produce an elevation of hepatic sinusoidal pressure which may have an adverse effect on hepatic tissue perfusion. There is, however, very little evidence in relation to this situation. Ligation of the common bile duct in the laboratory rat was shown by Hunt to produce a diminution in total hepatic perfusion, as measured by inert gas clearance techniques (Hunt 1979). There may, however, have been mechanical factors outwith the liver substance which were important in this model. Hall and his colleagues (1977) demonstrated no change in liver blood flow in dogs with biliary obstruction, as measured by the intraparenchymal injection of Xenon 133. Recent work in our own laboratory has examined hepatic arterial and portal venous blood flow by means of electro-magnetic flow meters during acute changes in bile duct pressure in the anaesthetised dog (Nagorney et al 1982). As the bile duct pressure increases above a threshold — around 25 mmHg (33 kPa) — there is a significant and marked increase in hepatic arterial blood flow, while portal venous flow remains constant. These changes occur very promptly, and when the bile duct pressure exceeds 50 mmHg (67 kPa) the arterial blood flow has increased to 250% of the resting value, contributing to a total hepatic blood flow increase of 30–40%. The mechanism of these acute changes remains obscure, and studies of chronic obstruction are clearly also required, as are studies of blood flow after relief of biliary obstruction in man. The situation in which chronic obstruction has led to fibrotic changes with secondary portal hypertension is a separate issue, and this is discussed below.

Pathological effects

Canalicular and ductular changes

There is much evidence to suggest that the pathological effects of bile duct obstruction are initiated at the canalicular level, and are largely mediated by high local concentrations of bile salts at the canalicular membrane due to stasis within the biliary tree (Schaffner & Popper 1979). Histologically there is dilatation of the centrilobular bile canaliculus, and bile thrombi are found within the lumen. Bile pigment granules may also be seen in the adjacent hepatocytes. Electron microscopy has shown that the earliest changes involve the microvilli of the dilated bile canaliculus, which become distorted and swollen, and appear to be absent in some areas. These changes are the forerunners of alteration in the cytoplasm of the hepatocytes bordering these microvilli, and the pathological changes at this level are essentially similar whether cholestasis is due to mechanical obstruction or to other metabolic or toxic factors producing 'intrahepatic cholestasis'. This partly explains the non-specificity of both morphological and biochemical parameters reflecting cholestasis, and the difficulty in distinguishing in borderline cases between intrahepatic and extrahepatic cholestasis.

In more prolonged cholestasis the bile ducts and ductules appear to be increased, probably both by lengthening and tortuosity, and by sprouting of the small bile ductules as a reaction to inflammation. These proliferated ductules are surrounded initially by inflammatory exudate, and eventually by increased deposition of collagen bundles. The stimulus for these alterations is poorly understood, but they can be reproduced by injection or feeding of lithocholate (Schaffner & Javitt 1966). Changes in the microcirculation in the portal tracts have also been proposed as a factor (Schaffner & Popper 1979).

Fibrotic changes
The 'cholangiolitis' resulting from cholestasis leads eventually to the deposition of collagen fibres in the periductular region. These are laid down first in the form of reticulin, and this is followed by the formation of hard collagen which causes fibrosis and scarring around the bile ducts and ductules. When these changes are severe they may lead to further mechanical interference with the ductular and ductal bile flow, and aggravate the cholestasis. The extrahepatic ducts are also subject to these changes, and particularly in the presence of infection a sequence of mucosal atrophy and squamous metaplasia may be followed by inflammatory infiltration and ultimately fibrosis in the subepithelial layers of the ducts. These changes lead ultimately to the grossly thickened bile ducts of long-standing obstruction.

These intrahepatic fibrotic changes may be sufficiently severe to produce mechanical obstruction to sinusoidal flow, with secondary portal hypertension (see below). Although often loosely referred to as 'secondary biliary cirrhosis', the lobular architecture of the liver is usually well preserved, and the marked perilobular fibrosis which may occur in long-standing cases rarely proceeds to a true cirrhotic pattern. This has important implications for therapy, since many of the changes are potentially reversible. We have observed a return to near normality of such a liver following relief of biliary obstruction (Blumgart 1978). Sclerosing cholangitis unassociated with previous biliary surgery or with gallstones (primary sclerosing cholangitis) may produce a picture which is histologically similar to the chronic pericholangitis of true biliary obstruction. Thus in this group of patients in whom it is difficult to establish a diagnosis operatively or radiologically, histological examination of liver biopsies may also fail to provide a precise distinction (Williams & Schoetz 1981).

Hepatocyte changes
The earliest changes are seen in the cytoplasm bordering the microvilli of the dilated bile canaliculi. Large vesicles are seen in the cells and the volume of both

rough and smooth endoplasmic reticulum is increased (Schaffner et al 1971). There is an increased number of lysosomes and other organelles around the biliary pole of the hepatocyte, associated with rarefaction of the cytoplasm, which is parallelled in intensity by the tissue content of bile salts (Greim et al 1972). This is in keeping with the general concept that local high concentrations of bile acids are responsible for the primary lesion in cholestasis. The concentrations of chenodedeoxycholate found in cholestasis are sufficient to produce detergent effects in vitro. Ligation of the common bile duct in the rat leads to intrahepatic concentration of dihydroxy bile acids sufficient to inhibit cytochrome P-450. This lesion also occurred in rat livers perfused with chenodeoxycholate, with transformation of P-450 into the inactive cytochrome P-420 (Schaffner & Popper 1979). Thus there is good evidence that the 'feathery degeneration' seen in the hepatocytes is due largely to cholestasis. In its most severe form destruction of the layer of hepatocytes around the portal tracts is seen, with associated leucocyte inflammation (biliary piecemeal necrosis). These changes produce marked effects on hepatocyte function and on biochemical markers.

Biochemical effects

Bilirubin

Although jaundice is the classical physical sign associated with biliary tract obstruction, the bilirubin level may be elevated only marginally, and in incomplete and intermittent obstruction repeated serum estimations may be necessary to detect an elevated level. Excluding haemolytic causes for mild jaundice is not usually a clinical problem, but it may be much more difficult to distinguish between minor degrees of hepatic dysfunction producing primarily hepatocellular jaundice and cases in which obstruction is the only cause of hyperbilirubinaemia. Indeed, in the complex cases with prolonged partial obstruction of the biliary tract a mixed biochemical picture is the rule, and distinction between these two entities becomes difficult. This fundamental diagnostic problem stems from the fact noted above that the basic lesion at the subcellular level is the same whether cholestasis is due to mechanical causes or to metabolic causes (Schaffner & Popper 1979).

Urinary bilirubin and urobilinogen are tests which are often unaccountably ignored by surgeons. The persistent absence of urobilinogen from the urine is strong evidence of obstructive jaundice, and bilirubin is usually present in the urine until secondary hepatocellular disease becomes advanced.

The mechanisms of transport of conjugated bilirubin within the hepatocyte and secretion into the canaliculus are incompletely understood. It has been proposed that in addition to the canalicular membrane transport processes the formation of mixed micelles at the canalicular surface or within the lumen may be an important determinant of the net hepatic bilirubin transport. A concentration gradient opposing transport of bilirubin into the canaliculus may be produced by the stasis at this level associated with biliary obstruction. The mechanism whereby conjugated bilirubin refluxes into the sinusoidal plasma in cholestasis also remains unclear. Although the secretory mechanisms for bile acids and for bilirubin and a variety of exogenous organic anions (such as BSP and some cholecystographic dyes) are functionally distinct, they do not appear to be functionally independent of each other. This may have important implications for management of patients with biliary obstruction and with external biliary fistulae (see bile salts below).

Bile acids

Complete biliary tract obstruction will ot course interrupt the enterohepatic circulation of bile salts. Serum bile acid levels may be very high, ranging from 4–60 times the normal level (Neale et al 1971). Nevertheless, the synthesis of bile acids is grossly impaired, with up to five-fold reduction in the levels of the rate limiting enzymes for bile acid synthesis (Salen et al 1975). There is an increased urinary excretion of bile acids, but this still amounts to a very small proportion of the normal faecal excretion (Heaton 1979). In addition abnormal bile acids are produced by the liver, including ursodeoxycholate, which are more easily excreted in the urine than the normal bile acids.

Pruritus in cholestasis is probably caused by the deposition of bile acids in the skin (Kirby et al 1974). Cholestyramine sequestrates bile acids in the intestine and promotes their excretion, and may be effective in the treatment of pruritus by lowering the circulating bile acid concentrations.

It has already been noted that stasis of bile acids at the canalicular level is responsible for at least part of the cellular damage caused by both extra- and intrahepatic cholestasis. Bile salt dependent canalicular flow can be measured experimentally by means of erythritol clearance. Lewis (1982) has shown that in the conscious dog external diversion of biliary flow leads to a decrease in the bile salt dependent canalicular flow within 30 minutes, which can be restored to normal by infusion of low levels of bile acids intravenously. This is consistent with the very rapid uptake and clearance of bile acids from the plasma, since 60–90% of bile acids are cleared by a single passage through the liver, giving half lives between 2 and 16 minutes (Heaton 1979). The work of Goresky (1974), demonstrating that stimulation of bile salt dependent canalicular flow by infusion of bile salts also produces more rapid excretion of bilirubin, assumes clinical importance in this context. Therapeutic drainage of the biliary tract in patients with obstruction leads to a prompt choleresis (McPherson et al 1981), but this may be short lived, and possibly associated with output of bile of a poor quality. Since external biliary drainage results in depletion of the bile salt pool, replacement of bile salts under these circumstances may have a beneficial effect on the clearance of bilirubin, and possibly of other moieties excreted by mechanisms dependent on the bile salt related canalicular flow. This important question is under investigation in our own unit at the present time.

Other important consequences of interruption of normal bile salt metabolism are considered below.

Alkaline phosphatase

Alkaline phosphatase is probably the most frequently used biochemical test of bile duct patency. A clear pitfall which requires no further emphasis lies in the existence of isoenzymes of alkaline phosphatase which originate from bone, and not from the liver. Other sources of the enzyme (intestine, kidney and placenta) are rarely a source of confusion. The hepatic enzyme occurs predominantly in the plasma membrane of the microvilli of the bile canaliculus (Price & Alberti 1979).

Certainly the highest levels of liver alkaline phosphatase are found in patients with complete biliary obstruction. Minor or intermittent degrees of obstruction, however, also produce significant elevations of alkaline phosphatase, and this may be an important biochemical sign raising suspicion of biliary pathology in the absence of jaundice or of any other derangement of liver function. In patients with hepatic malignancy the elevation of alkaline phosphatase is proportional to the extent of liver involvement (Baden 1971), and this may be an important differential diagnosis.

The return to normal of alkaline phosphatase after relief of biliary obstruction may be a good index of successful therapy in the majority of cases. However, it has been our experience that many patients with long-standing obstruction show a very slow return to normal and may have persistent elevations of this enzyme long after treatment, despite a clinically successful result. Lord Smith (1978) reported that of those patients with mucosal grafts for benign biliary strictures in whom sufficient data was available for analysis, up to 40% had persistent elevation of alkaline phosphatase throughout their follow-up. Way et al (1981) reported that 10 patients with good results following repair of benign biliary strictures had elevated alkaline phosphatase levels for more than three years after treatment. The reason for these findings is unclear. There are, however, at least two isoenzymes of the alkaline phosphatase produced by the liver, one derived from the liver cell and the other of biliary (possibly canalicular) origin, found only when there is obstruction to the flow of bile (Price & Sammons 1974). These workers have proposed that the elevation seen in patients with obstructive liver disease represents an overspill of the enzyme from the liver cell whose content is increased, combined with regurgitation of this biliary isoenzyme into the circulation. Price & Sammons (1976) have further proposed that quantitation of this 'biliary isoenzyme' may allow better differentiation of patients with complete or minimal biliary obstruction.

A simple practical application of the measurement of alkaline phosphatase is in the complex postoperative patient, particularly following biliary reconstruction or major hepatic trauma. Elevation of serum bilirubin in the absence of a rising alkaline phosphatase may indicate an intraperitoneal biliary collection, while parallel increases of bilirubin and alkaline phosphatase suggest a degree of obstruction. Although such changes must be interpreted with caution, this is a simple observation which we have found valuable in clinical practice.

Other enzymes
Gross elevation of the aminotransferases is an index of hepatocellular damage, and as an isolated biochemical finding may cast doubt upon a diagnosis of extra-hepatic obstruction. Minor elevation of aminotransferase activity is common, however, in extra-hepatic obstruction, and indeed the aminotransferase activity rises earlier than that of alkaline phosphatase in cases of acute obstruction. The levels fall to normal, or nearly so, within several days, despite deepening jaundice. In the later stages of prolonged obstruction, particularly in the presence of intrabiliary infection or invasive sepsis from suppurative cholangitis, the transaminases may be elevated again, and this is an adverse prognostic feature.

Gamma glutamyl transpeptidase tends to parallel alkaline phosphatase, and is sometimes used as an alternative to the isoenzyme fractionation of alkaline phosphatase.

It is doubtful whether other enzymatic tests of liver function are in themselves particularly helpful in assessment of proven or suspected biliary tract obstruction.

Other biochemical parameters

Serum protein abnormalities are often seen in patients with liver disease. Depression of serum albumin is a common feature in patients with malignant obstruction of the biliary tract, particularly when there has been prolonged nutritional impairment. Elevation of the globulins, particularly the IgG fraction, may be seen in patients with severe parenchymal liver disease due to long-standing obstruction. Because gross elevation of gamma globulins may be largely related to portal-systemic shunting (Benjamin et al 1976), this should also raise a strong suspicion of secondary portal hypertension.

Lipid metabolism is grossly altered by biliary obstruction though most changes are unhelpful because of lack of specificity. Cholesterol may be elevated in long-standing biliary obstruction. A more specific change is seen in the serum of patients with biliary obstruction in the appearance of an abnormal lipoprotein, lipoprotein-X (Magnani & Alaupovic 1976). This may give a better differentiation than alkaline phosphatase and other standard liver function tests between 'medical' and 'surgical' jaundice. Further studies are required to establish its clinical usefulness.

Functional effects

The standard tests of liver function based on serum estimations of bilirubin, enzymes etc, not only reflect the predictable physical effects of biliary tract obstruction, but may also be related to fundamental derangements of hepatocellular function. In addition there may be effects on other cellular elements within the liver, in particular the reticuloendothelial system (mononuclear phagocytic system).

Hepatocellular function

It has already been noted that one of the toxic effects of retained bile salts at the canalicular level is on the essential cellular component cytochrome P-450. Transformation into the inactive cytochrome P-420 has a profound effect on the metabolic activity of the hepatocyte. In addition, bilirubin itself has been shown to inhibit mono-oxygenase activity in vitro (Maines & Kappas 1975), so that cholestasis may cause both inhibition and destruction of cytochrome P-450. Disruption of mitochondrial function has also been demonstrated in biliary obstruction (Koyama et al 1981). These alterations have a marked effect on metabolic activity, including impairment of hepatic drug metabolism. This factor is invariably taken into account by clinicians who are treating patients with severe intrinsic parenchymal liver diseases, as cirrhotic changes of comparable magnitude may be seen in biliary obstruction.

The use of drug metabolism tests as a dynamic indicator of liver function may be a valuable adjunct to assessment of patients with biliary tract obstruction, particularly those who are candidates for major surgery involving liver resection.

We have investigated the clearance of antipyrine (a minor analgesic which is almost entirely oxidised in the liver) and paracetamol (which is conjugated to the glucuronide and sulphate esters in the liver), as parameters of liver function. The half-life and clearance of antipyrine from the plasma in patients with biliary obstruction was significantly impaired when compared with control subjects (McPherson et al 1982). The elimination of antipyrine in the jaundiced state showed a significant correlation with subsequent clearance of endogenous plasma bilirubin following relief of biliary obstruction. Antipyrine elimination appeared to have some predictive capability, in that patients with grossly impaired antipyrine clearance had worse results from biliary drainage, and a high mortality rate following subsequent surgery. Cytochrome P-450 content in the livers of these patients was comparable to that found in liver samples from patients with hepatitis and cirrhosis, and was only 33% of that present in normal liver. None of the other preoperative tests of liver function showed a significant correlation with the outcome of biliary drainage. This type of dynamic test requires further investigation to prove its value in the clinical setting, but appears to offer clear advantages over the standard laboratory tests of liver function.

Cholestasis also effects the rough endoplasmic reticulum, and the synthesis of proteins by the obstructed liver is altered. Lipoproteins appear to be particularly affected, and it has already been noted that an abnormal low density lipoprotein (lipoprotein-X) appears in the plasma of obstructed patients. While serum albumin levels may be reduced in patients with biliary obstruction, the control of albumin turnover in patients with liver disease is complex, and these levels may not necessarily reflect impaired hepatic synthesis. However, hepatic synthesis of proteins has been shown to be decreased early after bile duct ligation (Lee et al 1972).

Abnormal glucose tolerance is seen in the patient with impaired liver function. There is some evidence that this may be due to defects in the hepatic alanine cycle (Ansley 1978). Impaired gluconeogenesis has been reported after bile duct ligation in the rat (Lee et al 1972). These features have not been examined in patients with cholestasis, but may be important prognostic factors for surgical patients (Johnston 1981).

Reticuloendothelial function

The function of the hepatic Kupffer cells is known to be impaired in cirrhosis, and this makes a variable contribution to the hyperglobulinaemia of the cirrhotic patient (Benjamin et al 1976, Thomas et al 1976). In addition to the removal of microorganisms, macromolecules and immune complexes from the portal blood, the Kupffer cells have a major role in the inactivation of endotoxins, the abnormal lipopolysaccharides derived from the cell wall of Gram negative bacteria in the gut. Systemic endotoxaemia occurs in jaundiced patients before, during and after surgery, in contrast to non-jaundiced patients with disease of comparable severity (Wardle 1975, Bailey 1976). Drivas et al (1976) demonstrated impaired Kupffer cell phagocytosis of albumin microaggregates in patients with cholestasis. Ingoldby (1982) has demonstrated both increased absorption and decreased hepatic clearance of endotoxin in rats rendered jaundiced by bile duct ligation.

Since endotoxaemia is associated with postoperative renal failure in the jaundiced patient, these results have a most important therapeutic implication (Bailey 1976).

Secondary effects

Infection

The normal biliary tract is sterile. In the presence of gallstones, and following surgical intervention in the biliary tract, the incidence of bacteria in the bile increases (Keighley 1977). It is commonly believed that the biliary tract remains sterile in cases of primary malignant obstruction, but this is not so. Keighley (1977) reported a rate of 36% of biliary bacterial contamination, and our own studies have shown an initial positive bile culture rate of 32% for patients with obstruction due to this cause (McPherson et al 1982). Several of these patients had undergone multiple previous operations, however, and in no such patient was the bile sterile on initial needle puncture at PTC. In 73 patients undergoing repair of benign bile duct stricture, Lord Smith found bacteria in the bile in 80% of cases (Jackaman et al 1980): this group of patients also had the highest incidence of anaerobic biliary contaminants.

Although these patients may often have episodes of cholangitis, the bacterial contamination of the biliary tract in partial obstruction may not be clinically apparent. It does, however, assume clinical importance in patients undergoing surgery, since sepsis constitutes a major factor in postoperative complication and mortality rates.

The more florid condition of acute suppurative cholangitis is less commonly seen. However, Boey & Way (1980) reported suppurative cholangitis in 50% of their patients with malignant strictures, but the incidence was only 3% in those with benign stricture and 20% in gallstone obstruction.

The most common infecting organisms are *Escherichia coli* and *Streptococcus faecalis,* and in our experience anaerobic bacteria are rare as a primary finding. Following radiological intubation or surgical interference, the spectrum of bacteria may change due to exogenous acquisition of organisms (McPherson et al 1982). Apart from the danger of invasive sepsis following surgery, suppurative cholangitis almost certainly accelerates the progressive fibrotic changes of the obstructed biliary tract, and produces marked secondary changes in the small bile radicles which are readily appreciated radiologically. These changes may be indistinguishable from those of primary sclerosing cholangitis, both radiologically and histopathologically. Mucoid aggregates within the biliary tract may appear as filling defects on cholangiography, and are commonly associated with stenosed biliary-enteric anastomosis (Benjamin & Blumgart 1979).

Atrophy

The occurrence of lobar or segmental liver atrophy in association with a variety of liver pathologies has aroused sporadic comment in the radiological and surgical literature. However, the pathophysiology of liver atrophy remains poorly understood, and its clinical significance is only slowly emerging. The distribution of liver mass amongst the segments of the liver is regulated by a complex homeostatic balance, in which bile flow, portal venous inflow, and hepatic venous outflow are the principal regulators. Uniform liver atrophy will occur in the presence of malnutrition, or of partial occlusion of the main stem of the portal vein. Both the quantity and the quality of portal venous inflow are important in the maintenance of liver cell size and mass (Starzl et al 1973, Guest et al 1978). Factors which will produce segmental or lobar atrophy fall into three main categories:

(i) Portal venous occlusion
(ii) Bile duct occlusion
(iii) Proximity to a space-occupying lesion.

To these one must add the rare cases associated with unilobar veno-occlusive disease (Galloway et al 1973). Furthermore it is probable that bile duct occlusion achieves its effects by a secondary change in sinusoidal perfusion by portal venous blood in the chronically obstructed lobe.

The left lobe of the liver appears more susceptible to atrophy than the right (Ham 1979). The reason for this is not clear, although it has been suggested that compression of the left portal vein by dilatation of the long left hepatic duct may be responsible (Benz et al 1952). Unilobar atrophy is frequently associated with hypertrophy of the contralateral lobe, and this may present a clinical pitfall, in that a large palpable hypertrophied lobe of the liver may be a subtle indicator of pathology principally affecting the other lobe (Tzuzuki et al 1973). This situation arises through a gradual process, and in cases of hilar cholangiocarcinoma is due to asymmetrical and asynchronous involvement of the lobar hepatic ducts. This further emphasises that incomplete (lobar or segmental) obstruction may produce little in the way of physical signs or biochemical abnormalities when it is associated with an adequate functioning mass of unobstructed liver tissue.

The radiological signs of atrophy have been described, and can be determined by critical examination of isotope or CT scans (Thomas & Bernadino 1980, Makler et al 1980), and transhepatic cholangiograms (Myracle et al 1981). The existence of atrophy is important both to the radiologist and the surgeon, as it carries important implications for therapy (see below).

Hepatic fibrosis
Patients in whom biliary tract obstruction has progressed to established secondary biliary fibrosis represent a group at particularly high risk. Sedgwick and his colleagues (1966) reviewed 890 patients treated at the Lahey Clinic for biliary stricture. 19% of these patients showed some degree of portal hypertension, and although this usually took 4–5 years to develop from the onset of the stricture an interval of as little as two years was found in some cases. Eight of 59 patients (13.5%) reported by Way et al (1981) had 'biliary cirrhosis' during the course of treatment for biliary strictures. Five of these patients died, two associated with portal hypertension. We have seen several patients with hepatic fibrosis secondary to benign biliary strictures which has been sufficient to produce major stigmata of hepatocellular dysfunction, such as spider naevi, asterixis and portal systemic encephalopathy. The management of these patients is somewhat pragmatic, as there are few guidelines in the literature. It is crucial to determine whether the liver disease is entirely due to biliary pathology, since a staged procedure with simple relief of biliary tract obstruction as a primary approach may then lead to

sufficient regression of the liver disease to render definitive surgery safer. Conversely if there is a major component of primary hepatocellular disease (for example alcoholic cirrhosis) then the prognosis is poor, and it may be possible to take a decision to avoid major operative procedures.

When portal hypertension produces profuse haemorrhage at the time of surgery, simple tubal drainage of the biliary system may be followed by re-operation some weeks later to perform a portal-systemic shunt. Splenorenal shunting is more often technically possible in this situation than a direct approach to the portal vein in a scarred hilar region. In such patients the normal criteria for selection of patients for portal systemic shunting may be relaxed, since improvement in liver function may be anticipated following repair of the biliary stricture. This is supported by the results of Sedgwick and his colleagues (1966) in that only one of 18 such patients treated by spleno-renal shunting developed subsequent portal-systemic encephalopathy. Improved techniques of peroeso-phageal sclerotherapy for bleeding varices may provide a valuable temporising measure in these difficult cases.

Loss of bile salt circulation
Interruption of the normal enterohepatic circulation has been described above. In complete biliary obstruction this will produce steatorrhoea due to maldigestion of fatty foods, and this may also be aggravated by alteration of the bacterial flora of the upper small intestine in the absence of normal biliary secretion. Secondary to fat malabsorption there will be deficiencies of the fat soluble vitamins, so that parenteral administration of vitamin K_1 is mandatory to minimise coagulation disturbances.

Bailey (1976) highlighted the role of bile salts in protection of rats with obstructive jaundice from endotoxaemia and renal damage. Bile salts bind endotoxin, and prevent its absorption from the gut in the jaundiced animal (Ingoldby 1982). Endotoxaemia may exercise some of its effects on the kidneys by activation of microvascular thrombosis (Sagar & Shields 1980). Replacement of bile salts in the jaundiced patient, particularly after percutaneous transhepatic drainage, may thus be important in protecting against endotoxaemia and its consequences. This remains to be proven by controlled clinical study.

Clinical aspects

The clinical syndromes
It is clear from the foregoing account of the pathophysiological aspects of biliary obstruction that the clinical manifestations of this problem are protean in nature. The modes of presentation of biliary obstruction range from the simplest and most overt to the most complex and subtle, and this range may be challenging to the diagnostician. In this section the range of clinical presentations is reviewed.

Jaundice and its variants

The classical presentation of patients with malignant disease in the head of the pancreas or in the bile ducts is the abrupt onset of painless progressive jaundice. When combined with weight loss, and with other physical findings such as lymphadenopathy or an abdominal mass, such a presentation is usually diagnostic. It is not unusual, however, for malignant lesions to present with jaundice which is not continuous from onset, nor for an impacted gallstone to produce an unremitting jaundice. Similarly the presence or absence of pain is a rather unreliable sign in distinguishing between benign and malignant obstruction. Much of this diagnostic dilemma has been obviated by developments in radiological techniques of scanning and of cholangiography (see below).

In malignant obstruction, it is not only important to distinguish between tumours of the extrahepatic biliary tree and those of the head of the pancreas, but also to distinguish between cases of pancreatic adenocarcinoma and tumours affecting the periampullary region (distal bile duct, papilla of Vater and adjacent duodenum), since the prognosis and approaches to therapy are distinct in these three classes. A careful history is important, and fluctuating jaundice is more suggestive of a periampullary lesion than a pancreatic one. An intermittently palpable gallbladder is also described in association with periampullary tumours, in contrast to the constant enlarged non-tender gallbladder of complete malignant distal biliary tract obstruction (Blumgart & Kennedy 1973). However, the fallacy that a chronically inflamed gallbladder which is the seat of cholelithiasis is unlikely to distend secondary to calculous obstruction of the bile duct should not mislead the clinician (Smith 1978).

Biliary tract disease associated with the passage of small stones may produce intermittent jaundice with or without associated abdominal pain due to biliary colic or to acute pancreatitis, or to both. Although the serum amylase may be helpful, and possibly the amylase to creatinine clearance ratio (Lesser & Warshaw 1975), none of the laboratory tests is diagnostic. Even after the jaundice has faded, oral cholecystography may fail to reveal small stones, and intravenous cholangiography also gives a low diagnostic yield (Blumgart et al 1974, Goodman et al 1980). Gallstones may remain in the common duct for long periods before precipitating an episode of jaundice or cholangitis (Den Besten & Doty 1981). The occurrence of fever, rigors, and jaundice (the classical triad of Charcot) is highly suggestive of choledocholithiasis in the primary case, and of retained common duct stones or biliary stricture in the post-cholecystectomy patient. Nonetheless, the classical triad occurs in only three quarters of patients with acute cholangitis (Den Besten & Doty 1981). Although infection is commoner than has often been supposed in the presence of malignant biliary obstruction, severe cholangitis is not common as a primary presentation of these lesions.

It has already been noted that biliary tract obstruction may occur in the absence of jaundice. While liver function tests lack both sensitivity and specificity, careful attention should be paid to minor changes in difficult diagnostic cases. Elevated alkaline phosphatase may be an early indicator of biliary obstruction in patients with vague symptoms, and should lead to careful radiological investigation. It is more difficult to evaluate this finding in patients who have had biliary tract obstruction relieved surgically, as there is great variability in the return to normal of liver enzymes (see above).

Post-cholecystectomy patients pose a particular problem. In a group of 52 such cases referred to our unit for investigation, 17 presented with intermittent jaundice, eight with pancreatitis, five with cholangitis and the remaining 21 with vague symptoms of dyspepsia or 'biliary' pain (Blumgart et al 1977). Two of the patients with cholangitis were never jaundiced. It is clear that obstruction may promote the accumulation of debris within the bile duct without jaundice, and this phenomenon is probably related more to the duration than to the degree of obstruction (Benjamin & Blumgart 1978). This applies especially to patients with previous surgery to the bile duct, and most particularly to those with a stenosed sphincteroplasty or choledochoduodenostomy (Blumgart et al 1977).

The diagnosis of primary stenosis of the sphincter of Oddi or of biliary dyskinesia remains an extremely contentious one (Moody 1981). The chronic passage of small gallstones through the papilla is, however, a potent cause of secondary stenosing papillitis. This may produce a diagnostic problem since retrograde cannulation of the biliary tract may be impossible, while intravenous cholangiography may be unreliable or non-specific. Moody (1981) recommends examination of hepatic and gallbladder bile for calcium bilurubinate, cholesterol crystals and white blood cells as a test for occult biliary lithiasis.

Cholangiocarcinoma

Malignant lesions of the bile duct are not as uncommon as was formerly thought, the estimated incidence in the United States being some 4500 new cases per annum (Longmire 1976). Refined diagnostic techniques have led to an increasing awareness and also an increasing diagnostic rate for this cause of biliary obstruction. Of 37 patients referred to us at the Royal Postgraduate Medical School between January 1980 and May 1981, five had been surgically explored elsewhere and no diagnosis reached at laparotomy. However, of 21 patients in whom PTC was undertaken as an initial procedure, the diagnosis was achieved in every case (Voyles et al 1982). Nearly all patients present with obstructive jaundice, but because this is a slow-growing tumour it has often been present for a long period before presentation. Thus in the case of hilar tumours (the most common location) there may be unequal obstruction to the right and left hepatic ducts, and this may be of major importance for therapy. We have seen numerous cases in which there has been obstruction to the left hepatic duct of sufficient long-standing to produce severe atrophic changes. By the time jaundice occurs and PTC is undertaken, there is no communication between the right and left lobar ductal systems, and the left lobe of the liver has shown marked tissue atrophy, a large part of the shrunken left lobe being occupied by dilated and crowded bile ducts. The mechanisms for this situation and its importance for therapy are referred to elsewhere in this chapter.

Cholangitis is a feature of this disease, but is unusual as a presenting complaint. However, in cases of long-standing intermittent obstruction there may have been a period of several months of ill health with vague abdominal pain, pruritus, and occasional low grade fever, before the onset of overt jaundice. In some cases with this type of presentation differentiation from primary sclerosing cholangitis may be difficult and may not easily be resolved by radiology.

A pitfall in the presentation of cholangiocarcinoma lies in those patients who have had cholecystectomy for vague 'biliary' symptoms, and who may or may not have had cholelithiasis at the time of operation. If operative cholangiography has not been performed, or has been misinterpreted, then the patient's symptoms persist until the diagnosis of biliary stricture is made at subsequent radiology. In these cases the differential diagnosis is that of iatrogenic bile duct stricture, and unless a diagnosis can be reached preoperatively by means of cytology, laparotomy may be required to make this distinction.

Sclerosing cholangitis

Primary sclerosing cholangitis is a diffuse fibrosis of the wall of the biliary ducts resulting in compression and narrowing of the lumen to the point of almost complete occlusion. As such, this disease may be regarded as the classical example of chronic incomplete obstruction. The syndrome usually presents in the third to the fifth decade of life, with a male predominance in most series (Williams & Schoetz 1981). The classical presentation is with jaundice, often intermittent and mild but sometimes progressive, non-specific upper abdominal discomfort and pruritus. The history may range from months to years, and cholangitis may occur at a late stage in the course of the disease or may be a presenting feature. The association with inflammatory bowel disease is well known, and ulcerative colitis may be present in 20–30% of cases. We have seen patients in whom the sclerosing cholangitis was the presenting problem, and in whom ulcerative colitis has emerged some time after treatment of the biliary condition. The difficulty in diagnosing between sclerosing cholangitis and the diffuse form of cholangio-carcinoma has already been mentioned. However, we have also seen cases in which the radiological appearance at the hilus of the liver was highly suggestive of cholangiocarcinoma with a localised stricture and no diffuse involvement. In one case radical excision of the lesion and subsequent histology showed localised sclerosing cholangitis, and subsequently further benign strictures have been detected in the intrahepatic biliary tree.

Benign biliary strictures

In practice these are almost invariably a consequence of previous biliary surgery and iatrogenic injury to the bile duct. Patients who present soon after surgery with either a biliary fistula or jaundice are not a diagnostic problem, but commonly the presentation is delayed with a late onset of recurrent attacks of cholangitis with or without jaundice, following a cholecystectomy which has been considered by the surgeon to be uneventful (Maingot 1964). In Way's series (1981) the injury was recognised at the time of cholecystectomy in one quarter of patients, and within 30 days in an additional one third. The remaining patients presented with asymptomatic intervals ranging from 6 months to 26 years, the commonest late presenting feature being cholangitis with or without jaundice.

Percutaneous or retrograde cholangiography is almost invariably necessary to confirm the diagnosis and to determine the site and extent of the injury, as well as to plan the approach to treatment. Intravenous cholangiography has no place in the diagnosis of this lesion.

Following repair of a bile duct injury or stricture the success rate in the best hands may be as high as 70–80% (Smith 1978, Way et al 1981). Most recurrent strictures occur within three years of repair (Cattell & Braasch 1959). However, late recurrences do occur, and in any patient with a previous biliary stricture repair further attacks of cholangitis are due to this cause until proven otherwise. In some cases there may be an adequate anastomosis with obstruction by residual stones or intraductal debris causing recurrent attacks of cholangitis, and it is not always necessary to contemplate formal major reconstruction. We have seen such a stone which could not pass because of attachment to a suture.

A high serum bilirubin level which persists following repair of the biliary stricture indicates a bad result. On the other hand persistent elevation of alkaline phosphatase or other liver enzymes may be found in entirely asymptomatic patients (Way et al 1981). It is important to treat neither laboratory results nor radiographs, but to consider the patient's symptoms when assessing the need for further therapy.

Acute suppurative cholangitis
Charcot's triad (fever with rigors, jaundice, and pain in the right upper quadrant) was described over one hundred years ago, and this classical description of cholangitis has not been superceded. Reynolds and Dargan in 1959 added the features of shock and central nervous system depression to complete the clinical description of acute suppurative cholangitis (Reynolds & Dargan 1959). Although relatively uncommon in its most florid form this represents a most serious complication of biliary tract obstruction, conservative management of which is uniformly fatal (Chock et al 1981). Stones in the common bile duct are the most common cause, though almost any of the aetiologies of biliary tract obstruction may produce the syndrome. Even in patients with gallstone obstruction the syndrome is not common, and Boey & Way (1980) found suppuration at surgery in only 20% of such patients. Indeed these workers found that suppuration was present in 50% of patients with malignant obstruction.

A serious sequela of intraductal suppuration is the formation of intrahepatic abscesses scattered throughout the liver parenchyma. Once these abscesses become established the course of the disease is usually fatal. The normal pathogens of the biliary tree (*Escherichia coli, enterobacter* and *Streptococcus faecalis*) are the commonest causative organisms. A potent aggravating feature is surgery or instrumentation of the biliary tract, and in such cases the bacterial flora changes to include a significant number of exogenously acquired organisms (*Klebsiella* and *Pseudomonas* species: McPherson et al 1982).

Patients with this condition are usually elderly and severely ill, and apart from resuscitative measures with intravenous replacement and parenteral broad spectrum antibiotics, the usual recommended treatment is emergency surgery. This must be aimed at effective decompression of the biliary tree, and although cholecystostomy is attractive in its simplicity this may fail adequately to drain the bile duct. The safest course is wide bore T-tube drainage of the common bile duct. Percutaneous transhepatic drainage of the biliary tree is also in theory an attractive alternative. It is important to note, however, that the relatively fine-bore tubes used for transhepatic drainage may fail to drain ducts which contain thick pus. In one such patient who underwent percutaneous transhepatic biliary drainage for an obstructing periampullary cancer, large volumes of dilute hepatic bile drained from the catheter for 24 hours while the patient's condition failed to improve. Laparotomy showed that the common bile duct remained grossly distended with thick pus, and T-tube drainage produced a rapid improvement in his condition.

While urgent surgery is the essential and definitive treatment for this condition, Bismuth and his colleagues (1975) have stressed the importance of adequate resuscitation, fluid replacement and antibiotic treatment, and possibly renal dialysis, before operation. However, delay much beyond 24 hours leads to a marked increase in mortality, rising in one series from 17% of patients treated within 24 hours to 50% for those with a 24–72 hour delay (Welch & Donaldson 1976).

Biliary obstruction in pancreatitis

Biliary tract obstruction may be caused by benign diseases of the pancreas in three situations. Firstly some 10–15% of patients with acute pancreatitis have a degree of jaundice, and while this is usually due to the impaction or passage of a stone at the ampulla of Vater, this is not always so. Acute oedema of the pancreas during an attack may produce a mild obstructive picture. Secondly, patients who develop pancreatic cysts or pseudocysts in the region of the distal bile duct may become partially obstructed and even jaundiced, and this may occur with quite small cysts if they are immediately adjacent to the distal duct (McCollum & Jordan 1975).

The third and most important category consists of patients with chronic pancreatitis. Almost one third of patients with chronic pancreatitis suffer from episodes of obstructive jaundice (Sarles & Sahel 1978). Incomplete biliary tract obstruction may also occur, with normal serum bilirubin but elevated alkaline phosphatase (Snape et al 1976). This entity has been long overlooked as a feature of chronic pancreatitis, but has become more frequently recognised since the advent of endoscopic choledochography and pancreatography. The characteristic feature on cholangiography is a smooth tapering deformity of the retropancreatic bile duct, and in the presence of ERCP evidence of pancreatic duct abnormalities this is virtually diagnostic of chronic pancreatitis (Scott et al 1977). In a series of 210 patients referred to our unit over a period of five years for management of chronic pancreatitis, 16 required some form of biliary-enteric bypass for the relief of biliary tract obstruction. In six of these patients the biliary tract obstruction was the major cause of symptoms, and the main indication for surgical treatment of the chronic pancreatitis (I. S. Benjamin, data in preparation). The investigation of chronic incomplete or intermittent biliary tract obstruction should take account of this possible diagnosis, and conversely the surgical management of chronic pancreatitis must take account of the possible need for biliary diversion.

Therapy

When obstruction is complete the outcome of therapy has a very clear endpoint, and is evident in the clearance of jaundice. In the more subtle forms of obstruction the endpoint of therapy is less clear-cut, and it is partly for this reason that prolonged follow-up is necessary to determine the clinical outcome in patients undergoing surgery for biliary strictures. We have noted already that the majority of recurrent strictures will occur within three years of repair (Cattell & Braasch 1959), so that a satisfactory follow-up at five years is often taken as a cure. Certainly patients with a good result at two years have a 90% chance of a satisfactory long-term cure (Way & Dunphy 1972). Sandblom, however, found a 20% incidence of recurrent symptoms in a large series of benign strictures followed for 10 years, and regards a follow-up period of three to five years as inadequate for the assessment of long-term results (in discussion of Lane et al 1973).

In all but the simplest cases of biliary obstruction, therapy relies upon some form of biliary-enteric anastomosis. For high strictures and tumours this may be a hepatico- or cholangiojejunostomy, while for low obstructions or recurrent choledocholithiasis the choice may lie between a side-to-side choledochoduodenostomy or a sphincteroplasty.

Choledochoduodenostomy and sphincteroplasty

There is much sterile debate between the enthusiasts for these techniques, and almost certainly each has its place. A sphincteroplasty correctly performed is a terminal choledochoduodenostomy, and should produce a stoma equal in calibre to the widest part of the common duct (Jones 1973). As such it should adequately fulfil the requirement of free dependent drainage of the biliary tree. The operation carries the potential complication of pancreatitis, and in some series this carries a high mortality (Imrie et al 1978). Side-to-side choledochoduodenostomy suffers the theoretical disadvantage of the 'sump syndrome' caused by debris remaining or accumulating within the infraduodenal bile duct above a distal obstruction. However, existing evidence would suggest that if a stoma of adequate size (> 2 cm) is made in a duct which is dilated and thick-walled, then long-term patency will be maintained and this syndrome should not occur (Johnson & Stevens 1969). When stasis within the bile duct is produced by late stenosis of either a choledochoduodenostomy or a sphincteroplasty, then debris accumulates and ascending cholangitis will occur due to chronic incomplete obstruction. Bacteria harboured in the poorly-drained biliary tract may encourage the formation of primary gallstones by the deconjugation of bilirubin by glucuronidase (Thomas, in discussion of Saharia et al 1977). The message is clearly that whatever drainage procedure is performed must be adequate and remain adequate if recurrent symptoms are to be avoided.

Reversal of chronic changes in the biliary tract even after adequate drainage may be very slow. Lygidakis (1981) examined choledochoduodenostomies in 100 patients in a follow-up study ranging over 10 years. The patency of the stoma was assessed by serial barium studies, and all stomata were found to be adequate. Despite this, abnormal emptying of the small intrahepatic ducts was found in many patients, with retention of barium for four days to one month after ingestion. Although this emptying time returned to normal during follow-up in the majority, this took in some cases more than one year after operation. Many of these patients had had common bile duct stones of very long standing, and moreover had proven intrabiliary infection and secondary cholangiolitic changes shown on operative liver biopsy. These studies serve further to emphasize the deep-seated damage rendered to the biliary tract by prolonged incomplete obstruction, and the necessity of adequate drainage for a return to normal. They also provide a morphological counterpart to the very slow return to normal of liver function tests following drainage (vide supra).

Hepaticojejunostomy

This type of drainage may be the procedure of choice in many cases of biliary obstruction, particularly high benign or malignant strictures or tumours of the head of the pancreas. While the traditional teaching for relief of jaundice due to pancreatic cancer has been a cholecystojejunostomy this technique carries the hazard of tumour encroachment on the cystic duct and subsequent failure of decompression, and may also be compromised by a narrow and tortuous or fibrotic cystic duct. Hepaticojejunostomy to a loop of jejunum in continuity carries the risk of reflux of intestinal content into the biliary tree, and is usually combined with a distal side-to-side enteroanastomosis. There is radiological evidence, however, that this does not adequately defunction the isolated loop of jejunum, and we prefer to use the Roux-en-Y technique. It is our current practice to make such a Roux loop at least 50 cm long in order to prevent reflux.

Segmental obstruction and atrophy

The occurrence of segmental obstruction, particularly in hilar cholangio-carcinomas, has already been discussed. This may pose a therapeutic dilemma, both in terms of preliminary biliary decompression and of definitive surgery. Drainage of a segment of liver which is obstructed and atrophied may produce a poor clearance of jaundice because of irreversibly impaired hepatocellular function in this segment. On the other hand, the presence of infection in such a closed segment may demand drainage as a therapeutic manoeuvre. When there is no communication between the right and left intrahepatic ductal systems, as a general rule drainage of one or other lobe will be satisfactory for the clearance of jaundice, and the technically easier side (usually the right) may be selected. However, if subsequent liver resection and biliary-enteric anastomosis is contemplated, then it may be advantageous to drain the lobe which is to be resected, since a collapsed ductal system presents a greater technical problem at the time of surgery than does a lobe with a dilated biliary tree. These are subtle considerations which have been brought to light by advances in both radiological and surgical techniques.

The presence of infection as well as atrophy may be of crucial therapeutic importance. In a recent series of 37 patients with hilar cholangiocarcinoma treated over an 18-month period, 25 patients had tumours which on cholangiographic grounds alone were considered for further investigation of resectability. In four of these patients hepatic resection would have been required for tumour clearance, but the potential hepatic remnant was compromised by segmental atrophy in two cases, and by gross infection with intrahepatic abscess formation in a further two. These findings were confirmed at laparotomy for a palliative drainage procedure (Voyles et al 1982).

Tubal drainage of the biliary tract

Intubation of the biliary tract may be performed either for relief of obstruction as a preliminary to definitive surgery, or as definitive treatment for irresectable tumours or benign strictures. In either case the insertion of a tube into the biliary tract carries hazards as well as benefits, and these hazards should not be underestimated or taken lightly.

Staged surgery for jaundice

The increased risk of surgery in patients with obstructive jaundice has been recognised for many decades. In patients undergoing surgery for carcinoma of the pancreas, Braasch and Gray (1977) demonstrated that the major complications of haemorrhage and renal failure were related to the depth of jaundice at the time of surgery. The original resection of the pancreatic head described by Whipple was a two-stage procedure, to relieve jaundice and allow recovery of liver function and prevent the inevitable haemorrhagic problems (Whipple et al 1935). Although this approach has waned in popularity since that time, a number of surgeons have continued to practise two-stage procedures in order to reduce mortality from some of the reversible side effects of obstructive jaundice. Some of these reversible factors (infection, endotoxaemia, renal impairment, hypoalbuminaemia and coagulation disturbances) have already been discussed. However, the evidence for reduction of mortality by use of such a staged approach is difficult to determine. Monge and his colleagues (1964) reported a reduced mortality rate in high risk patients when treated by two-stage surgery. Maki and his colleagues (1966) described a fall in mortality from 50% for the ten years ending in 1959, to 8% for the following five years, and attributed this to adoption of a two-stage method. There are no controlled studies to support these findings, however.

Two-stage surgery in its classical form, with laparotomy and temporary cholecystojejunostomy or external T-tube drainage, has some obvious disadvantages which have reduced its popularity. Firstly, the initial laparotomy in itself in the jaundiced patient carries a significant mortality. In eight reported series between the years 1970 and 1979, 1699 patients were treated by simple biliary bypass for irresectable pancreatic and periampullary cancers. The pooled mortality rate for these cases was 21.9% (Benjamin 1981). Avoidance of even this minimal procedure would therefore be valuable, and for this reason the advent of a non-operative method for decompression of the biliary tract was particularly welcome.

Percutaneous transhepatic catheter drainage

This technique was first proposed as early as 1962, but the earliest series of patients successfully treated by the technique was that of Molnar & Stockum in 1974. Since then there have been a large number of reports which stress the low complication rate and uniform success in relieving jaundice which may be achieved. The technique has been adopted with enthusiasm in a large number of centres, and yet there has been no formal report of a controlled trial demonstrating clearly the benefits of preliminary percutaneous drainage. Nakayama and his colleagues reported 49 patients with malignant disease who came to second-stage surgery after preliminary percutaneous drainage, with an operative mortality of 8.2%. They compared this with a retrospective control group of 148 patients undergoing single-stage surgery, with an operative mortality of 28%. This study suffers not only from the use of a retrospective group of controls, but also from the complete absence of any statement of the criteria for drainage. Considerable technical advances have now been made in this area without any direct evidence for the benefit of the technique, and still without controlled studies. However, several trials are now in progress in centres around the world, and the results of these trials are awaited. Present available unpublished data from these studies shows no significant difference in post-operative mortality for patients undergoing percutaneous drainage. Dooley and his colleagues (1979) reported an operative mortality of 24% in a small group of patients who underwent surgery following drainage.

We have carefully studied a prospective series of patients with malignant obstruction of the biliary tract who have undergone percutaneous drainage for carefully defined criteria (McPherson et al 1982b). Some of these patients have formed part of a prospective randomised controlled study. Thirty-three of the first 37 patients so reported underwent definitive surgery, and eight of these died without leaving hospital. At the time of writing the controlled study is at an early stage, but so far there is no apparent difference in major complications or survival between the drained and undrained patients. Percutaneous drainage was successful in relieving jaundice in almost all cases. Patients with impaired renal function showed an improvement in creatinine clearance during drainage, but despite an intensive intravenous feeding regimen it was not always possible to improve nutritional status during drainage, thus negating one of the aims of the staged procedure.

Such success as we have enjoyed has been bought at a price of several major complications. Biochemical abnormalities due to excessive electrolyte losses and problems with mechanical dislodgement of the tubes have been encountered. However, the most important complication was that of bacterial contamination. A study of serial specimens of bile from the drainage catheters and collecting bags shows rapid acquisition of environmental bacteria during the first few days of drainage. 40% of bile cultures were positive at the start of drainage, all with single organisms. By 20 days after insertion of the drain every catheter grew bacteria, and 79% showed a polymicrobial growth (McPherson et al 1982a). We subsequently found that it was possible to prevent this exogenous contamination by the use of povidone iodine as an antiseptic 'lock' in the taps and bags of the drainage system. A new closed drainage system has since been designed and implemented, which may further reduce this problem (Blenkharn & McPherson 1981).

Infection of these catheters is not merely an insignificant bacterial contamination, but has produced serious invasive sepsis. Two of the eight patients who died following surgery were found at autopsy to have intrahepatic abscess cavities in association with the track of the transhepatic catheter. Similar cases have been reported from the Mayo Clinic (Berquist et al 1981). Serious hazards of this type must be carefully considered when electing to treat the obstructed biliary tract with techniques of this type.

Physiological considerations of biliary drainage

Following relief of obstruction by percutaneous catheter there is a major choleresis, and bile volumes of four or more litres per day have been observed. The electrolyte content of this bile is such that hyponatraemia, hypokalaemia and acidosis may readily develop. This volume can often be replaced orally, but may sometimes require intravenous replacement. It is our own practice to administer an electrolyte solution which contains a volumetric replacement of the lost electrolytes in concentrated form, the flavour being disguised by blackcurrant juice.

The bile which is produced during the first few days of biliary drainage is of poor 'quality', so that excretion of an adequate bilirubin and bile salt load is achieved by high volumes of bile with low concentration of these constituents. There are several reasons for this. The impaired liver is unable to return immediately to normal function after relief of obstruction. Moreover, loss of the recirculation of bile salts leads to diminution of bile salt dependent canalicular flow.

This latter factor may be of therapeutic relevance. Since bile salts are lost through the external fistula the total bile salt pool becomes rapidly depleted by loss of entero-hepatic circulation. For this reason oral bile replacement has been recommended, although it is not always possible to persuade patients to drink their own bile. Replacement in capsule form may be more palatable. The evidence has been presented above for the important role of bile salts in prevention of endotoxaemia. Additionally replacement of bile salts and improvement of canalicular flow may carry bilirubin as a 'passenger', and possibly also encourage elimination of other toxic substances from the circulation.

Drainage systems which obviate the external electrolyte and bile losses may have major physiological advantages. The operatively placed transhepatic U-tube (Saunders & Louw 1972) offers this advantage, as does advancement of a percutaneous drain through the biliary obstruction with drainage holes above and below the lesion. Percutaneous insertion of an endoprosthesis which has no communication with the outside is also attractive. This technique has been strongly recommended for bile duct carcinomas which are proven to be irresectable, but the technique carries a significant mortality (Dooley et al 1981), and access to the prosthesis if it becomes dislodged or blocked is difficult. For patients with malignant strictures in whom transhepatic tubes are to be placed operatively we have used a technique ('exo-endoprosthesis') in which the end of the tube brought out through the abdominal wall is buried in a subcutaneous pocket instead of exiting from the skin (Blumgart et al 1981). This technique offers the advantage of having no external tube to be managed, or to become infected, while retaining ready access to the tube as a minor procedure should jaundice recur, or the tube become blocked or infected.

References

Ansley J D, Isaacs J W, Rikkers L F, Kutner K H, Nordlinger B M, Rudman D 1978
   Quantitative tests of nitrogen metabolism in cirrhosis in relation to other manifestations of liver disease. Gastroenterology 75: 570–579

Baden H, Anderson H, Augestenborg G, Hanel H K 1971 Diagnostic value of gamma-glutamyl transpeptidase and alkaline phosphatase in liver metastases. Surgery, Gynecology and Obstetrics 133: 769–773

Bailey M E 1976 Endotoxin, bile salts, and renal function in obstructive jaundice. British Journal of Surgery 63: 774–778

Benjamin I S, Ryan C J, McLay A L C, Horne C H W, Blumgart L H 1976 The effects of portacaval shunting and portacaval transposition on serum IgG levels in the rat. Gastroenterology 70: 661–664

Benjamin I S, Imrie C W, Blumgart L H 1977 Liver biopsy in 'difficult' jaundice. British Medical Journal 2: 578

Benjamin I S, Blumgart L H 1979 Biliary bypass and reconstruction. In: Wright R, Alberti K G M M, Karran S, Millward-Sadler G D T (eds) Liver and biliary disease: pathophysiology, diagnosis, management. Saunders, London, ch 54

Benjamin I S 1981 Tumour and host: aims and decisions in pancreatic cancer. In: Cohn I Jr, Hastings P R (eds) Pancreatic cancer. U.I.C.C., Geneva

Benz E J, Baggenstoss A H, Wollaeger E E 1952 Atrophy of the left lobe of the liver. Archives of Pathology 53: 315–330

Berquist T H, May G R, Johnson C M, Adson M A, Thistle J L 1981 Percutaneous biliary decompression: internal and external drainage in 50 patients. American Journal of Roentgenology 136: 901–906

Bismuth H, Kuntziger H, Corlette M B 1975 Cholangitis with acute renal failure: priorities in therapeutics. Annals of Surgery 81: 881–887

Blenkharn J I, MacPherson G A D 1981 An improved system for external biliary drainage. Lancet 2: 781–782

Blumgart L H, Kennedy A 1973 Carcinoma of the ampulla of Vater and duodenum. British Journal of Surgery 60: 33–40

Blumgart L H, Carachi R, Imrie C W, Benjamin I S, Duncan J G 1977 Diagnosis and management of post-cholecystectomy symptoms: the place of endoscopy and retrograde choledochopancreatography. British Journal of Surgery 64: 809–816

Blumgart L H, Salmon P R, Cotton P B 1974 Endoscopy and retrograde choledochopancreatography in the diagnosis of the patient with jaundice. Surgery, Gynecology and Obstetrics 138: 565–570

Blumgart L H, Voyles C R, Smadja C 1981 Exo-endoprosthesis for relief of obstructive jaundice. Lancet 2: 306–307

Boey J H, Way L W 1980 Acute cholangitis. Annals of Surgery 191: 264

Braasch J W, Gray B N 1977 Considerations that lower pancreatoduodenectomy mortality. American Journal of Surgery 133: 480 — 484

Cattell R B, Braasch J W 1959 General considerations in the management of benign strictures of the bile duct. New England Journal of Medicine 261: 929–933

Chock E, Wolfe B M, Matolo N M 1981 Acute suppurative cholangitis. Surgical Clinics of North America 61: 885–892

DenBesten L, Doty J E 1981 Pathogenesis and management of choledocholithiasis. Surgical Clinics of North America 61: 893–907

Dooley J S, Dick R, Irving D, Olney J, Sherlock S 1981 Relief of bile duct obstruction by the percutaneous transhepatic insertion of an endoprosthesis. Journal of Radiology 32: 163–172

Dooley J S, Olney J, Dick R, Sherlock S 1979 Non-surgical treatment of biliary obstruction. Lancet 2: 1040–1043

Galloway S, Casarella W J, Price J B 1973 Unilobar veno-occlusive disease of the liver. American Journal of Roentgenology 119: 89–94

Goodman M W, Ansel H J, Vennes J A et al 1980 Is intravenous cholangiography still useful? Gastroenterology 79: 642

Goresky C A, Haddad H H, Kluger W S, Nadleau B E, Bach G G 1974 The enhancement of maximal bilirubin excretion with taurocholate-induced increments in bile flow. Canadian Journal of Physiology and Pharmacology 52: 389–403

Greim H, Trulzsch D, Czygan P, Rudick J, Hutterer F, Schaffner F, Popper H 1972 Mechanism of cholestasis: 6. Bile acids in human livers with or without biliary obstruction. Gastroenterology 63: 846–850

Guest J, Ryan C J, Benjamin I S, Blumgart L H 1978 Portacaval transposition and subsequent partial hepatectomy in the rat: effects on liver atrophy, hypertrophy and regenerative hyperplasia. British Journal of Experimental Pathology 58: 140–146

Hall L, Bergen A, Henriken J E 1979 Blood flow in normal and cholestatic dogs as measured by intraparenchymal injection of Xenon-133. European Surgical Research 9: 357–363

Ham J 1979 Partial and complete atrophy affecting hepatic segments and lobes. British Journal of Surgery 66: 333–337

Heaton K W 1979 Bile salts. In: Wright R, Alberti K G M M, Karran S, Millward-Sadler G D T (eds) Liver and biliary disease: pathophysiology, diagnosis, management. Saunders, London, ch 12

Hunt D R 1979 Changes in liver blood flow with development of biliary obstruction in the rat. Australian and New Zealand Journal of Surgery 49: 733–737

Imrie C W, Mackay A J, Benjamin I S, Blumgart L H 1978 Secondary acute pancreatitis: aetiology, prevention, diagnosis and management. British Journal of Surgery 65: 399–402

Ingoldby C J H 1982 Changes in endotoxin handling in obstructive jaundice in rats. British Journal of Surgery (in press)

Jackaman F R, Hilson G R F, Lord Smith of Marlow 1980 Bile bacteria in patients with benign bile duct stricture. British Journal of Surgery 67: 329–332

Johnson A G, Stevens A E 1969 Importance of the size of the stoma in choledochoduodenostomy. Gut 10: 68–70

Johnston I D A 1981 Indications for nutritional therapy prior to major surgery. In: Hill G C (ed) Nutrition and the Surgical Patient. Churchill Livingstone, Edinburgh, ch 4

Jones S A 1973 Sphincteroplasty (not sphincterotomy) in treatment of biliary tract disease. Surgical Clinics of North America 53: 1123–1137

Keighley M R B 1977 Microorganisms in the bile: a preventable cause of sepsis after biliary surgery. Annals of the Royal College of Surgeons of England 59: 328–334

Kirby J, Heaton K W, Burton J L 1974 Pruritic effect of bile salts. British Medical Journal 4: 693–695

Knill-Jones R P, Cochrane K M, Sokhi G S, Russell R I, Blumgart L H 1975 Early diagnosis of jaundice. A computer and clinical study. British Journal of Surgery 62: 654–655

Koyama K, Takagi Y, Ito K, Sato T 1981 Experimental and clinical studies on the effect of biliary drainage in obstructive jaundice. American Journal of Surgery 142: 293–299

Kune G A 1972 Current practice of biliary surgery. Little, Brown, Boston

Lance P, Bevan P G, Hoult J G, Paton A 1977 Liver biopsy in 'difficult jaundice'. British Medical Journal 2: 236

Lane C E, Sawyers J L, Riddell D H, Scott H W 1973 Long-term results of Roux-en-Y hepatocholangiojejunostomy. Annals of Surgery 177: 714–722

Lee E, Ross B D, Haines J R 1972 The effect of experimental bile duct ligation on critical biosynthetic functions of the liver. British Journal of Surgery 59: 564–568

Lesser P B, Warshaw A L 1975 Differentiation of pancreatitis from common bile duct obstruction with hyperamylasaemia. Gastroenterology 68: 636–641

Lygidakis N J 1981 Histological changes and intrahepatic biliary abnormalities in extrahepatic biliary tract obstruction. Surgery, Gynecology and Obstetrics 153: 532–536

Lynn J A 1979 Physiology of the extrahepatic biliary tree. In: Wright R, Alberti K G M M, Karran S, Millward-Sadler G D T (eds) Liver and biliary disease: pathophysiology, diagnosis, management. Saunders, London, ch 11, p 228

Magnani H N, Alaupovic P 1976 Utilization of the quantitative assay of lipoprotein-X in the differential diagnosis of extrahepatic obstructive jaundice and intrahepatic diseases. Gastroenterology 71: 87–93

Maines M D, Kappas A 1975 The degradative effect of porphyrins and heme compounds on components of the microsomal mixed function oxidase system. Journal of Biological Chemistry 250: 2363–2369

Maingot R 1964 Injuries of the biliary tract. In: Smith R, Sherlock S (eds) Surgery of the gallbladder and bile ducts. Butterworth, London

Maki T, Sato T, Kakizaki G 1966 Pancreatoduodenectomy for periampullary carcinomas. Appraisal of two-stage procedure. Archives of Surgery 92: 825

Makler P T, Lewis E, Cantor R, Charkes N D, Malmud L S 1980 Nonvisualization of the left lobe of the liver due to atrophy or aplasia. Clinical Nuclear Medicine 5: 163–165

McCollum W B, Jordan P H Jr 1975 Obstructive jaundice in patients with pancreatitis without associated biliary tract disease. American Journal of Surgery 182: 116–120

McPherson G A D, Benjamin I S, Boobis A R, Brodie M J, Hampden C, Blumgart L H 1982b Antipyrine elimination as a dynamic test of hepatic functional integrity in obstructive jaundice. Gut (in press)

McPherson G A D, Benjamin I S, Habib N A, Bowley N B, Blumgart L H 1982c Percutaneous transhepatic drainage in obstructive jaundice: advantages and problems. British Journal of Surgery (in press)

McPherson G A D, Blenkharn J I, Nathanson B, Bowley N B, Benjamin I S, Blumgart L H

1982a Significance of bacteria in external biliary drainage systems: a possible role for antisepsis. Journal of Clinical Surgery 1: 22–26

McPherson G A D, Echetebu Z O, Moss D W, Blumgart L H 1981 Studies of human bile during tube drainage of the obstructed biliary tree. British Journal of Surgery 68: 36

Molnar W, Stockum A E 1974 Relief of obstructive jaundice through a percutaneous transhepatic catheter — a new therapeutic method. American Journal of Roentgenology 122: 356–367

Monge J J, Judd E S, Gage R P 1964 Radical pancreatoduodenectomy: a 22-year experience with the complications, mortality rate and survival rate. Annals of Surgery 160: 711

Moody F G 1981 Surgical applications of sphincteroplasty and choledochoduodenostomy. Surgical Clinics of North America 61: 909–922

Myracle M R, Stadalnik R C, Blaisdell F W, Farkas J P, Matin P 1981 Segmental biliary obstruction: diagnostic significance of bile duct crowding. American Journal of Roentgenology 137: 169–171

Nagorney D, Mathie R T, Lygidakis N J, Blumgart L H 1982 Effects of increased bile duct pressure on hepatic blood flow in the dog (Submitted for publication)

Nakayama T, Ikeda A, Okuda K 1978 Percutaneous transhepatic drainage of the biliary tree. Gastroenterology 74: 554–559

Neale G, Lewis B, Weaver V, Panveliwalla D 1971 Serum bile acids in liver disease. Gut 12: 145–152

Price C P, Alberti K G M M 1979 Biochemical assessment of liver function. In: Wright R, Alberti K G M M, Karran S, Millward-Sadler G D T (eds) Liver and biliary disease: pathophysiology, diagnosis, management. Saunders, London, ch 17

Price C P, Sammons H G 1974 The nature of the serum alkaline phosphatases in liver disease. Journal of Clinical Pathology 27: 392–398

Price C P, Sammons H G 1976 An interpretation of the serum alkaline phosphatase isoenzyme patterns in patients with obstructive liver disease. Journal of Clinical Pathology 29: 976–980

Reynolds B M, Dargan E L 1959 Acute obstructive cholangitis: a distinct clinical syndrome. Annals of Surgery 150: 299

Ryan C J, Benjamin I S, Blumgart L H 1974 Portacaval transposition in the rat: a new model and its effects on liver and body weight. British Journal of Surgery 61: 224–228

Sagar S, Shields R 1980 Fibrinogen in the 'hepato-renal syndrome': an experimental study. British Journal of Surgery 67: 562–564

Saharia P C, Zuidema G D, Cameron J L 1977 Primary common duct stones. Annals of Surgery 185: 598–604

Salen G, Nicolau G, Shefer S, Mosbach E H 1975 Hepatic cholesterol metabolism in patients with gallstones. Gastroenterology 69: 676–684

Sarles H, Sahel J 1978 Cholestasis and lesions of the biliary tract in chronic pancreatitis. Gut 19: 851–857

Schaffner F, Javitt N B 1966 Morphologic changes in hamster livers during intrahepatic cholestasis induced by taurolithocholate. Laboratory Investigation 15: 1783–1792

Schaffner F, Bacchin P G, Hutterer F, Scharnbeck H H, Sarkozi L L, Denk H, Popper H 1971 Mechanism of cholestasis: 4 structural and biochemical changes in the liver and serum in rats after bile duct ligation. Gastroenterology 60: 888–897

Scott J, Summerfield J A, Elias E, Dick R, Sherlock S 1977 Chronic pancreatitis: a cause of cholestasis. Gut 18: 196–201

Sedgwick C E, Poulantzas J K, Kune G A 1966 Management of portal hypertension secondary to bile duct stenosis: review of 18 cases with splenorenal shunt. Annals of Surgery 163: 949–953

Smith, Lord 1978 Injuries of the liver, biliary tree and pancreas. British Journal of Surgery 65: 673–677

Smith, Sir Rodney 1978 Cancer of the pancreas — Thom Bequest Lecture. Journal of the Royal College of Surgeons of Edinburgh 23: 133–150

Snape W J, Long W B, Trotman B W, Marin G A, Czaja A J 1976 Marked alkaline phosphatase elevation with partial common bile duct obstruction due to calcific pancreatitis. Gastroenterology 70: 70–73

Starzl T E, Francavilla A, Halgrimson C G et al 1973 The origin, hormonal nature, and action of hepatotrophic substances in portal venous blood. Surgery, Gynecology and Obstetrics 137: 179–199

Strasberg S M, Dorne B C, Redinger R N, Small D N, Egdall R H 1971 Effect of alteration of biliary pressure on bile composition — a method for study: primate biliary physiology. V. Gastroenterology 61: 357–362

Terblanche J, Saunders S J, Louw J H 1972 Prolonged palliation in carcinoma of the main hepatic duct junction. Surgery 71: 720–731

Thomas H C, Ryan C J, Benjamin I S, Blumgart L H, MacSween R N M 1976 The immune response in cirrhotic rats. Gastroenterology 71: 114–117

Thomas J L, Bernardino M E 1980 Segmental biliary obstruction: its detection and significance. Journal of Computer Assisted Tomography 4: 155–158

Tsuzuki T, Hoshimo Y, Uchiyama T, Kitazima M, Mikata A, Matsuki S 1972 Compensatory hypertrophy of the lateral quadrant of the left hepatic lobe due to atrophy of the rest of the liver appearing as a mass in the left upper quadrant of the abdomen. American Journal of Surgery 177: 406–410

Wardle E N 1975 Endotoxaemia and the pathogenesis of acute renal failure. Quarterly Journal of Medicine 44: 389–395

Way L W, Dunphy J E 1972 Biliary stricture. American Journal of Surgery 124: 287–295

Way L W, Bernhoft R A, Thomas J M 1981 Biliary stricture. Surgical Clinics of North America 61: 963–972

Welch J P, Donaldson G A 1976 The urgency of diagnosis and surgical treatment of acute suppurative cholangitis. American Journal of Surgery 131: 527

Whipple A O, Parsons W B, Mullins C R 1935 Treatment of carcinoma of the ampulla of Vater. Annals of Surgery 102: 763

Williams L F Jr, Schoetz D J Jr 1981 Primary sclerosing cholangitis. Surgical Clinics of North America 61: 951–962

11 Carcinoma of the gallbladder and biliary ducts

RONALD K. TOMPKINS

Introduction

Less heralded, but far more lethal and challenging to manage than biliary lithiasis, are the malignant tumours of the gallbladder and biliary ducts. These lesions demand the anatomical knowledge and technical expertise of the diagnostic radiologist, gastroenterologist and surgeon. Increasing experience with these tumours in many medical centres around the world has led to a concerted evaluation and rethinking of older plans of management of these frustratingly difficult lesions. This chapter will be an attempt to present the current state of our knowledge and to point out some avenues by which we may advance in our treatment in the future.

Cancer of the gallbladder

Natural history

Since its description by Stoll in 1777, carcinoma of the gallbladder has been a highly lethal but difficult-to-diagnose disease. The incidence is not clearly established but estimates range between 0.4% of all gallbladder operations in Sweden (Welton et al 1979) and 0.08% of all patients admitted to the M.D. Anderson hospital and Tumor Institute over a 36-year period (Perpetuo et al 1978). If the figure of 500 000 cholecystectomies annually in the United States is accepted then it would be expected that there would be about 2000 cases of gallbladder cancer discovered at operation each year.

Patients with gallbladder cancer are on the average in their seventh decade and about six times more likely to be female than male. Only 2% do not have gallstones. The median survival in a group of well-studied patients was 5.2 months (Perpetuo et al 1978). Mildly or moderately symptomatic patients survived a median of 6.5 months and patients treated with chemotherapy survived a median of 5.8 months versus a median of 4 months for those with no chemotherapy. A five year survival figure of 2–3% is the expectation (Fig. 11.1).

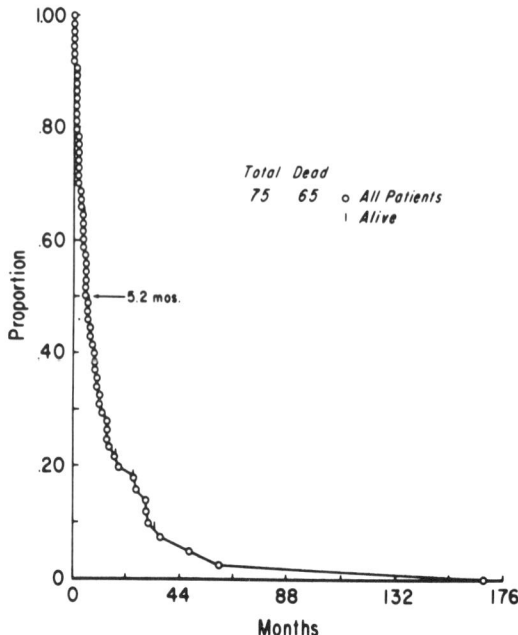

Fig. 11.1 Survival of patients with gallbladder cancer from diagnosis. (Reproduced with permission from Perpetuo et al 1978.)

Etiologic factors

a) Gallstones

While virtually all patients with gallbladder carcinoma have gallstones, certainly the vast majority of patients with gallstones do not develop carcinoma. Some authors have suggested that the chronic irritation of gallstones predisposes to malignant degeneration while others have taken the obverse view that stones occur as a consequence of the tumour. In this connection it is interesting to note that, since 1968, the total deaths and total crude mortality rates for gallbladder cancer have fallen in the U.S. This has been largely due to a decline in these figures for white women (Table 11.1).

During the same time, the number of cholecystectomies performed in the U.S. rose (at a yearly rate) from 1.9 to 2.1 per 1000 population (Diehl 1980). This is suggestive but not conclusive data that an increasing incidence of chole-cystectomies (which tend to be done in a more affluent segment of the society) has lowered the risk of dying from gallbladder cancer. This assumption requires validation, however, as the two observations may be coincidental.

b) Racial-ethnic influences

While differing rates among various countries might be influenced by different diagnostic practices and recording characteristics, the data from the U.S. show that there are racial differences in the incidence of gallbladder cancer. Whites in the U.S. have an incidence of gallbladder cancer which is 50% higher than that of

Table 11.1 Total deaths and crude mortality by sex and race for patients with gallbladder cancer (156.0), United States, 1968–1975. (Reproduced with permission from Diehl et al 1980.)

Parameter	Year							
	1968	1969	1970	1971	1972	1973	1974	1975
Total deaths	2777	2742	2555	2545	2518	2494	2476	2397
Crude mortality*								
White males	0.8	0.7	0.7	0.7	0.7	0.7	0.6	0.6
White females	2.2	2.1	2.0	1.9	1.9	1.8	1.8	1.8
Non-white males	0.4	0.3	0.3	0.4	0.3	0.3	0.5	0.4
Non-white females	1.0	0.9	0.8	0.9	0.8	1.0	0.9	0.9
Total	1.4	1 4	1.3	1.2	1.2	1.2	1.2	1.1

*Per 100 000. *Source*: Vital Statistics of the United States, vol. II (Mortality), part A, table 1-23 for 1969–1975; table 1-22 for 1968.

blacks. In the American Southwest the rate of gallbladder cancer was 1.4 per 100 000/yr in Caucasians; 10.5 per 100 000/yr in Spanish-Americans; and 21.1 per 100 000/yr in American Indians. This trend was similar for males as well as females (Diehl 1980).

Thus it is apparent that sex, ethnicity and cholelithiasis are among the most frequently observed risk factors in the development of gallbladder cancer (Fig. 11.2).

c) Carcinogens and other factors

Administration of dimethylnitrosamine to hamsters was found to result in gallbladder carcinoma if the hamsters had previously been implanted with a 'gallstone' (cholesterol pellet) (Kowaleski & Todd 1971). The proposal was made that gallstones damage the mucosa, making it more susceptible to the action of the carcinogen. In this respect, chemical analogues of bile salts, such as 3.methyl-cholanthrene as well as aflatoxin B_1 and other chemical agents have been shown to induce carcinoma in gallbladders of experimental animals. As yet, no human carcinogen has been identified. Other risk factors which have been proposed, but on less convincing data, are radiation, bacterial degradation of bile salts, toxins in industry, and a variety of associated medical conditions.

Research into etiologic factors may well advance along cell isolation lines. The recent establishments of a cell-line from human gallbladder carcinoma (Koyama et al 1980) should facilitate this type of experimentation.

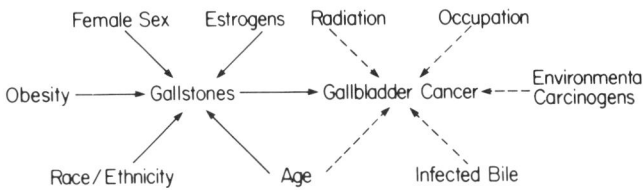

Fig. 11.2 Schema for epidemiology of gallbladder cancer. Solid arrows indicate established associations; broken arrows indicate unconfirmed relationships. (Reproduced with permission from Diehl 1980.)

Treatment

Since most gallbladder cancers are not diagnosed preoperatively and have hopelessly involved the liver and/or the structures in the porta hepatis at the time of operation, only biopsy or palliative manoeuvres are usually carried out. The tendency of carcinoma of the gallbladder to be locally invasive until late in the course of the disease is well described (Fahim et al 1962). Lymphatic spread occurs to the cystic and common duct nodes, then to the pancreatico-duodenal nodes and thence to para-aortic nodes. Venous drainage is to the quadrate lobe of the liver. Papillary type tumours spread within the ducts but account for less than 20% of all gallbladder cancers.

When the results of treatment of gallbladder cancer are reviewed, a helplessness invades the surgeon's spirit. However, several analyses have demonstrated that the group of patients who are able to be treated by cholecystectomy with or without extension of resection to adjacent areas may have a better result than average.

Moosa et al (1975) have retrospectively analysed the experience over 30 years at the University of Chicago in treatment of 82 patients with gallbladder cancer. Four patients survived for five years (4.9%). However, 40 of the 82 patients underwent no treatment at all. When the remaining 42 patients were considered, the five-year survival increased to 9.5%. Further, when only the 28 patients who underwent cholecystectomy were considered, the four five-year survivors constituted a 14.3% five-year survival rate. Thus, when discussing the long-term results, it is necessary to analyse the effects of surgical therapy in the small group of patients in whom an operative resection can be done.

Bergdahl (1980) analysed the survival of 32 patients who had been discovered to have carcinoma microscopically in removed gallbladders. Eleven of these patients had carcinoma confined to the mucosa and submucosa and were in Group A. Group B (21 patients) carcinomas involved the entire gallbladder wall. Group B had an operative mortality of 14.3% and the remainder were dead of carcinoma within 2 years 5 months, including one patient who was re-operated and underwent a right hepatic Lobectomy. Group A patients fared much better, however, with a five-year survival of seven of the 11 patients (63.6%) and a 10-year survival of five of 11 (45.5%). Clearly, the stage of the carcinoma relates directly to prognosis (Fig. 11.3). The author recommended that patients with microscopic carcinomas be re-operated with a wedge resection of 3–5 cm of normal liver and dissection of the regional lymph nodes.

Similar findings were reported by Nevin et al (1976) who retrospectively analysed their cases by stages: I = intramucosal only; II = involvement of mucosa and muscularis; III = all three layers involved; IV = all three layers and cystic lymph node; V = direct extension or metastases to liver or other organ. They found that six of seven patients (86%) with Stage I tumour who survived the operation of cholecystectomy lived five years or more. In addition the authors surveyed the literature and found 399 cases which could be classified histologically and by stage and found similar results (Table 11.2).

While these authors recommended simple cholecystectomy only for Stage I and II lesions, they favored radical cholecystectomy for Stage III and IV tumours in hopes of providing better survival. Stage V tumours are usually not treatable by surgical or any other means.

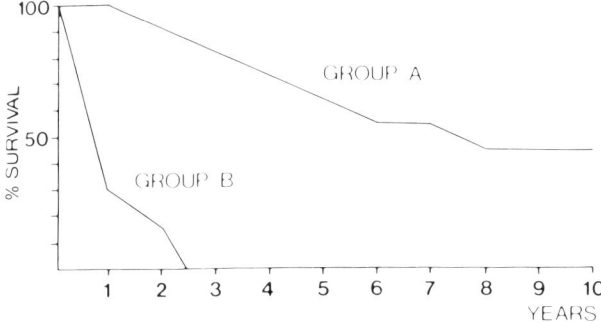

Fig. 11.3 Percentage survival in different groups of patients. Group A = carcinoma confined to mucosa and submucosa. Group B = carcinoma infiltrating all layers of the gallbladder wall. (Reproduced with permission from Bergdahl 1980.)

The enthusiasm for radical surgical procedures is not shared by Evander & Ihse (1981) nor by Ong's group (Koo et al 1981) in Hong Kong. Neither group was able to attribute any longer survival to the use of radical procedures for carcinoma of the gallbladder.

It is my approach to perform so-called radical excision of the gallbladder (with adjacent wedge of liver tissue and regional lymphatics) in those cases where the tumour is small and appears localised to the gallbladder (Nevin's Stages I, II and III). In more advanced lesions palliative decompressions are performed and the radiotherapist and medical oncologist are consulted regarding postoperative adjuvant therapy. It is estimated, from reviewed case material, that only approximately 12% of patients will fall into the Stage I or II groups, 16% into Stage III or IV group and 72% into the advanced category where only palliative procedures are possible (Piehler & Crichlow 1978).

Current recommendations

It is evident that earlier diagnosis and treatment can have a marked effect on survival. The only way to diagnose lesions at the Stage I or II level is by early cholecystectomy for stone disease. Yet the risk of dying from cholecystectomy is approximately the same as that of developing a carcinoma of the gallbladder in most population groups. Therefore it is not scientifically valid to recommend cholecystectomy for the prevention of possible carcinoma. The physician and surgeon can find much more statistical support when they recommend early

Table 11.2 Comparison between stage of lesion and survival of patients: analysis of 399 patients reported in the literature. (Reproduced with permission from Nevin et al 1976.)

Stage	No. of patients	Survival in years				
		1	2	3	4	5
I	8					8
II	32					32
III	91	37	27	13	8	6
IV	3					3
V	265	265				

elective cholecystectomy for the prevention of possible gallstone complications, such as jaundice, pancreatitis or acute cholecystitis, which have a higher incidence and a higher associated mortality risk in most populations of gallstone patients.

Surgeons should open all gallbladders and inspect the lining following removal. Consultation with the pathologist should be carried out in any suspicious case. In cases in which an early carcinoma of the gallbladder is identified in the operating room, consideration should be given to radical excision. This is much preferred over the delayed finding of carcinoma several days later and then agonising discussion as to whether the patient should be re-operated.

The rationale for performing right hepatic lobectomy in such cases appears weak when it is remembered that the gallbladder lies in the anatomical plane between right and left lobes of the liver. If one is going to embark on such radical procedures, then an extended right hepatic lobectomy, removing the medial segment of the left lobe of the liver, would be the minimum procedure necessary to remove all potential local invasion of tumour. Such a procedure may carry an inordinate risk of mortality when compared to wide wedge excision of the liver in the gallbladder fossa.

Adjunctive therapy

Treadwell and Hardin from the Scott and White Memorial Hospital in Texas have reviewed their experience with 43 patients with gallbladder cancer treated between 1950 and 1974 (Treadwell & Hardin 1976).

Carcinoma occurred in 1.2% of gallbladders removed from 3511 patients during that period. Females outnumbered males 2.6:1 and only 5% of the patients had no gallstones. Adenocarcinoma was found in 40 patients and three patients had a combination of squamous and adenocarcinoma. Cholecystectomy alone was done in 25 patients and was combined with wider resection of lymph nodes or liver tissue in three others. Exploration and biopsy was done in 14 patients. One patient died before operation. Five-year survival was 17% overall, but of 21 patients in whom the operation was done for cure, the survival was 33%. More extensive operations did not significantly prolong the patients' lives but the numbers were small. Histology of the tumour had no effect on survival. 15 patients received some type of adjunctive therapy (either radiation or chemotherapy or a combination) and they survived significantly longer than did the non-treated group. When patients with extensive disease outside the gallbladder were considered the

Table 11.3 Interval to death in patients with primary carcinoma of the gallbladder. (Reproduced with permission from Treadwell & Hardin 1976.)

Interval (yr)	No with adjunctive therapy	No without adjunctive therapy
<0.5	2(13%)	15(58%)
0.5–1	6(40%)	4(15%)
1—2	5(33%)	0
2–5	1(7%)	1(4%)
>5	1(7%)	6(23%)
Total	15	26

Table 11.4 Interval to death in patients with primary carcinoma of the gallbladder by extent of disease at operation. (Reproduced with permission from Treadwell & Hardin 1976.)

Interval (yr)	Widespread disease		No obvious disease	
	No with adjunctive therapy	No without adjunctive therapy	No with adjunctive therapy	No without adjunctive therapy
<0.5	4(44%)	12(75%)	0	1(10%)
0.5–1	2(22%)	4(25%)	1(17%)	2(20%)
1–2	3(33%)	0	3(50%)	0
2–5	0	0	1(17%)	1(10%)
>5	0	0	1(17%)	6(60%)
Total	9	16	6	10

longer than in previous reports. The authors feel more trials with mitomycin C are indicated (Table 11.5).

At present, there is no good data to indicate whether postoperative radiation and/or chemotherapy have any effect on prognosis in gallbladder cancer. adjunctive therapy seemed to be of more value. The nontreated patients were all dead within one year whereas two patients receiving treatment out of nine (22%) survived longer than one year (Tables 11.3 and 11.4).

Smoron, from Northwestern University (1977), analysed their results in radiotherapy of patients with unresectable carcinoma of the gallbladder and bile ducts. Of five patients with gallbladder cancer only one responded, but four of eight patients with bile duct cancer had response to treatment. Survivals were difficult to analyse in these two groups because of the small number of cases.

Von Eyben and associates (1980) have treated 10 patients with advanced gallbladder cancer (two Stage III and eight Stage V) with celiac or hepatic artery infusions of chemotherapeutic agents in seven and intravenous infusions in the others. Although no objective remissions occurred, the survival was somewhat

Table 11.5 Doses and results of mitomycin C in gallbladder carcinoma. (Reproduced with permission from von Eyben et al 1980.)

Case No.	Mitomycin C treatment				Overall total dose (mg/m^2)	Response	Survival (in months)	
	Intraarterially		Intravenously				After diagnosis	After mitomycin C
	No. of courses	Total dose (mg/m^2)	No. of courses	Total dose (mg/m^2)				
1	—	—	1	10	10	TF	7	1
2	—	—	1	10	10	TF	2	1
3	3	28	7	52	80	NC	10	10
4	3	32	5	33	65	NC	35+	23+
5	3	27	15	62	89	NC	66	13
6	3	30	—	—	30	PD	4	3
7	3	17	3	13	30	NC	6	5
8	—	—	6	53	53	PD	8	5
9	2	16	—	—	16	NC	2	1
10	5	41	—	—	41	PD	3	2

NC = stationary disease. PD = progressive disease. TF = treatment failure

Carcinoma of the cystic duct

This rare lesion is almost always found incidentally at operation for obstruction of the gallbladder or discovered in the specimen removed at cholecystectomy. In its advanced state, it is indistinguishable from carcinoma arising in the mid-portion of the bile ducts or in the gallbladder. The criteria for diagnosis of cystic duct carcinoma which were outlined by Farrar have been those applied to most of the 20 or so cases reported in the literature. These criteria are: a) the growth must be restricted to the cystic duct b) there is no neoplastic process in the gallbladder, hepatic or common duct c) histological examination must confirm carcinoma.

In a review of 25 cases by Nishimura et al (1975) cholecystectomy and removal of the entire cystic duct was the treatment in 52% of cases, whereas partial resection of the common duct was added in 32% of cases. The remaining 16% were diagnosed at autopsy. The tumours ranged in size from 0.4 cm to 3.2 cm in diameter with an average size of 1.3 cm. The prognosis is not entirely clear from the collected cases. Six patients died within one month after operation. Four patients died one to 11 months after operation. Nine patients were alive at 12–52 months after operation. No follow-up was available in the remaining patients.

Patients have been treated in a variety of fashions, with some receiving chemotherapy and/or postoperative irradiation.

Only 33% of the cases had associated gallstones (a figure quite similar to that seen in extrahepatic bile duct carcinoma). 81% of patients had right upper quadrant pain attacks, and a palpable mass was present in 41%, but 84% had distended gallbladders at operation (Manabe & Sugie 1978).

Operative removal of the gallbladder, entire cystic duct and periductal lymphatics is the treatment for localised lesions. If the adjacent common duct is involved, radical resection of the duct from the hilum to the pancreas is indicated, with reconstruction by a Roux-Y jejunal limb. In certain cases a Whipple procedure may be necessary to remove the tumour completely. The data to support adjuvant therapy is not convincing.

Bile duct cancer

The ideal treatment of the frustratingly small, yet most often unresectable bile duct cancers continues to elude the best efforts of biliary tract surgeons and oncologists. To add to the feeling of urgency surrounding the diagnosis and treatment of these lesions, there is evidence from a number of sources (Broden et al 1978, Cohn 1978, Tompkins et al 1981) that the incidence of the disease is increasing.

Natural history

The carcinomas of the bile ducts differ in a number of ways from those of the gallbladder. Firstly, they afflict males equally or more than females. Secondly, only a fraction (10–30%) are associated with stones. Thirdly, the course of bile duct cancer is more prolonged than that of gallbladder cancer.

Etiology

There are several relationships, though no proven causality, between toxins and bile duct cancer and between associated diseases such as ulcerative colitis and the development of biliary malignancy.

Aflatoxins have been incriminated in the causation of tumours in biliary ducts of animals but have not been established as a cause of the disease in humans (Tilak 1975).

Infestation with *Clonorchis sinensis* is found more frequently in patients with intrahepatic cholangiocarcinoma in the Orient (Murray-Lyon 1979) than in matched controls.

The possibility of sex hormones causing these lesions has been raised by reports of cholangiocarcinoma in young women taking oral contraceptives (Ellis et al 1978, Littlewood et al 1980) and in a young man taking high doses of anabolic steroids (Strohmeyer et al 1979).

The association between ulcerative colitis and cancer of the bile ducts seems to be more than just a chance relationship. Akwari et al (1975) have analysed their experience, and that in the literature, and concluded that: the onset of bile duct cancer is earlier in patients with ulcerative colitis; prior removal of the colon or successful medical management does not prevent the later occurrence of the biliary cancer; the tumour seems more aggressive in ulcerative colitis patients.

Finally, a recent study by Welton et al from New York (1979) has found that chronic typhoid carriers in that city died of hepatobiliary cancer six times more often between 1922 and 1975 than their matched controls. They theorised that bacterial degradation of bile salts might be the etiology although their findings did not exclude the possibility that the cancer had preceded the typhoid infection.

The association between cystic dilatation of the biliary system and carcinoma is being reported more frequently. Choledochal cyst involving the extrahepatic biliary tree is a well-known risk factor for development of carcinoma. Flanigan (1977) reported a case and found 24 cases reported in the literature up to 1977. Bloustein in the same year analysed the association of carcinoma with various cystic conditions of liver and bile ducts. He reported that carcinoma in solitary non-parasitic cysts of the liver or in polycystic liver disease was distinctly rare (Bloustein 1977). Carcinoma arose in frequencies of approximately 1% in congenital hepatic fibrosis, 4% in choledochal cyst and 7% in congenital cystic dilatation of the intrahepatic ducts (Caroli's disease).

By mid-1978, Kagawa et al were able to collect 47 cases of carcinoma associated with congenital duct dilatation, both intra- and extrahepatic (Kagawa et al 1978). Dayton et al (in press), from UCLA, have recently reported four cases of carcinoma associated with Caroli's disease from their experience and reviewed an additional 138 cases of Caroli's disease from the literature. The overall incidence of carcinoma in that review was 7%.

Symptoms

Virtually all the patients reported have been diagnosed because of the onset of jaundice, either clinically or chemically determined. In a recent review of the UCLA experience (Tompkins et al 1981), it was found that 91% of patients with bile duct cancer had bilirubin levels over 2.0 mg/100 ml, and 50% of the patients had serum bilirubin levels greater than 13.0 mg/100 ml. Serum alkaline phosphatase and transaminase levels were uniformly abnormal in all patients. Only about 29% of patients present with pain of biliary origin.

Weight loss, steatorrhea, pruritus and anemia are seen in varying frequencies among the patients. Cholangitis due to tumour obstruction does occur and tumour should be considered among the possible causes of obstruction in jaundiced patients with fever and pain.

Diagnosis
Cholangiography is necessary to make the diagnosis preoperatively. Our approach has been to utilise ultrasound first to determine whether or not the intrahepatic ducts are dilated in the jaundiced patient. If they are, a 'skinny' needle cholangiogram is done to determine the anatomical site of obstruction. If, for some reason, the ducts are not dilated, the initial attempt at cholangiography is made by endoscopic retrograde cannulation of the bile duct.

Site of lesion
Our experience (Tompkins et al 1981), as that of others, has shown that the vast majority of these tumours occur in the difficult hilar region at the confluence of the right and left hepatic ducts, often arising in one or the other duct and spreading down to the bifurcation (Fig. 11.4).

In addition, as the use of the operative cholangioscope has become routine in our institution, we have discoverd multicentric bile duct cancers in about 7% of our cases (Tompkins et al 1976, Tompkins & Berci 1981).

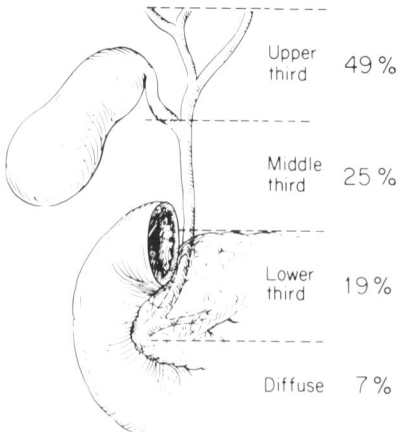

Fig. 11.4 Anatomic distribution of extrahepatic bile duct tumours. (Reproduced with permission from Tompkins et al 1981.)

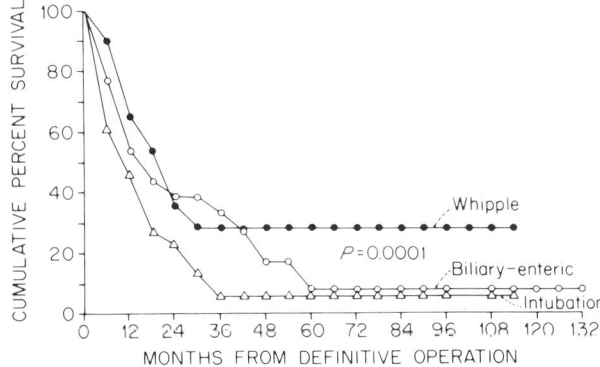

Fig. 11.5 Postoperative survival curves according to type of operation performed. When Whipple's procedure could be done for middle or lower third lesions, survival was significantly better. (Reproduced with permission from Tompkins et al 1981.)

Treatment

The ideal management of these tumours is complete surgical excision and this is possible in most of the patients with lesions arising in the middle or lower third of the bile duct. The UCLA experience has been that Whipple's procedure could be done with an overall operative mortality rate of 8% and a statistically superior long-term survival rate (Tompkins et al 1981) (Fig. 11.5).

In the technically difficult lesions of the upper third, however, resection often fails to remove all tumour, or is not possible because of early involvement of the portal vein and/or hepatic artery (Williamson et al 1980). Resection rate for these hilar tumours range in the literature from 5% (Bismuth & Corlette 1975) to 58% (Launois et al 1979) with mortality rates for the operation from zero (Akwari & Kelly 1979) to 50% (Fortner et al 1976). In our experience (Tompkins et al 1981), resection was carried out in 47% of patients with upper third lesions, with an operative mortality of 23% (Table 11.6) and a slightly longer, but not statistically better, survival as compared to those patients treated with tube bypass of the lesions (Fig. 11.6).

Terblanche has stated (1979) that he does not believe that resection should be done for lesions in the main hepatic duct junction area. He prefers to intubate

Table 11.6 Results of operations. (Reproduced with permission from Tompkins et al 1981.)

Location	Patients	Resected		Palliated		
		Number	Mortality rate	Number	Mortality rate	Total mortality rate
Upper third	47	22	23%	25	16%	19%
Middle third	24	16	0	8	0	0
Lower third	18	12	8%	6	0	6%
Diffuse	6	0	0	6	16%	16%
	95*	50	12%	45	11%	12%

*One patient died before operation.

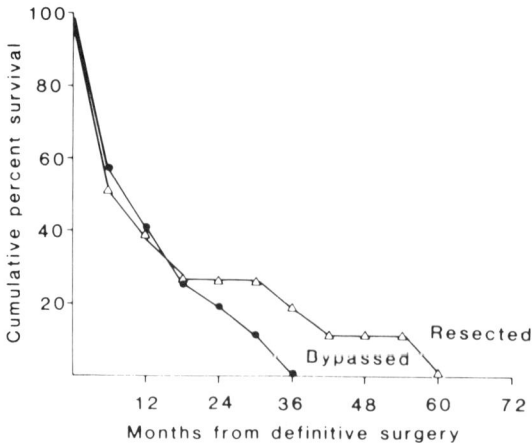

Fig. 11.6 Postoperative survival for upper third lesion patients showed a slightly better, but statistically insignificant, result for resection versus bypass. (Reproduced with permission from Tompkins et al 1981.)

these tumours with a U-tube and to treat them with radiotherapy. In a recent update of his experience (Terblanche 1981), he reported that two of 15 patients so treated have survived eight years and 10 years. Of the 13 who died, the longest survivor was five years. Assuming that the lesions treated were all indeed biopsy-proved carcinomas of the bile duct, these are results which compare very favourably to those of resection of the hilar lesions. Care to prove the diagnosis by biopsy must be taken, however. We have found the cholangioscopically directed punch biopsy of these lesions to be much more reliable than the older method of currettage of the lesion. One recent patient was seen in whom the cholangiogram and operative findings were consistent with a hilar tumour. The biopsy specimens removed by punch forceps, however, were not consistent with carcinoma and a tube was placed through the obstruction. The patient showed progressive clearing of the obstruction over the ensuing six to nine months and the tube was removed at 1.5 years. He is currently alive and well almost three years postoperatively. On clinical grounds alone this would have been a successful 'palliation' of a bile duct cancer.

Current recommendations

We continue to practise resection of all bile duct cancers, including those in the hilar region, when exploration indicates that the tumour can be *completely removed surgically*. Undoubtedly this criterion will not be satisfied as often in those patients with hilar lesions as in those with lesions in the middle or distal thirds of the ducts. We expect to see more of our hilar tumour patients undergoing intubation and some form of adjunctive therapy than has been the case in the past, when many hilar lesions were partially resected to relieve obstruction (i.e. 'palliative resections').

There is anecdotal experience in our group to show that radiation and/or chemotherapy may be of benefit in such patients. Reports of benefit in small and heterogeneous groups of patients (Kopelson et al 1977, Pilepich & Lambert 1978) also give some hope of benefit from radiation therapy in prolonging the survival of these patients. Extension of this therapy to the use of intraoperative radiation by one group has been associated with some improved palliation (Todoroki et al 1980). What is needed are results of prospective, collaborative, multicentre trials of adjuvant therapy in randomized patients to prove or disprove the value of adjunctive radiation and/or chemotherapy.

Clearly, future advances in the treatment of bile duct cancer will depend upon earlier cholangiographic diagnosis based upon a heightened suspicion of the lesion in patients with unexplained itching, subclinical jaundice or unexplained elevations of alkaline phosphatase.

References

Akwari O E, Kelly K A 1979 Surgical treatment of adenocarcinoma — location: junction of the right, left and common hepatic biliary ducts. Archives of Surgery 114: 22–25
Akwari O E, van Heerden J A, Foulk W T, Baggenstoss A H 1975 Cancer of the bile ducts associated with ulcerative colitis. Annals of Surgery 181: 303–309
Bergdahl L 1980 Gallbladder carcinoma first diagnosed at microscopic examination of gallbladders removed for presumed benign disease. Annals of Surgery 191: 19–22
Bismuth H, Corlette M B 1975 Intrahepatic cholangioenteric anastomosis in carcinoma of the hilus of the liver. Surgery, Gynecology and Obstetrics 140: 170–178
Bloustein P A 1977 Association of carcinoma with congenital cystic conditions of the liver and bile ducts. American Journal of Gastroenterology 67: 40–46
Broden G, Ahlberg J, Bengtsson L, Hellers G 1978 The incidence of carcinoma of the gallbladder and bile ducts in Sweden 1958 to 1972. Acta chirurgica scandinavia supplementum 482: 24–25
Cohn I Jr 1978 Gastrointestinal cancer. Surgical survey of abdominal tragedy. American Journal of Surgery 135: 3–11
Dayton M, Longmire W P Jr, Tompkins R K (in press) Is Caroli's disease a pre-malignant condition? American Journal of Surgery
Diehl A K 1980 Epidemiology of gallbladder cancer: a synthesis of recent data. Journal of National Cancer Institute 65: 1209–1214
Ellis E F, Gordon P R, Gottlieb L S 1978 Oral contraceptives and cholangiocarcinoma. Lancet 1: 207
Evander A, Ihse I 1981 Evaluation of intended radical surgery in carcinoma of the gallbladder. British Journal of Surgery 68: 158–160
von Eyben F, Hellekant C, Mattsson W, Ljungquist V, Jonsson K 1980 Mitomycin C in advanced gallbladder carcinoma. Acta Radiologica 19: 81–84
Fahim R B, McDonald J R, Richards J C, Ferris D O 1962 Carcinoma of the gallbladder: a study of its modes of spread. Annals of Surgery 156: 114–122
Farrar D A T 1951 Carcinoma of the cystic duct. British Journal of Surgery 39: 183–185
Flanigan D P 1977 Biliary carcinoma associated with biliary cysts. Cancer 40: 880–883
Fortner J G, Kallum B O, Kim D K 1976 Surgical management of carcinoma of the junction of the main hepatic ducts. Annals of Surgery 184: 68–73
Kagawa Y, Kashihara S, Kuramoto S, Maetani S 1978 Carcinoma arising in a congenitally dilated biliary tract. Gastroenterology 74: 1286–1294
Koo J, Wong J, Cheng F C Y, Ong G B 1981 Carcinoma of the gallbladder. British Journal of Surgery 68: 161–165
Kopelson G, Harisiadis L, Tretter P, Chang C H 1977 The role of radiation therapy in cancer of the extrahepatic biliary system. International Journal of Radiation Oncology, Biology, Physics 2: 883–894
Kowalewski K, Todd E F 1971 Carcinoma of the gallbladder induced in hamsters by insertion of cholesterol pellets and feeding dimethylnitrosamine. Proceedings of the Society for Experimental Biology and Medicine 136: 482–486

Koyama S, Yoshioka T, Mizushima A, Kawakita I, Yamagata S, Fukutomi H, Sakita T, Kondo I, Kikuchi M 1980 Establishment of a cell line (G-415) from a human gallbladder carcinoma. Gann: Japanese Journal of Cancer Research 71: 574–575

Launois B, Campion J P, Brissot P, Gosselin M 1979 Carcinoma of the hepatic hilus. Annals of Surgery 190: 151–157

Littlewood E R, Barrison I G, Murray-Lyon I M, Paradinas F J 1980 Cholangiocarcinoma and oral contraceptives. Lancet 1: 310–311

Manabe T, Sugie T 1978 Primary carcinoma of the cystic duct. Archives of Surgery 113: 1202–1204

Moosa A R, Anagnost M, Hall A W, Moraldi A, Skinner D B 1975 The continuing challenge of gallbladder cancer. Survey of thirty years experience at the University of Chicago. American Journal of Surgery 130: 57–62

Murray-Lyon I M 1979 Biliary tract disorders — cholangiocarcinoma. British Journal of Hospital Medicine 21: 478–481

Nevin J E, Moran T J, Kay S, King R 1976 Carcinoma of the gallbladder. Cancer 37: 141 148

Nishimura A, Mayama S, Nakano K, Seki Y, Tamaka N 1975 Carcinoma of the Cystic duct: case report. Japanese Journal of Surgery 5: 109–117

Perpetuo M D C M O, Valdivieso M, Heilbrun L K, Nelson R S, Connor T, Bodey G 1978 Natural history study of gallbladder cancer. Cancer 42: 330–335

Piehler J M, Crichlow R W 1978 Primary carcinoma of the gallbladder. Surgery, Gynecology and Obstetrics 147: 929–942

Pilepich M V, Lambert P M 1978 Radiotherapy of the extrahepatic biliary system. Radiology 127: 767–770

Smoron G L 1977 Radiation therapy of carcinoma of gallbladder and biliary tract. Cancer 40: 1422–1424

de Stoll M 1929 Rationis medendi in noscomio practico vindobonensi. Quoted in Rolleston H D, Mc Nee J S Disease of the liver, gallbladder and bile ducts, 3rd edn. MacMillan, London, p 691

Strohmeyer F W, Smith D H, Ishak A G 1979 Anabolic steroid therapy and intrahepatic cholangiocarcinoma. Cancer 43: 440–443

Terblanche J 1979 Carcinoma of the proximal extrahepatic biliary tree — definitive and palliative treatment. Surgery Annual 11: 249–265

Terblanche J 1981 Discussion of paper. Annals of Surgery 194: 455–456

Tilak T B G 1975 Induction of cholangiocarcinoma following treatment of a rhesus monkey with aflatoxin. Food and Cosmetics Toxicology 13: 247–249

Todoroki T, Iwasaki Y, Okamura T et al 1980 Intraoperative radiotherapy for advanced carcinoma of the biliary system. Cancer 46: 2179–2184

Tompkins R K, Berci G 1981 Operative cholangioscopy. Surgical Rounds 4: 20–28

Tompkins R K, Johnson J, Storm F K, Longmire W P Jr 1976 Operative endoscopy in the management of biliary tract neoplasm. American Journal of Surgery 132: 174–182

Tompkins R K, Thomas D, Wile A, Longmire W P Jr 1981 Prognostic factors in bile duct carcinoma. Annals of Surgery 194: 447–457

Treadwell T A, Hardin W J 1976 Primary carcinoma of the gallbladder: the role of adjunctive therapy in its treatment. American Journal of Surgery 132: 703–706

Welton J C, Marr J S, Friedman S M 1979 Association between hepatobiliary cancer and typhoid carrier state. Lancet 1: 791–794

Wenckert A, Robertson B 1966 The natural course of gallbladder disease: Eleven year review of 781 non-operated cases. Gastroenterology 50: 376–381

Williamson B W A, Blumgart L H, McKellar N J 1980 Management of tumors of the liver. Combined use of arteriography and venography in the assessment of resectability, especially in hilar tumors. American Journal of Surgery 139: 210–215

12 Biliary, pancreas and papilla of Vater interrelationships

FRANK G. MOODY

It is understandable that there should be a close relationship between events, both normal and abnormal, within the hepatobiliary tree and pancreas since their major ducts in man share a common opening at the papilla of Vater. Surprisingly, these relationships have been difficult to define and their associated pathophysiology is poorly understood. An important factor in this ignorance is the as yet undefined functions of the papilla of Vater and its sphincter of Oddi as they contribute to and are influenced by diseases within the hepatobiliary tree and pancreas. Necessarily, the documentation of my points of view will be incomplete, but it is consistent with what is known or has been subjected to critical analysis.

Embryology and functional anatomy

Embryogenesis
The bile and major pancreatic ducts in man share a common anlage from the primordial foregut (Boyden 1926). These relationships at six weeks of gestation are revealed in Fig. 12.1. Because of this common origin, the termini of the bile and major pancreatic ducts join within the papilla of Vater a few millimetres from its opening into the duodenum. The dorsal pancreas in the developing embryo is drained by the duct of Santorini. The duct of Wirsung, which joins the duct of Santorini prior to gestation, becomes the major pancreatic duct after birth, and the duct of Santorini is relegated the role of a subsidiary or minor conduit. This relationship is shown schematically in Fig. 12.2.

Congenital anomalies
There are numerous ways in which the development of the hepatopancreatic ductal system might go astray, thereby contributing to congenital malformations within the biliary tree, pancreatic ductal system or papilla (Dawson & Langman 1961). One of the more common anomalies within the pancreas is a failure of fusion of the ducts of Wirsung and Santorini (Millbourn 1960). This anomaly is called a pancreatic divisum or isolated ventral pancreas. It is present in about 10% of autopsy specimens of the pancreas and is observed in 3–5% of endoscopic

197

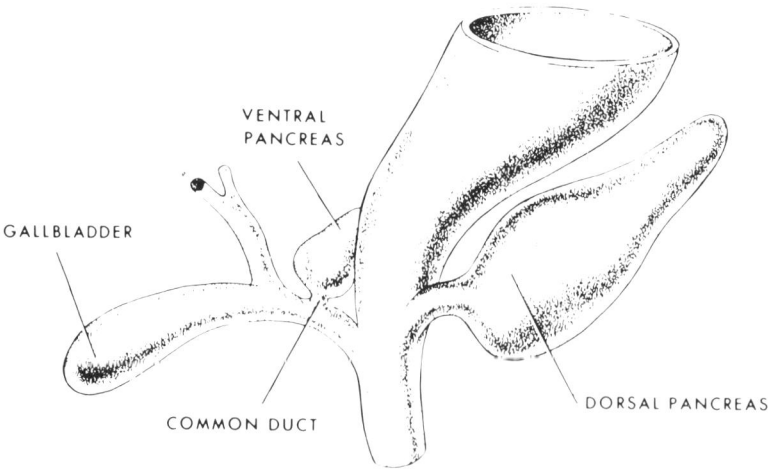

Fig. 12.1 Pancreas at approximately six weeks of gestation (modified after Arey) (Reproduced with permission from Brandborg 1978.)

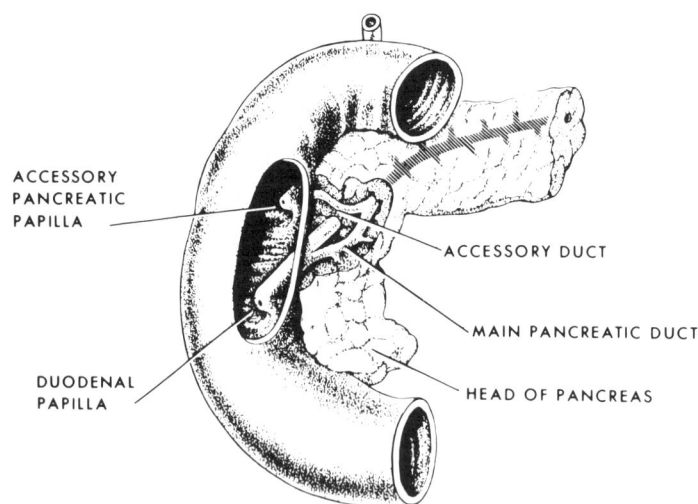

Fig. 12.2 Pancreas at birth (modified after Arey) (Reproduced with permission from Brandborg 1978.)

retrograde pancreatograms performed on patients with primary biliary tract disease (Cotton 1980). In this condition the duct of Santorini becomes the major conduit for egress of pancreatic juice. There is controversy as to whether this anomaly is merely a variant of ductal anatomy to be appreciated when interpreting pancreatograms, or whether it is the source of pancreatic disease (Rosch et al 1976, Gregg 1977, Mitchell et al 1979, Thompson et al 1981). Since most patients with the anomaly are without symptoms, the minor duct in their case must be adequate to handle the flow of pancreatic juice. The ventral pancreas must also have adequate drainage through the duct of Wirsung. In some patients the duct of

Wirsung is atretic and serves an underdeveloped ventral lobe that probably contributes little to pancreatic exocrine secretion.

A less common anomaly relates to the relationships of the opening of the duct of Wirsung to the opening of the papilla of Vater. In most people, the duct of Wirsung terminates on the inferior lip of the papilla just within its opening (about 80% of cases). Occasionally it lies several millimetres within the lumen of the papilla or is other than on its inferior lip. These aberrations are important to recognize, for at the time of exploration of the papilla the duct of Wirsung may be overlooked or injured in the course of sphincteroplasty.

Papillary anatomy

The intimate anatomy of the Vaterian complex is shown in Fig. 12.3. Note that the duct of Wirsung is separated from the bile duct by a thin veil of tissue called the transampullary septum. This septum in essence obliterates the common channel or ampulla found in lower mammalian species, an arrangement of important clinical significance. For example, the transpapillary passage of even the smallest gallstone would impinge on the septum and lead to obstruction of the pancreatic outflow tract. There is no possibility that a stone could lodge at the papilla in such a way that bile would be forced into the pancreatic ductal system under pressure, thereby producing pancreatitis. Opie's 'common channel' theory lacks not only experimental verification but even a reasonable anatomic possibility (Opie 1901). On the other hand, it is easy to see how oedema of the septum from pancreatitis might lead to obstruction to the flow of bile and transient jaundice. These notions, however, are highly speculative since even the normal role of the septum has yet to be elucidated. It is conceivable that it exists to monitor the flow of bile and pancreatic juice into the duodenum, while preventing the reflux of either secretion into the opposite channel. The margins of the septum also serve as an attachment

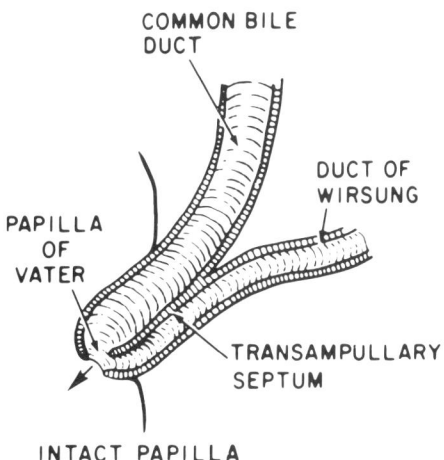

Fig. 12.3 Schematic details of the human papilla of Vater. Note the prominent septum that separates the duct of Wirsung from the terminal end of the bile duct (Reproduced with permission from Moody et al 1977.)

for the sphincter of Oddi and thereby provide an anchor for that portion of the sphincter that surrounds the duct of Wirsung.

Sphincter of Oddi

Possibly no structure has received more attention and unsubstantiated notoriety than the sphincter of Oddi. Boyden (1957) has contributed in a classic way to our appreciation of the elegant nature of this potentially important sphincter (Fig. 12.4). There is now general agreement that the sphincter of Oddi in man is a unique cluster of smooth muscle fibres that can be distinguished from the adjacent smooth muscle of the wall of the duodenum within which it is contained. The purpose of the sphincter of Oddi is not well understood. It appears to meter the rate of flow of bile and pancreatic juice into the duodenum and prevents the reflux of duodenal contents into either ductal system. A high pressure zone within the transpapillary portion of either ductal system has been demonstrated by retrograde transpapillary cannulation by Geenen and his colleagues (1980) and by antegrade cannulation at operation by Potts and myself as shown in Fig. 12.5. These mechanical functions of the sphincter are likely not critical, since its

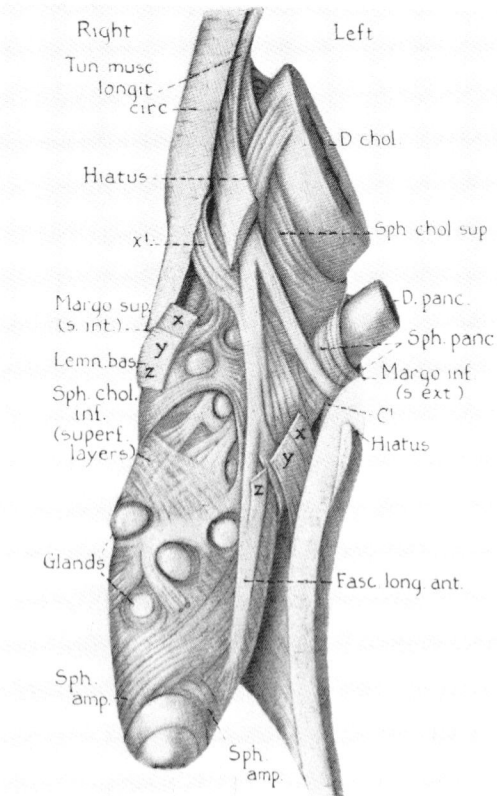

Fig. 12.4 Intimate details of the muscular components of the sphincter of Oddi (Reproduced with permission from Boyden 1957.)

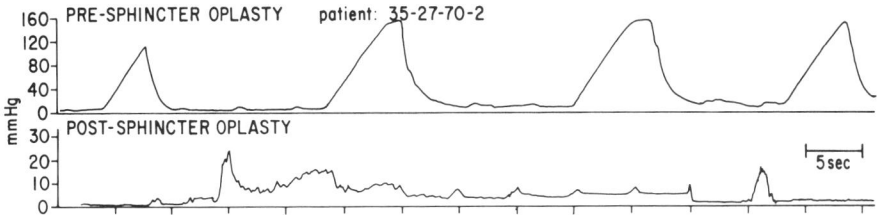

Fig. 12.5 Cyclical high pressure waves within the papilla of Vater recorded from a 1.7 mm Teflon catheter inserted through the cystic duct prior to sphincteroplasty. The wave forms were interrupted by a 2 cm transduodenal sphincteroplasty.

ablation or bypass is not followed by serious sequelae. This is surprising in view of the elegance of its structure and function.

The hormonal responses of the sphincter of Oddi are currently receiving a great deal of attention (Becker et al 1981). Clearly, the normal human sphincter relaxes in response to endogenous and exogenous cholecystokinin. But not all species respond in this way. The sphincter of Oddi of opposum, rabbit and prairie dog contract in response to cholecystokinin (Becker et al 1980, Sarles et al 1976, Doty et al 1981). In fact, cholecystokinin may be an agonist for the sphincter of Oddi of dog and even man under appropriate experimental conditions (Watts & Dunphy 1966, Toouli & Watts 1972).

It has been postulated that the varying interspecies responses of the sphincter of Oddi may relate to the activity of an inhibitory nerve (Behar & Biancani 1980, Toouli et al 1981). This is pure speculation, since little is known about neural influences upon sphincter function. Tansy & Kendall (1975) have recently summarized what is known in this area. In a word, the vagus appears to modulate a variety of humoral stimuli and is responsible for the intrinsic rhythmic contractions and tone of the sphincter. There is great need for a better understanding of neurohumoral influences on sphincter function. For example, it is possible that the sphincter of Oddi of man in some situations may respond in an adverse fashion to cholecystokinin, thereby contracting at the time of vigorous gallbladder emptying, leading to a true instance of biliary dyskinesia. No such situations have as yet been identified, but there is clear evidence that myoelectric activity within the sphincter region of the papilla of Vater in man is associated with contraction of the sphincter of Oddi and cessation of bile flow (Ono et al 1968, Becker et al 1981).

The papilla and biliary-pancreatic disease

Gallstones
There has been recurring speculation that the papilla of Vater may contribute to stone formation within the gallbladder as well as the biliary tree. This may have a rational based on the papilla's role in controlling the flow of bile, both into the duodenum as well as in and out of the gallbladder. The earthy stones that form within the dilated, thick-walled bile duct in papillary stenosis or distal bile duct stricture may well be a clinical example of how the papilla can contribute

to common duct stones. Recently, Hutton and his colleagues (1981) have shown that sphincteroplasty will prevent cholesterol gallstone formation within the gallbladder of prairie dogs fed a hypercholesterol diet. This may be a more relevant experimental finding, for it implicates the papilla of Vater in the pathogenesis of gallstones in this model. The result, in fact, is unexpected, since it is contrary to previous studies which suggest that sphincteroplasty renders canine gallbladder bile lithogenic (Cohn et al 1979). I am reluctant to suggest that sphincteroplasty may revert a lithogenic tendency in the human; the prairie dog experiments make this provocative thought a possibility. But at this point in time there is no evidence to support a primary role of the papilla in the etiology of biliary lithiasis. Papillary stenosis may contribute to stone formation as a consequence of obstruction to bile flow, but in this situation the stenosis is probably secondary to pre-existing stone disease.

Acute pancreatitis

Does the papilla of Vater play a role in the pathogenesis of acute pancreatitis? This has been a popular notion over the years in view of the strategic relationship of the terminal ends of the bile and pancreatic ducts within the papilla (Nardi & Acosta 1966). The studies of Opie at the turn of the century contributed to an extensive investigation of the possibility that biliary reflux into the pancreatic duct, especially in the presence of a stone within the papilla, might be a cause of pancreatitis. Unfortunately, little scientific evidence has been put forth to support the theory. As pointed out above, man does not usually have an ampulla or a significant length of a common channel. Clinical observation would suggest that gallstone pancreatitis is secondary to obstruction of the opening of the duct of Wirsung by compression of the transampullary septum as a stone traverses the papilla of Vater (Acosta & Ledesma 1974, Acosta et al 1978). Possibly pancreatitis associated with alcohol may also be a consequence of obstruction to the pancreatic duct within the papilla as a result of oedema or spasm of the sphincter of Oddi. This possibility has not been subjected to systematic study. Work thus far suggests that alcohol, even in high concentrations, has little effect on the sphincter of Oddi. It is possible, however, that it may influence transpapillary resistance by inducing an inflammatory response within the papilla. The resulting increased blood flow and oedema could contribute to a reduction in the diameter of the terminus of the duct of Wirsung (Tansy et al 1975). One final speculation relates to the association between hyperlipidemia and pancreatitis. Possibly an increased secretion of biliary lipids could lead to inflammation within the papilla and pancreatitis on the basis of outflow obstruction. As will be discussed below, submucosal cholesterol deposits can occur within the papillary portion of the bile duct in a manner similar to that seen in cholesterolosis of the gallbladder.

Biliary dyskinesia

There has been a sustained interest in the possibility that an intense contraction of the sphincter of Oddi may be associated with episodic upper abdominal pain (Dahl-Iversen et al 1958). It is presumed that such pain is either from the papilla itself or from distention of either the bile or pancreatic ducts as their secretions are impeded by prolonged occlusion of the papilla. Dyskinesia implies that the papilla would be closed at a time when it should be open, such as during contraction of the gallbladder or active secretion of pancreatic juice. The cholecystokinin test, when positive, may reproduce a patient's pain on this basis (Freeman et al 1975). A similar explanation might be provided for the Nardi test in which the sphincter of Oddi is induced to contract by the intramuscular injection of morphine (10 mg), and pancreatic secretion is activated by the administration of prostigmine (1 mg) (Nardi & Acosta 1966). Unfortunately, these tests have a very low specificity and therefore are not useful clinically (Steinberg et al 1980). It is possible, however, that when they initiate upper abdominal pain, the pain is related to spasm of the sphincter of Oddi. This hypothesis cannot be tested until methods are available for assessing papillary function in the awake, unsedated subject during exposure to provocative stimuli.

Diseases of the papilla of Vater

Classification
The papilla of Vater may be the site of congenital, neoplastic, inflammatory or motor abnormalities (Table 12.1, Moody 1981). Each entity provides a diagnostic and therapeutic challenge. In fact, there exists considerable scepticism as to whether the papilla is the site of unique pathology, or whether it is merely a victim of its strategic relationship to the biliary tree and pancreas.

Recent advances in radiographic and ultrasonic imaging have provided a means for more precise identification of hepatobiliary and pancreatic disease. While endoscopic cholangiopancreatography has been helpful in evaluating the size and configuration of the bile and pancreatic ducts, it has been less useful in providing information on abnormalities of the papilla (Blumgart et al 1977). Possibly this paradox relates to the fact that primary diseases of the papilla, other than infiltrating or ulcerating neoplasms, cause little distortion of its external appearance. Stenotic lesions would be missed, since the catheter used to instill radio contrast material would be inserted through the lesion. An inability to cannulate either ductal system might represent the presence of inflammation or

Table 12.1 Abnormalities of the papilla of Vater

Congenital anomalies
Ectopic papilla
Pancreatic divisum

Neoplasms
Papilloma
Carcinoma

Inflammation
Cholesterolosis
Stenosing papillitis
Gallstones
Pancreatitis
Peptic ulcer

Motor dysfunction

fibrosis (Gregg et al 1980). Antegrade biliary manometry, and more recently endoscopic retrograde transpapillary biliary and pancreatic manometry, have also been employed in an attempt to identify patients with abnormal resistances and pressures within the papilla of Vater (Geenen et al 1980). Unfortunately the interpretation of these studies is inconclusive, and the results of therapies based on them are difficult to assess because of lack of controls.

We have carried out a prospective, non-randomized study over the past 10 years of 82 patients with chronic, addictive upper abdominal pain, presumed to be due in part to dysfunction of their papilla of Vater. Each patient was subjected to an extensive medical evaluation to include endoscopic retrograde cholangio-pancreatography when it became available in our institution in 1974. Patients with neoplastic disease were excluded from the study. Each patient underwent an exploratory laparatomy and transduodenal sphincteroplasty and transampullary septectomy as previously described (Moody et al 1977). The clinical-pathological findings are presented in Table 12.2.

Congenital anomalies

Pancreatic divisum, a common variant of the pancreatic ductal system, is observed in about 5% of endoscopic retrograde pancreatograms. One must presume that patients studied in this way have symptoms of upper gastrointestinal disease. Cotton (1980) has observed rather extensive changes within the dorsal pancreatic duct of patients who have recurrent episodes of acute pancreatitis and this specific anomaly. Others have found the dorsal, as well as ventral, ducts to be normal, even when hyperamylasemia accompanies the clinical pain syndrome (Mitchell et al 1979). There is still a serious question as to whether either the opening of the duct of Santorini or the duct of Wirsung is abnormal in this entity. Division of the opening of the minor or major ducts has not been uniformly successful in relieving the severe pain experienced by some patients with this entity. I have been impressed with the atretic nature of the duct of Wirsung in two of the three cases that I have treated by sphincteroplasty and transampullary septectomy. I also performed, with reluctance, a plastic procedure upon the duct

Table 12.2 Clinical-pathologic correlations in 82 patients who underwent transduodenal sphincteroplasty and transampullary septectomy.

Clinical status	
Prior cholecystectomy	68
Prior choledochotomy	16
Prior sphincteroplasty	16
Recurrent acute pancreatitis	23
Chronic pancreatitis	2
Papillary findings	
Fibrosing septitis	31
Papillary stenosis	19
Papillary cholesterolosis	9
Papillitis	6
Ectopic Wirsung	3
Papillary web	3
Pancreatic divisum	3
Normal papilla	8

of Santorini in the third case, since the opening was small in contrast to the more distal duct. There are too few cases thus far studied to be certain of whether this is a clinical entity worthy of surgical intervention.

The opening of the duct of Wirsung is usually on the inferior lip of the papilla. Occasionally it may have a separate opening at any point on the circumference of the papilla, or at a point caudad from it. These variations are not associated with pathological change, but one must be aware of them, lest the opening of the major duct be injured or occluded at the time of papillary surgery. In two cases of the present series, the opening of the duct of Wirsung entered low on the inferior lip of the papilla, thereby presenting a long narrow channel into the major duct. Following its division anteriorly and excision of the ampullary septum, access was gained to a duct at least four times its more distal diameter. In an additional three cases, a mucosal web was encountered overlying the opening of the papilla. Since there was no evidence of inflammation to account otherwise for the pinpoint opening in this area, one must assume that the mucosal covering was a congenital defect or an inconsequential finding.

Inflammatory lesions

As can be seen from the above discussion, stenosing papillitis and ampullary septitis and fibrosis are the more common abnormalities of the papilla. Their association with cholelithiasis raises the possibility that they may be a consequence of injury from the transpapillary passage of gallstones. A confusing feature of papillitis relates to its tendency to occur years after cholecystectomy. The diagnosis of stenosing papillitis is obvious in the advanced case where there is dilatation of both the bile duct and the duct of Wirsung. In most cases, however, the ductal systems are normal by radiologic criteria. The major changes are within the papilla of Vater.

The operative findings in this disease usually include a normal appearance of the papilla on gross inspection. The opening of the papilla may allow passage of only a small urethral filiform from above (<2 mm), but the most striking finding relates to the opening of the duct of Wirsung, which may allow passage of only the smallest lacrimal probe. The presence of scar tissue is usually obvious as one cuts the anterior portion of the papilla to perform a sphincteroplasty and incises the transampullary septum prior to septectomy. These findings do not come as a surprise when ERCP shows dilation of the bile and pancreatic ducts as shown in Fig. 12.6. Such findings, however, are difficult to explain when the radiographs of the ductal system are normal. Furthermore, histologic verification of fibrosis and inflammation is difficult to obtain. For some reason, the fibrosis is associated with only minimal signs of inflammation, such as œdema or cellular infiltrate. The presence of dense collagen is not helpful, since the normal papilla and septum is composed primarily of collagen and smooth muscle. Occasionally, the fibrosis is overt and associated with a dense round cell infiltration on histologic examination. Acosta and his colleagues (1967) encountered a variety of pathologic findings in their histologic study of biopsies of the papilla of Vater obtained during transduodenal sphincterotomy. However, no histologic abnormalities were found in 42% of the specimens studied.

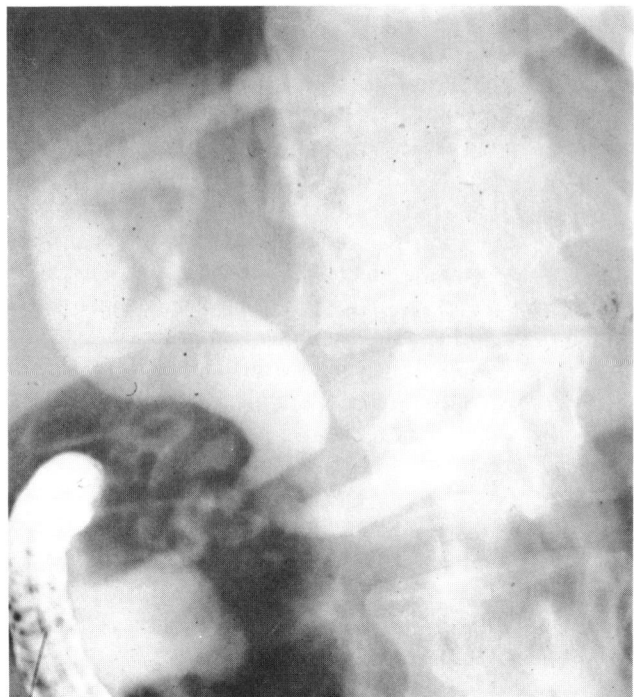

Fig. 12.6 This endoscopic retrograde cholangiopancreatogram reveals a dilated bile and major pancreatic duct in a patient with stenosing papillitis.

Cholesterolosis of the papilla is also a potential cause of stenosing papillitis. Possibly an entity that as yet has not been fully described should not be discussed in the context of this writing, but not to do so would detract from the theme of my hypothesis. I have classified nine of the 82 cases of papillary disease in this category. The reason for doing so is the finding of yellow submucosal deposits within the papillary portion of the bile duct, a 'strawberry papilla' if you will. In this entity, the papilla is usually hypertrophic and edematous, and the transampullary septum is greatly thickened. It is possible that the cholesterol deposits in this disease are secondary to injury incurred by the transpapillary passage of stone. Three of the nine cases in my experience had gallstones at cholecystectomy; three patients had cholesterolosis of the gallbladder without stones. Three patients in whom the pathology within the gallbladder is not known may have had either cholesterolosis or cholelithiasis, or both.

Chronic pancreatitis may also be associated with inflammation and fibrosis of the papilla of Vater. This can only be stated with assurance in two cases in this series in which the degree of stenosis within the papilla was accompanied by extensive fibrosis within the pancreas. Sphincteroplasty and septectomy did not provide pain relief in these patients, and this approach has been abandoned in patients with this disease. Possibly recurrent episodes of acute pancreatitis also produce sclerosis within the papilla. Twenty-three cases were placed in this category in my series in view of the episodic nature of the pain syndrome, and its association with hyperamylasoemia.

It would be premature to advise sphincteroplasty for chronic abdominal pain by either the endoscopic or transduodenal route at this point in time and understanding of papillary function. The study described above was presented to each patient as an attempt to find out what was wrong with them and not as a therapeutic panacea. Clearly, the results of the study thus far have directed our attention to the septum that lies between the bile and major pancreatic ducts. In addition, the primary role of the transpapillary passage of gallstones in inflammatory lesions of the papilla has been reinforced. It now remains to find an explanation for the severe epigastric pain experienced by these patients. Is it biliary, pancreatic or papillary in its origin? We lean towards a source either within the papilla or its septum, but spasm of the sphincter of Oddi cannot be excluded at this time. Unfortunately, there is no way to assess the presence of the latter during an episode of pain. My own personal view from working with such patients during the past decade both in and out of the operating room is that they have a problem with their papilla of Vater. Until better ways are developed to define papillary function, it is best not to disturb its role as gateway to and from the biliary and pancreatic ductal systems by indiscriminate biliary enteric bypass or sphincteroplasty.

References

Acosta J M, Ledesma C L 1974 Gallstone migration as a cause of acute pancreatitis. New England Journal of Medicine 290: 484–487

Acosta J M, Civantos F, Nardi G L, Castleman B 1967 Fibrosis of the papilla of Vater. Surgery, Gynecology and Obstetrics 124: 787–794

Acosta J M, Rossi R, Galli O M R, Pellegrini C A, Skinner D B 1978 Early surgery for acute gallstone pancreatitis: Evaluation of a systemic approach. Surgery 83: 367–370

Becker J M, Moody F G 1980 The dose/response effects of gastrointestinal hormones on the opossum biliary sphincter. Current Surgery January-February: 60–62

Becker J M, Duff W M, Moody F G 1981 Myoelectric control of gastrointestinal and biliary motility: A review. Surgery 89: 466–467

Behar J, Biancani P 1980 Effect of cholecystokinin and the octapeptide of cholecystokinin on the feline sphincter of Oddi and gallbladder. Journal of Clinical Investigation 66: 1231–1239

Blumgart L H, Carachi R, Imrie C W, Benjamin I S, Dunan J G 1977 Diagnosis and management of post-cholecystectomy symptoms: the place of endoscopy and retrograde choledochopancreatography. British Journal of Surgery 64: 809–816

Boyden E A 1926 The accessory gallbladder — an embryological and comparative study of aberrant biliary vesicles occurring in man and the domestic mammals. American Journal of Anatomy 38: 177–231

Boyden E A 1957 The anatomy of the choledochoduodenal junction in man. Surgery, Gynecology and Obstetrics 104: 641–652

Brandborg L L 1978 Anatomy, embryology, and developmental anomalies. In: Sleisenger M H, Fordtran J S (eds) Gastrointestinal Disease: Pathophysiology, Diagnosis, Management, 2nd Edn. Saunders, Philadelphia, ch 89, p 1389

Cohn M S, Schwartz S I, Faloon W W, Adams J T 1979 Effect of sphincteroplasty on gallbladder function and bile composition. Annals of Surgery 189: 317–321

Cotton P B 1980 Congenital anomaly of pancreas divisum as cause of obstructive pain and pancreatitis. Gut 21: 105–114

Dahl-Iversen E, Sorensen A H, Westengaard E L 1958 Pressure measurement in the biliary tract in patients after cholecystolithotomy and in patients with dyskinesia. Acta chirurgica scandinavica 114: 181–190

Dawson W, Langman J 1961 An anatomical-radiological study on pancreatic duct pattern in man. Anatomical Record 139: 59–68

Doty J E, Pitt H A, Kuckenbecker S L, DenBesten L 1981 The effect of gallbladder filling and cholecystokinin on the prairie dog sphincter of Oddi. Surgical Forum 32: 148–150

Freeman J B, Cohen W N, DenBesten L 1975 Cholecystokinin cholangiography and analysis of duodenal bile in the investigation of pain in the right upper quadrant of the abdomen without gallstones. Surgery, Gynecology and Obstetrics 140: 371–376

Geenen J E, Hogan W J, Dodds W J, Stewart E T, Arndorfer R C 1980 Intraluminal pressure recording for the human sphincter of Oddi. Gastroenterology 78: 317–324

Gregg J A 1977 Pancreas divisum: its association with pancreatitis. American Journal of Surgery 134: 539–543

Gregg J A, Clark G, Barr C, McCartney A, Milano A, Volcjak C 1980 Postcholecystectomy syndrome and its association with ampullary stenosis. American Journal of Surgery 139: 374–378

Hutton S W, Sievert C E Jr, Vennes J A, Duane W C 1981 The effect of sphincterotomy on gallstone formation in the prairie dog. Gastroenterology 81: 663–667

Millbourn E 1960 Calibre and appearances of the pancreatic ducts and relevant clinical problems. A roentgenographic and anatomical study. Acta chirurgica scandinavica 118: 286–303

Mitchell C J, Lintott D J, Ruddell W S J, Losowsky M S, Axon A T R 1979 Clinical relevance of an unfused pancreatic duct system. Gut 70: 1066–1071

Moody F G 1981 Surgical applications of sphincteroplasty and choledochoduodenostomy. Surgical Clinics of North America 61: 909–922

Moody F G, Berenson M M, McCloskey D 1977 Transampullary septectomy for post-cholecystectomy pain. Annals of Surgery 186: 415–423

Nardi G L, Acosta J M 1966 Papillitis as a cause of pancreatitis and abdominal pain: role of evocative test, operative pancreatography and histologic evaluation. Annals of Surgery 164: 611–621

Ono K, Watanabe N, Suzuki K, Tsuchida H, Sugiyama Y, Abo M 1968 Bile flow mechanism in man. Archives of Surgery 96: 869–874

Opie E L 1901 Etiology of acute hemorrhagic pancreatitis. Bulletin of the Johns Hopkins Hospital 12: 182–188

Rosch W, Koch H, Schaffner O, Demling L 1976 The clinical significance of the pancreatic divisum. Gastrointestinal Encoscopy 22: 206–207

Sarles J C, Bidart J M, Devaux M A, Eichinard L, Gastagnini A 1976 Action of cholecystokinin and caerulein on the rabbit sphincter of Oddi. Digestion 14: 415–423

Steinberg W M, Salvato R F, Toskes P P 1980 The morphine-protigmin provocative test — is it useful for making clinical decisions? Gastroenterology 78: 728–731

Tansy M F, Kendall F M 1975 Choledochoduodenal junction. In: Friedman M H F (ed) Functions of stomach and intestine. University Park Press, Baltimore. pp 93–120

Tansy M F, Salkin L, Innes D L, Martin J S, Kendall F M, Litwack D 1975 The mucosal lining of the intramural common bile duct as a determinant of ductal opening pressure. Digestive Diseases 20: 613–625

Thompson M H, Williamson R C N, Salmon P R 1981 The clinical relevance of isolated ventral pancreas. British Journal of Surgery 68: 101–104

Toouli J, Watts J M 1972 Actions of cholecystokinin/pancreazymin, secretin and gastrin on extra-hepatic biliary tract motility in vitro. Annals of Surgery 175: 439–447

Toouli J, Dodds W J, Honda R, Hogan W J 1981 Effect of histamine on motor function of opossum sphincter of Oddi. American Journal of Physiology 241: G122–G128

Watts J M, Dunphy J E 1966 The role of the common bile duct in biliary dynamics. Surgery, Gynecology and Obstetrics 122: 1207–1218

13 Postoperative strictures of the bile duct

HENRI BISMUTH

Iatrogenic injuries represent the most frequent etiology of benign bile duct strictures. Inflammatory stenosis related to biliary lithiasis and associated with acute calculous cholecystitis is less frequent; other causes such as primary sclerosing cholangitis and congenital diaphragm of the bile duct are exceptional. In our experience, more than 90% of benign strictures of the common bile duct are secondary to previous surgery.

Postoperative biliary strictures may be encountered following two different circumstances.

1. Accidental trauma to the common bile duct during cholecystectomy, which is the most frequent situation.
2. Common bile duct surgery: choledochotomy, biliary enteric anastomosis or sphincterotomy. In this situation the development of a bile duct stricture is generally related to technical failure.

Etiology

In a recent French National Enquiry (Bismuth & Lazorthes 1981) 643 cases of postoperative biliary stricture were analysed. It appeared that 93.6% were related to a surgical procedure on the biliary tract. The remaining 6.4% occurred after non-biliary operations; gastrectomy, liver surgery (hepatectomy and surgery of hydatid cyst) and finally following portacaval shunt. Since 1970 there has been a striking decrease in the frequency of post-gastrectomy biliary trauma. This is probably due to the replacement of partial gastrectomy by a more conservative approach to the ulcer disease. During the same time, the development and more extensive use of portal and liver surgery has brought its share of biliary trauma.

Cholecystectomy accounts for 92% of the injuries which occur during two particular steps of the operation; firstly, dissection of the cystic duct and secondly, of the gallbladder neck (Bismuth & Lazorthes 1981). Inflammatory adhesions and fibrosis following acute or chronic cholecystitis are without doubt a predisposing factor for common bile duct injury. The frequency rate of biliary trauma during cholecystectomy seems to be similar in European countries where a National Enquiry on this subject was made: 0.2% in Sweden (Rosenquist & Myrin 1960),

Finland (Viikari 1960) and Germany (Gutgemann et al 1965) and 0.15% in France (Bismuth & Lazorthes 1981).

After bile duct injury, two patterns may be observed. In the first, the common bile duct has been repaired during the first operation, usually by direct suture over a stent. In 50% of the cases (Bismuth & Lazorthes 1981), this repair fails and biliary stricture appears progressively after removal of the tube. In the second, there has been no attempt at immediate repair, usually due to a failure to appreciate that injury has occurred.

In general, the clinical presentation is of three kinds. Firstly, progressive jaundice, clinically obvious on the second or third postoperative day, reflecting ligation of the bile duct. Secondly, external biliary fistula along the abdominal drainage tube which, after some days or weeks, gives place to jaundice. Finally, bile peritonitis may occur and is the most serious manifestation leading to immediate re-operation in order to treat the peritonitis and place abdominal drains. There is usually no attempt at biliary repair and an external biliary fistula is either created or develops along a drain track. Irrespective of the bile duct injury mechanism (section or ligation, with or without attempt at repair) biliary stricture is the common end point.

Pathology

The cicatrical process which characterizes the postoperative biliary stricture comprises three main features which must be appreciated by the surgeon since they are fundamental to surgical repair.

1. Sclerosis of the ductal wall at the level of the trauma. This is proportionate to the degree and type of the injury. If the biliary injury has been a simple ligation of the bile duct, the stricture may be limited to a fibrous nodule without neighbouring inflammatory changes. On the other hand, when there has been a biliary fistula or a subhepatic abscess, and one or more re-operations, the sclerosing process is more extensive, involving not only the bile duct but also the periductal tissue. This intense inflammatory reaction increases the difficulty of the biliary repair.
2. The second factor is retraction of the biliary stump. At the site of trauma, the lumen of the duct disappears and is replaced by fibrosis. The cut ends of the bile duct become separated over a variable distance. The inferior end retracts towards the pancreas and, particularly important for repair, the superior end retracts upwards towards and into the hilus. The length of the superior biliary stump is one of the most important elements in assessing the difficulty and the outcome of the subsequent biliary repair.
3. Dilatation of the upper part of the bile duct is the third factor. It appears rapidly when there is simple ligation of the bile duct but is less marked after biliary fistula or when longstanding cholangitis leads to chronic inflammation of the biliary wall.

Since the length of the superior biliary stump is a determinant factor in biliary repair, a classification of postoperative biliary strictures according to the level where healthy biliary mucosa can be found may be proposed. Cholangiography is indispensable to precise knowledge of the level of the stricture. We have classified postoperative strictures of the common bile duct into five types (Fig. 13.1).

Type 1. Low common hepatic duct stricture: the hepatic stump is longer than 2 cm.

Type 2. Middle common hepatic duct stricture: the hepatic stump is less than 2 cm.

Type 3. High stricture or hilar stricture preserving the biliary confluence: the hepatic duct does not exist any more. The stricture reaches the confluence of the right and left hepatic ducts but communication between the two branches is preserved across the confluence.

Type 4. Hilar stricture interrupts the confluence: communication between the left and right branches no longer exists. If the fibrotic scar joining the two branches is thin, then they may remain in continuity, but if the process has destroyed an important part of the ductal tissue, the right and left hepatic ducts may be separated by 1–2 cm.

Type 5. When the trauma has involved an anomalous distribution of the segmental right branches ('convergence étagée'*), one of these two ducts can be separated from the biliary tract by the stricture.

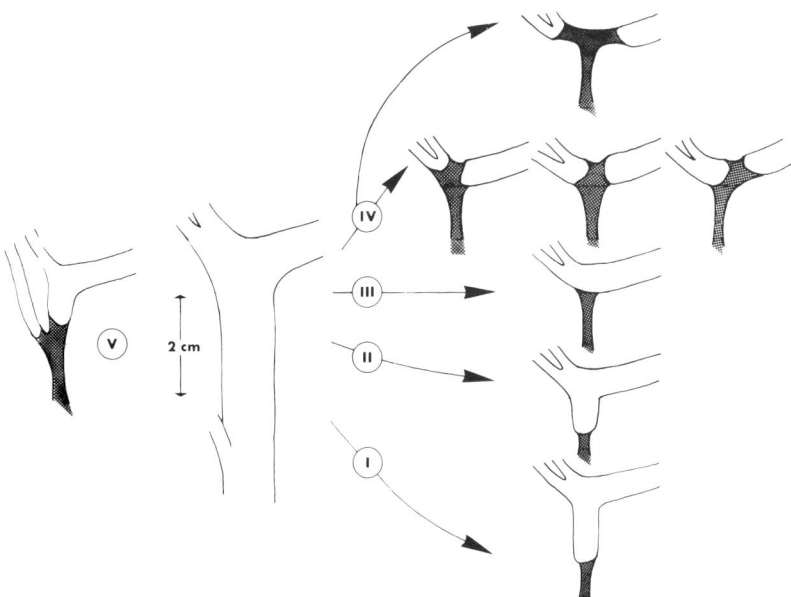

Fig. 13.1 The different types of postoperative strictures classified according to the length of the superior end. Three landmarks are used: 2 cm under the biliary confluence, the inferior level of the confluence, the roof of the confluence. Type 1: Low stricture. Type 2: Middle stricture. Type 3: High stricture (hilar stricture) preserving the biliary confluence. Type 4: High stricture (hilar structure) interrupting the biliary confluence. Type 5: Apart, stricture on an anomalous union of the sectorial right branches.

*Separate junction of posterior right sectorial duct below the major confluence.

Clinical symptomatology

Jaundice and cholangitis are the main and usually the only symptoms. The timing of appearance of cholangitis varies. Usually, bouts of cholangitis become more frequent and more severe as time passes. Without treatment, there is a risk of the process evolving, more or less rapidly, towards secondary biliary cirrhosis.

Preoperative investigations

The purpose of pre-operative investigations is to document precisely the characteristics of the stricture, to foresee the difficulties of biliary repair and to plan therapy. The most important factors are:

1. The level of the biliary stenosis
2. The degree of dilatation of the hepatic stump and of the hepatic branches
3. The influence of cholestasis on the liver and the presence of liver hypertrophy or of secondary biliary cirrhosis

In addition to the usual biological tests, liver ultrasound is a necessary investigation to evaluate the degree of dilatation of the bile ducts and the size of the liver. In some cases, endoscopy is indicated to look for oesophageal varices, especially if biliary cirrhosis is considered likely or for assessment of a spontaneous biliary enteric fistula. Because of the high rate (approximately 40%) in cases of bile duct injury of an associated hepatic arterial injury, usually of the right branch, selective coeliac arteriography may be indicated. Percutaneous transhepatic cholangiography is more debatable. It is, without doubt, the best means of demonstrating, before operation, the exact location of the stricture, but it exposes the patient to the risk of severe cholangitis. Therefore it should not be a routine exploration but can be done immediately before laparotomy in some particular patients in whom hypertrophy of the liver, by modifying the location of the hilus, may influence the surgical approach. Endoscopic retrograde cholangiography is useless, since the inferior stump of the bile duct is not used for biliary repair.

Treatment

Principles of biliary repair

The basic principle of the operation of biliary repair is to reestablish mucosal continuity between the biliary tract and the digestive mucosa. This mucosa-to-mucosa 'bord à bord' is the best approach to prevent recurrence of the stricture, and requires on one hand normal biliary mucosa and on the other the necessity to bring this biliary mucosa in close apposition to another healthy mucosal surface. The latter is relatively easy to achieve. It can be obtained by using the inferior end of the strictured bile duct or by bringing up a segment of bowel. The use of the inferior stump of the bile duct to perform an end-to-end anastomosis was used for a long time by some authors (Cattel & Brasch 1959, Lahey & Pyrtek 1950). However, the difficulty in obtaining a good mucosa-to-mucosa approximation without undue tension probably explains why long-term results with this technique appear worse than those of a biliary enteric anastomosis (Warren et al

1971). In our experience, it is best to bring up a Roux-en-Y jejunal loop to the prepared biliary mucosal stump (Bismuth et al 1978).

Realization of the first objective, (that is, the exposure of a healthy biliary mucosa at the level of the superior stump of the severed bile duct) is the principal aim of biliary repair procedures and constitutes the most important step in the operation. Difficulties in defining the level of the biliary stump are resolved by intraoperative cholangiography.

In low strictures (Type 1), exposure of the biliary mucosa is easy and the biliary stump is long enough to allow straightforward performance of hepaticojejuno-stomy. When the stricture is higher, simple dissection of the hepatic pedicle is not sufficient to allow exposure of a wide biliary stoma lined by normal mucosa, and it is necessary to open the bile duct at the junction between the right and left branches. This is achieved using the manoeuvre described by Hepp & Couinaud (1956) whereby the hilar plate is dissected and lowered and the left hepatic duct approached. The hilar plate (Fig. 13.2) is constituted by the thickening of Glisson's capsule at the level of the hilus and covers, as a ceiling, the hilar structures, the highest of which are the hepatic ducts, the left duct for two-thirds of the width of the hilus and the right for one-third. For this anatomical reason, the branch exposed by lowering of the hilar plate is the left one. The manoeuvre for lowering the hilar plate consists in incision of Glisson's capsule at the anterior edge of the hilus, that is, at the posterior edge of the quadrate lobe, immediately at the union between the quadrate lobe and the anterior surface of the heaptic pedicle (Fig. 13.3). This incision gives access to the superior surface of the hilar plate which can be separated from the liver parenchyma. By lowering the hilar plate, the hepatic duct is exteriorized and progressively turns anteriorly so that its superior part becomes anterior. Even in high biliary strictures, the left branch approach allows access to the biliary mucosa above the stricture and will provide a biliary stoma with normal mucosa for performance of bilio-enteric suture anastomosis.

In most instances, lowering of the hilar plate is sufficient to expose the bile duct widely. Sometimes, however, other manoeuvres must be additionally employed:

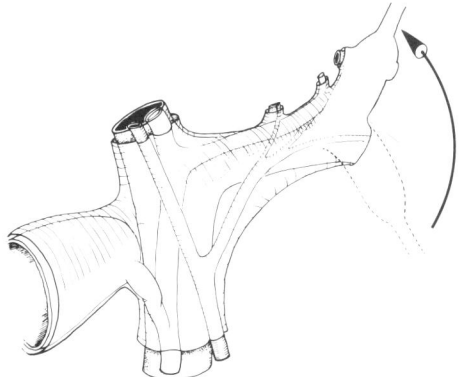

Fig. 13.2 Anatomy of the hilus. The hilar plate, represented in hatched lines, covers the hilar structures and is in continuity to the right with the gallbladder's plate and to the left with the umbilical plate. The biliary confluence is the superior and anterior element.

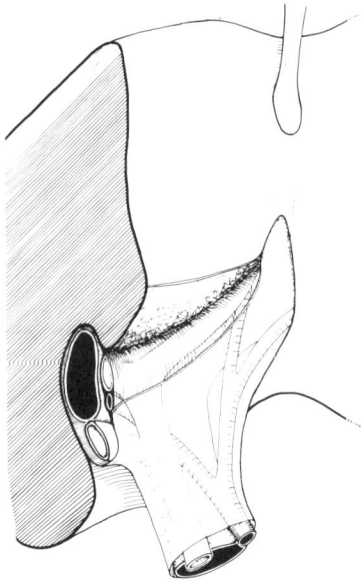

Fig. 13.3 The lowering of the hilar plate and the left branch approach.

1. To the left — section of the parenchymatous bridge between the left lateral and left medial parts of the left hemi-liver located at the inferior part of the round ligament, allows enlargement of the left hepatic duct approach (Champeau & Pineau 1964).
2. To the right — opening of the fibrous and retractile scar of the gallbladder bed.

In *very high strictures*, also called lesions of the biliary confluence, difficulties are more significant. In such cases the sclerotic scar of the wounded bile duct involves one or both branches and opening of the convergence alone is not enough to allow access to mucosa. Furthermore, communication between the two branches may be interrupted and opening the left branch does not give access to the entire intrahepatic biliary tract, the right branch remaining obstructed. Two situations may be encountered.

Firstly, the union between the right and left branches may be destroyed but the two ducts are close together, the lack of mucosa involving the roof of the confluence or the stoma of only one branch, usually the right.

Secondly, the two ducts may be separated by a large band of sclerosis, there being two isolated stumps buried in fibrotic tissue.

Intraoperative cholangiography by direct puncture of the biliary stump is mandatory to study these lesions. Sometimes the confluence is reduced to a small hole between the two branches. Sometimes, however, only one branch is opacified and search for the missing branch by puncturing the area of sclerosis in the hilus is indispensable. When the two branches are found and opened, a second and separate cholangiography of each branch is individually performed in order to verify that no intrahepatic duct is missing.

The manoeuvre for lowering the hilar plate is conducted here further to the left, comprising necessarily a section of the parenchymatous bridge under the round ligament (vide supra) and further to the right by opening the scar of the gallbladder bed. The technique of repair itself differs according to the proximity of the two branches. If the two are close together, it is possible to create a single stoma for the anasomosis but if distant, with a large band of fibrous scar between them, it is better to perform two separate anastomoses on the same Roux-en-Y loop of jejunum. The indication for one or two-anastomotic stents depends upon the quality of the mucosa at the level of the biliary stoma.

Results of biliary repair by hepatico-jejunostomy to the left hepatic duct (left branch approach)

There are, in the literature, few reports on series of patients operated on by the left branch approach (Fernandez 1980). Since the description of the technique in 1956 (Hepp & Couinaud 1956), we have operated on 186 patients by this type of operation (the majority by Dr Hepp). Most of these patients (70%) have had one or more re-operations before coming to us and had associated lesions which complicated operation and compounded the difficulty of the biliary repair. These lesions were mainly intrahepatic stones above the stricture, or external biliary fistulae, but hepatic hypertrophy or atrophy/hypertrophy and secondary biliary cirrhosis were also common. The frequency of these complications is listed in Table 13.1. Despite such complications, these patients were operated on by a mucosa-to-mucosa suture as described above. In our experience since 1956, the left branch approach has been possible in all but four patients, three early in the series (between 1956 and 1964) and one with a very high biliary stricture destroying the confluence, who was operated on by an intrahepatic cholangiojejunostomy. The results observed in this series are analysed below.

Table 13.1 Difficulties in biliary repair. 186 patients with a mucosa-to-mucosa hepaticojejunostomy

Previous attempted biliary repair	70%
Hilar strictures interrupting the biliary confluence	24%
Intrahepatic stones	44%
External biliary fistulas	12%
Spontaneous bilio-digestive fistulas	10%
Associated arterial lesions	39%
Hepatic hypertrophy and atropho-hypertrophy	5%
Secondary biliary cirrhosis	8%

Immediate results

Operative mortality (intraoperative and immediate postoperative mortality) was one (0.6%). Morbidity was significant with 18 complications (9%), mainly wound infections (4.3%), transitory external biliary fistulae without necessitating re-operation (1.5%). Two patients required re-operation, one for intestinal obstruction and the other for leakage from the jejunal loop.

Late results

There is in the literature a large variability in the criteria chosen to assess long-term results of biliary repair operations. The follow-up usually reported is from two to three years after operation. Smith (1979) considers two years' follow-up is long enough for a precise evaluation of the results of operation and that a good result at two years tends to be maintained. Braasch (1973) advocates a three-year follow-up and defines as a good result patients without trouble or with, at the most, two episodes of fever each year. Walters (1980) maintains that a good result is obtained when there are episodes of pain and fever with slight jaundice, and satisfactory results when these episodes are more frequent but allow the patient to work. We consider a follow-up of two to three years too short and have observed failure of the operation in patients in whom symptoms appeared more than three or even five years after surgery. In addition, any kind of persistent biliary symptomatology cannot be considered a good result. In our series of patients of hepaticojejunostomy (according to the technique described above) we have chosen a 10-year follow-up.

Of the 186 patients, 141 had been operated on between 1956 and 1970 and were recently studied for assessment of late results. (Bismuth & Lazorthes 1981). Fourteen patients, most of them from foreign countries, were lost to follow-up (11%). Seven died from non-biliary causes less than 10 years after the operation. One hundred and twenty patients were reassessed recently and have a 10 to 20 year follow-up period. Of these, 88% (106 patients) have an excellent result defined by absence of any biliary troubles and affirmation by the patient that he feels cured.

5% (6 patients) have a satisfactory result defined by occurrence during the interval of follow-up of troubles, probably related to the operation, which appeared shortly after operation, were transitory and did not need re-operation. Presently these six patients are symptom-free.

7% (8 patients) have unsatisfactory results. Three have recurrent stenosis and required re-operation, with good results, and five patients died who were operated on at the stage of secondary cirrhosis, development of which was not modified by the operation. The technique of repair used here must be compared with other types of biliary repair.

End-to-end anastomosis

This is the true biliary repair in the proper meaning of the term. This technique was the first reported for biliary repair and was widely used, chiefly in the United States of America. Initially it appeared as the ideal technique of repair since it reconstitutes the normal anatomy of the common bile duct and limits the re-operation to the previous operative area. In fact, this operation is not as simple as it may look. Firstly, finding the inferior biliary stump is difficult and, secondly, discrepancy in calibre between the inferior and superior stumps and the distance between the two renders anastomosis difficult. In the most recent series reported from the Lahey Clinic (Warren et al 1971), long-term results of biliary repair using an end-to-end anastomosis appeared less satisfactory than those obtained with a hepatico-jejunostomy. These considerations may explain why end-to-end anastomosis, which has always been rarely employed in France, falls progressively into disfavour.

Other types of biliary-enteric anastomosis

1. *Hepaticoduodenostomy* has no advantage compared with hepaticojejunostomy and is not always technically possible.

2. *Other types of hepaticojejunostomy* — that is to say, without mucosa-to-mucosa approximation — expose the patient to recurrent stenosis. It is possible to calibrate the anastomosis using a long-term transanastomotic stent in order to obtain healing by secondary intention without stenosis. The best procedure derives from the studies of Praderi (1974) and consists in a U-tube with a double outlet, one superior and transhepatic, the other inferior and transjejunal. This procedure permits the replacement of the tube if it is obstructed or if a larger tube becomes necessary.

The procedure proposed by Smith (1969) consists of a 'jejunal mucosal graft'. The jejunal mucosa is pulled up through the stenosis and up to the biliary lumen without exposing the biliary mucosa itself. The results recently reported by Smith (1980) using this technique are apparently similar to those obtained with our technique of hepaticojejunostomy (85% of the patients remain asymptomatic, 15% are failures). However, it should be noted that these results were obtained at a two-year follow-up and that contraindications for this technique are frequent and include biliary cirrhosis, severe infection of the bile ducts and stones above the stricture. Furthermore, the technique is not easy if the ducts are narrow. Two points must be debated concerning this method. Firstly, the basic principle is related to the fact that the biliary mucosa is inaccessible for suture so that it becomes necessary to lift the jejunal mucosa. In fact, even for very high strictures the biliary mucosa is usually accessible provided that the approach to the hilar area is sufficient and that the hilar plate is lowered. Secondly, the performance of the mucosal graft leads to an imperfect mucosa-to-mucosa approximation due to the haphazard positioning of the mucosal graft and the absence of visual control, with potential risk of intra-hepatic duct obstruction. This procedure should be considered as a 'makeshift' technique in patients in whom the biliary mucosa is really inaccessible despite a deep adequate dissection.

Conclusion

Post-operative strictures of the bile duct are a most serious condition and there is a risk of evolution towards secondary biliary cirrhosis. To prevent this we advocate early repair. This repair should be an elaborate mucosa-to-mucosa suture hepaticojejunostomy to a Roux-en-Y loop. Even for high strictures, exposure of the biliary stump mucosa can be achieved by lowering the hilar plate which allows approach to the left hepatic duct.

References

Bismuth H, Lazorthes F 1981 Les traumatismes opératoires de la voie biliaire principale. Masson Ed, Paris, Vol 1

Bismuth H, Franco D, Corlette M B, Hepp J 1978 Long term results of Roux-en-Y hepaticojejunostomy. Surgery, Gynecology and Obstetrics 146: 161–167

Braasch J W 1973 Current consideration in the repair of the bile ducts strictures. Surgical Clinics of North America 53: 423–433

Cattel R B, Braasch J 1959 Primary repair of benign strictures of the bile duct. Surgery, Gynecology and Obstetrics 109: 351–538

Champeau M, Pineau P 1964 Voie d'abord élargie trans-hépatique due canal hépatique gauche. Mémoires de l'Academie de Chirurgie 90: 602–613

Fernandez M 1980 Treatment of benign strictures of the bile ducts. World Journal of Surgery 4: 479–482

Gutgemann A, Schrieffers K H, Philipp R, Wulfing D 1965 Zur rekonstruktiven Chirurgie des verletzten und strikturierten grossen Gallenganges. Bruns' Beiträge zur klinschen Chirurgie 210: 129–150

Hepp J, Couinaud C 1956 L'abord et l'utilisation du canal hépatique gauche dans les réparations de la voie biliaire principale. Presse médicale 64: 947–948

Lahey F H, Pyrtek L J 1950 Experience with operative management of 280 strictures of the bile ducts. Surgery Gynecology and Obstetrics 91: 25–26

Praderi R 1974 Twelve years' experience with transhepatic intubation. Annals of Surgery 179: 937–940

Rosenquist H, Myrın S O 1960 Operative injury to the bile ducts. Acta chirurgica scandinavica 119: 92–107

Smith R 1969 Strictures of the bile ducts. Proceedings of the Royal Society of Medicine 62: 131–137

Smith R 1979 Obstructions of the bile duct. British Journal of Surgery 66: 69–79

Smith R 1980 Le traitement chirurgical des sténoses des voies biliaires. Chirurgie 106: 318–321

Viikari S J 1960 Operative injuries to the bile ducts. Acta chirurgica scandinavica 119: 83–92

Warren K W, Mountain J C, Middel A I 1971 Management of strictures of the biliary tract. Surgical Clinics of North America 51: 711–731

14 *Infection and the biliary tree*

M. R. B. KEIGHLEY

Introduction

Infection is still one of the most serious complications of operations on the biliary tract. Some of these infections may seem to be trivial, such as those confined to a drain site or the wound, but other infections, particularly septicaemia are responsible for mortality. The serious complications of septicaemia include liver abscess, chronic liver failure, disseminated intravascular coagulation, renal failure and endotoxaemia. It is these complications which threaten the life of patients having surgical treatment for biliary disease.

Not only is infection a complication of surgical treatment, but sepsis is often the presenting feature of biliary disease. Infection may thus manifest itself by Charcot's triad of intermittent fever, pain and jaundice. Alternatively patients with biliary disease may present for the first time with an episode of endotoxaemia, circulatory collapse and oliguria. Acute cholecystitis and pyogenic abscess usually presents with clinical signs of infection, local pain, fever and occasionally rigors. Infection may also be responsible for some of the radiological features of biliary disease: such as gas from gas producing *Escherichia coli*, *Klebsiella* sp or *Clostridium* sp in the gallbladder or bile ducts.

Infection may also be a serious complication of certain diagnostic radiological procedures on the biliary tract. Fatal septicaemia has been recorded after percutaneous transhepatic cholangiography and after endoscopic cholangiography. In both, the pathogenesis of septicaemia appears to be due to introducing contrast material under pressure into a heavily infected biliary tract.

The purpose of this chapter is to review the microflora of the biliary tract and to examine the relationship between infection in bile and septic complications occurring after operation and interventional radiology. Having defined high risk groups and the organisms responsible for sepsis an attempt will be made to provide a rational approach to the choice and use of antibiotics for treatment and prophylaxis. The chapter will conclude with a survey of the results of a policy of antibiotic cover in patients requiring surgical treatment for obstructive jaundice.

219

Aetiology of infection in biliary surgery

Morphology and counts of bacteria in infected bile

Most accounts of the bacterial isolates of patients with infected bile concur with one another (Keighley 1977, Mason 1968, Edlund et al 1959). The predominant organisms in bile are *Escherichia coli*, *Klebsiella* sp and *Streptococcus faecalis* (Table 14.1). There is however some discrepancy in the literature on the isolation rate of anaerobes from bile. The reason for these differences can be partly explained by the techniques used to culture strict anaerobes and also by the selection of patients studied. Strict anaerobes, particularly *Bacteroides fragilis*, *Bifido-bacterium* sp and *Fusobacterium* sp appear to be extremely uncommon in Europe and in North America from patients with stones. On the other hand *Bacteroides fragilis* is commonly recovered after a previous biliary-intestinal anastomosis, particularly if there is a recurrent stricture (Elliott 1980). Anaerobes also seem to be more common in Asiatic cholangiohepatitis and from liver abscesses of biliary origin. Microaerophilic organisms such as *Peptococcus* and *Peptostreptococcus* sp are more common and *Clostridium* sp is well recognised as a frequent pathogen in acute acalculous cholecystitis and in chronic cholecystitis.

The bile is usually colonised by more than one organism, and in our experience a single bacterial species was isolated in only 38% of patients with a positive bile culture. Two species were identified together in 29%, three species in 20%, four species occurred together in 12% and in a small proportion (1%) more than four different isolates were recovered from the bile.

Table 14.1 Bacteria in the bile

	Malignant obstruction	Cholelithiasis	Stricture	Previous bypass
Aerobic:				
Gram positive:				
Streptococcus faecalis	4 (9%)	30 (15%)	3 (8%)	5 (15%)
Beta-haemolytic streptococci	1	4	2	2
Streptococci viridans	2	1	1	2
Staphylococcus aureus	3	3	0	0
Staphylococcus albus	1	4	0	3
Gram negative:				
Escherichia coli	10 (23%)	77 (38%)	12 (31%)	7 (21%)
Klebsiella aerogenes	7 (16%)	22 (11%)	2 (5%)	2 (6%)
Enterobacter spp	3	8	1	0
Proteus spp	2	13	3	1
Pseudomonas aeruginosa	2	4	2	1
Acinitobacter spp	1	4	0	0
Serratia spp	0	2	0	0
Aeromonas spp	0	2	0	0
Anaerobic:				
Gram positive:				
Clostridium welchii	4 (9%)	16 (8%)	3 (8%)	3 (9%)
Anaerobic streptococci	2	7		2
Gram negative:				
Bacteroides spp	0	2 (1%)	7 (18%)	5 (15%)
Total	43	199	36	33

The counts of bacteria in bile vary from 10^9 organisms per ml to 10^4 bacteria per ml. The highest counts are usually found in the common bile duct, but similar numbers of bacteria are recovered from infected T-tube bile as well (Fig. 14.1).

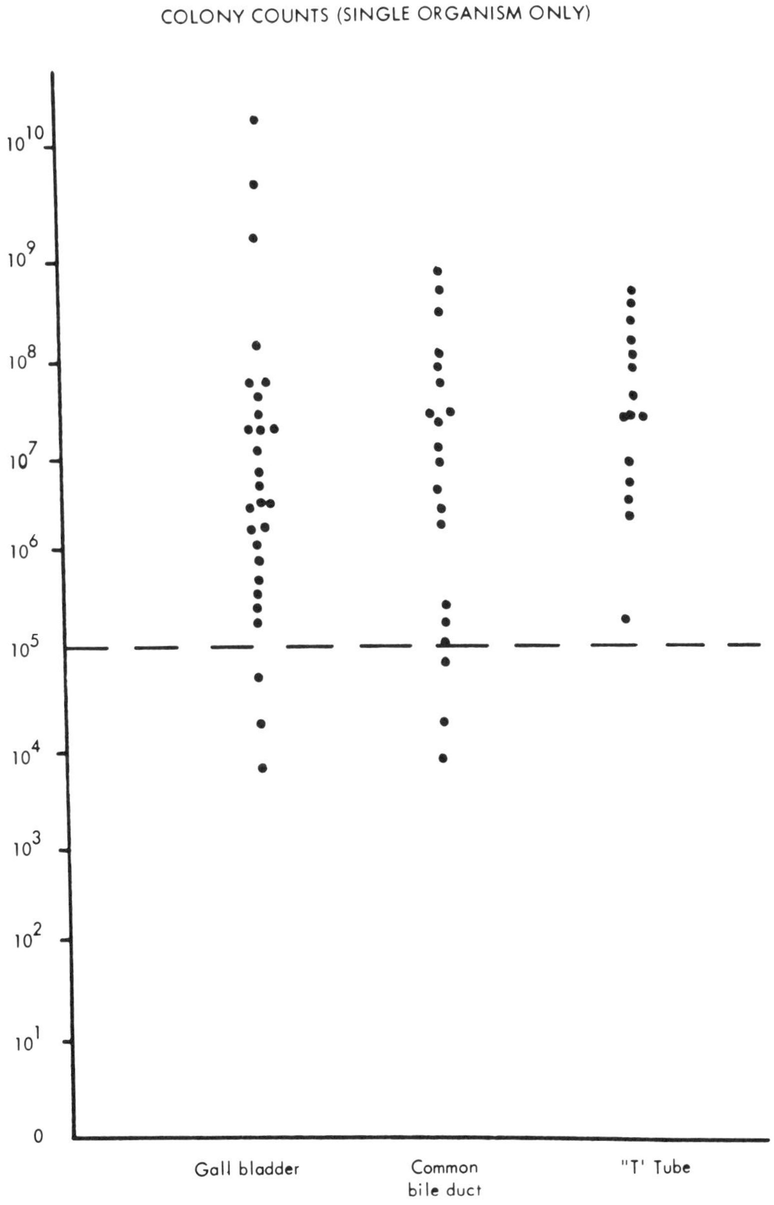

COLONY COUNTS (SINGLE ORGANISM ONLY)

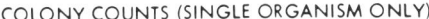

Fig. 14.1 Counts of bacteria (organisms per ml) from gallbladder common bile duct and T-tube bile

Table 14.2 Incidence of bacteria in the bile according to biliary disease and age

Bilary pathology	% Positive bile cultures by age in decades							
	<20yrs	20–30	30–40	40–50	50–60	60–70	70–80	>80
Uncomplicated gallstones (n=412)	18	10	0	7	14	17	33	50
Acute cholecystitis (n=55)	0	0	—	23	36	70	33	100
Common duct stones, no jaundice (n=36)	—	66	66	25	80	55	0	66
Common duct stones and jaundice (n=29)	—	0	0	20	50	—	100	100

Incidence of bacteria in the biliary tract

The reported incidence of bacteria in the bile is extremely variable ranging from 8–42% (Elliott 1980, Watson 1969, Anderson & Priestley 1951, Elkeles & Mirrizi 1942, Flemma et al 1967, Maddocks et al 1973, Engstrom et al 1971). The reason for this enormous variation includes the types of patient being studied and the use of antibiotics preoperatively. It is now well established that micro organisms are more common in the bile if the patient is jaundiced, particularly if the obstruction is due to stones or a stricture in the bile duct. Infection is also more common in elderly patients and if there has been a recent acute attack of cholecystitis (Table 14.2). Bacteria are invariably present if there is an anastomosis between the bile ducts and the bowel. We were able to perform a comprehensive microbiological survey on the incidence of bacteria in the bile from patients who had been receiving no antibiotic cover (Table 14.3). The greatest incidence of bacterial proliferation in the biliary tract occurred in patients with resolving acute cholecystitis, choledocholithiasis, stricture, high bile duct obstruction from malignancy and a previous choledochoduodenostomy.

We have also tried to assess the incidence of bacteria throughout the biliary tree by sampling material for microbiological study from the bile ducts, liver biopsies, gallbladder wall, cystic lymph node and from needle aspirates of duodenal contents (Fig. 14.2). When the lumen of the gallbladder was infected the bile ducts were invariably colonised by the same bacteria. In patients with bacteria in the gallbladder, organisms were also recovered from 80% of liver biopsy specimens,

Table 14.3 Incidence of bacteria in the bile (author's series)

		n	% positive bile cultures
Acute cholecystitis (emergency operation)		29	82
Resolving acute cholecystitis		41	48
Mucocoele of the gallbladder		17	29
Empyema of the gallbladder		14	34
Normal gallbladder with stones	< 50 years	42	11
	50–70 years	37	13
	> 70 years	42	17
Stones in the common bile duct		70	84
Stricture of the bile duct		8	(100%)
Tumours of the distal bile duct		31	34
High bile duct obstruction from malignancy		8	(50%)
Previous choledochoduodenostomy		3	(67%)
Previous choledochojejunostomy (Roux Y)		3	(100%)

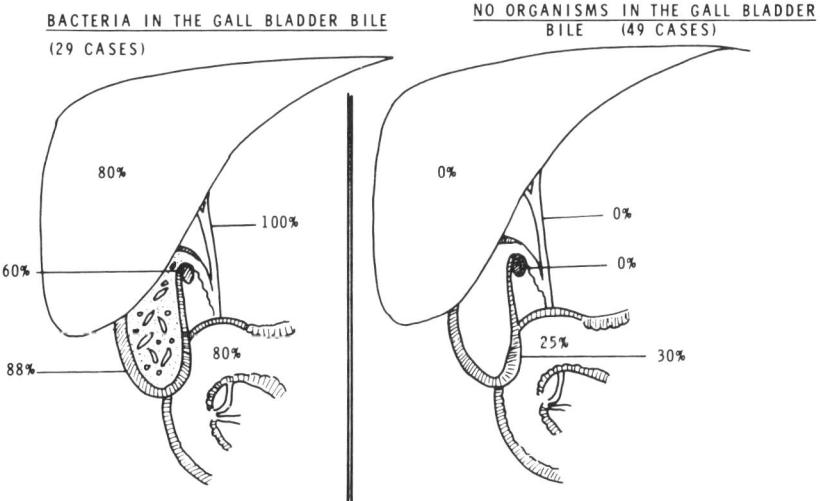

Fig. 14.2 Incidence of bacteria throughout the biliary tract in relation to the presence of infected gallbladder bile

from 80% of duodenal aspirates, from the wall of the gallbladder in 88% of cases and from the cystic lymph node in 60%. Conversely, when the gallbladder bile was sterile so were all other sites in the biliary tract with the exception of the duodenum and the gallbladder wall (colonised by bacteria in 52% and 30% respectively).

The relationship between infected bile and post-operative sepsis
The close association between organisms in bile and infection after biliary surgery has been observed by many groups (Mason 1968, Edlund et al 1959) who have investigated the pathogenesis of post-surgical sepsis. The close correlation between bile cultures and the morphology of organisms recovered from infected wounds and positive blood cultures was demonstrated conclusively from this hospital before prophylactic antibiotics were routinely used in biliary surgery (Fig. 14.3). 64% of wound infections and 90% of the episodes of septicaemia occurring after biliary surgery were caused by an organism previously identified in the bile. When organisms were found in the bile at operation, the incidence of wound sepsis (39%) and septicaemia (20%) was significantly greater than in patients with sterile bile (11% and 3% respectively). Most of the wound infections in patients in whom the bile was sterile were staphylococcal and therefore presumably exogenous in origin. The episodes of septicaemia in patients with sterile bile were either anaerobic and associated with incidental appendicectomy or they occurred as a complication of T-tube drainage.

Incidence of postoperative sepsis
The principal reasons for postoperative morbidity are wound sepsis, abscess and septicaemia. Respiratory infection is common but cannot be regarded as a specific complication of biliary surgery. The incidence of wound sepsis and septicaemia in

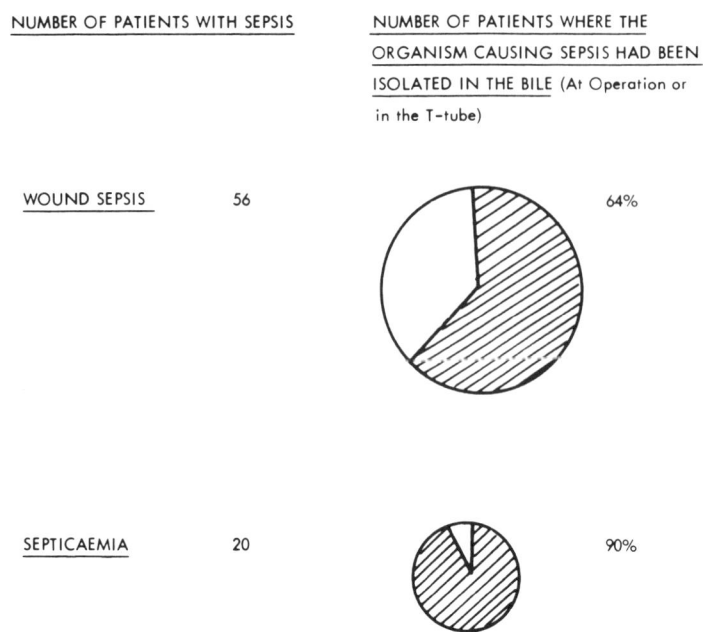

NUMBER OF PATIENTS WITH SEPSIS

NUMBER OF PATIENTS WHERE THE
ORGANISM CAUSING SEPSIS HAD BEEN
ISOLATED IN THE BILE (At Operation or
in the T-tube)

WOUND SEPSIS   56   64%

SEPTICAEMIA   20   90%

Fig. 14.3 Incidence of wound sepsis and septicaemia according to whether the bile contained bacteria at the time of operation: no antibiotics given

this hospital when no antibiotic cover was used is listed according to the underlying pathology and to the incidence of infected bile. (Table 14.4).

The overall incidence of wound sepsis was 20% and there was a significantly higher incidence of wound sepsis after emergency surgery (41%) than after elective operation (18%). In elective operations the incidence of wound sepsis was three times greater after choledochotomy than after cholecystectomy alone. The incidence of septicaemia during elective operations was significantly higher after exploration of the bile duct (12%) than after cholecystectomy alone (1%). Septicaemia was recorded before or after biliary surgery in 27 (6.2%) of 436 patients who were not receiving antibiotic cover. Five patients developed septicaemia within six hours of transhepatic cholangiography and two after endoscopic retrograde cholangiography. Septicaemia was also recorded in two patients after choledochoscopy and in two other patients in whom an operative cholangiogram had demonstrated cholangiovenous reflux due to an impacted calculus in the distal bile duct. There were also seven episodes of rigors and cholangitis after T-tube cholangiography. Of the 27 patients with septicaemia, nine developed endotoxic shock, complicated by acute renal failure in six, and five died. This represents an overall mortality from septicaemia in patients undergoing biliary surgery of 1.5%. The bacteria responsible for septicaemia and those isolated from the bile in the same patients are listed in Table 14.5.

Abscess occurred in only five of 181 patients (2%), two cases occurred after emergency cholecystectomy for empyema, one after a routine elective chole- cystectomy and the remaining two after choledochotomy for stones.

Table 14.4 The correlation between organisms in the bile and the incidence of wound sepsis and septicaemia

		Organisms in the bile	Wound sepsis	Septicaemia
17	Emergency operation	16 (94%)	7 (41%)	3 (18%)
164	Elective operation	41 (25%)	29 (18%)	9 (6%)
101	Cholecystectomy alone	12 (12%)	10 (10%)	1 (1%)
63	Choledochotomy	29 (46%)	19 (31%)	8 (12%)
23	Stones	16 (69%)	8 (35%)	5 (22%)
13	Carcinoma	3 (23%)	4 (31%)	1 (8%)
27	No stones	10 (37%)	7 (26%)	2 (7%)
TOTAL	181	57 (31%)	36 (20%)	12 (7%)

Presence of bacteria in bile after external biliary drainage

There has been recent interest in the place of external biliary drainage for patients with obstructive jaundice, since it has been claimed that preoperative drainage may reduce the mortality in patients with profound jaundice. Postoperative decompression with T-tubes has been widely used and claimed to be the safest procedure for patients in whom the common bile duct is explored. However, both of these procedures involve creating an external biliary fistula with a foreign body in the bile ducts. Some years ago we showed that postoperative sepsis was more common following T-tube drainage and that many of these infections may have originated from bacteria in the external drainage system (Keighley & Graham 1971). Furthermore septicaemia is still an occasional complication of T-tube cholangiography, particularly if contrast material is introduced into the biliary tract under high pressure. For these reasons it is appropriate to consider the problems of bacteria in bile after external biliary drainage.

a) T-Tube bile

The microflora of T-tube bile after choledochotomy was studied in 50 patients. Although the bile was infected in only 24 cases (48%) at the time of the operation, by the fifth postoperative day organisms were recovered from the T-tube in 40

Table 14.5 Aetiology of septicaemia

	Organisms isolated from blood cultures	Same organism in the bile
Escherichia coli	28	26
Klebsiella spp	7	7
Streptococci faecalis	3	3
Pseudomonas aeruginosa	1	1
Serratia spp	2	2
Clostridium welchii	2	2
Bacteroides fragilis*	3	1
	46	42 (93%)

* two patients had appendicectomy

(80%). The bacteria recovered from the T-tube frequently differed from those found at the time of the operation. The bile remained sterile in only 10 cases (20%), 'new' organisms were recovered from the T-tube in 25 (50%) and in only 15 cases (30%) did the T-tube contain the same organisms as those previously isolated at operation. The 'new' bacteria found in the T-tube were intestinal organisms and not surface pathogens, and it is probable that these new organisms were introduced through the drainage system. In our study, we found that once bacteria colonised the T-tube they remained in the bile even though appropriate antibiotics were given. Hence once an external biliary drainage system becomes infected,

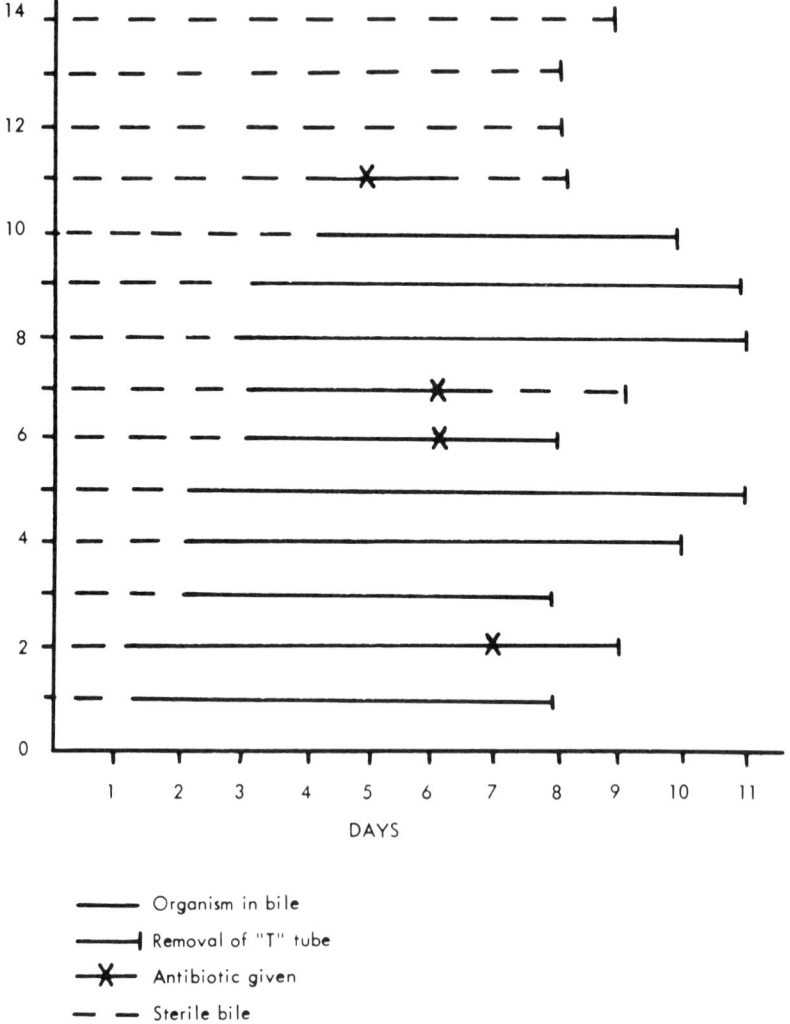

Organism in bile
Removal of "T" tube
Antibiotic given
Sterile bile

Fig. 14.4 Daily cultures of T-tube bile in patients whose bile was sterile at operation: solid line represents bacterial colonisation: dotted line indicates sterile bile. A cross represents use of antibiotics to which the biliary organisms were sensitive

these organisms are likely to persist until the drainage tube is removed. The results of daily cultures from T-tube bile in patients in whom the bile was sterile at operation are shown in Fig. 14.4. The majority became infected by the fifth post-operative day and remained so until they were removed.

b) External drainage for malignant bile duct obstruction

At least two thirds of patients with malignant bile duct obstruction have a sterile biliary tract. Nevertheless, transhepatic drainage tubes often become infected. Colonisation of the biliary tract is a serious problem since the bacteria recovered from transhepatic drains are commonly resistant to many available antibiotics and species such as *Pseudomonas, Proteus, Serratia, Enterobacter* and *Aerobacter*, not usually present in infected bile, proliferate. Furthermore these bacteria may be responsible not only for episodes of septicaemia, but have also been implicated as the cause of intrahepatic abscess following transhepatic drainage. Although careful attention to aseptic handling of the drain site and an entirely closed drainage system has reduced the incidence of colonisation (McPherson et al 1982), one must seriously question the use of preoperative drainage, since in half of these patients pre-operative decompression is likely to convert a sterile biliary tract to one colonised by highly pathogenic bacteria.

Antibiotics in biliary surgery

Principles of antibiotic therapy

It is important to differentiate antibiotic therapy from antibiotic prophylaxis. The term prophylaxis is quite inappropriate if there is established infection, for instance in patients requiring operations for acute cholecystitis, cholangitis and subhepatic or intrahepatic abscess associated with biliary disease. By contrast, patients having operations where bacteria may be disseminated from the biliary tract deserve to be protected from the postoperative infections which may occur as a consequence of operative endogenous bacterial contamination. The dose, timing and duration of antibiotic administration for prophylaxis differ from the use of antibiotics as therapy for established infection, and for this reason they will be considered separately.

a) Therapy

For therapeutic purposes, an antibiotic must penetrate inflamed tissues and there should be a normally functioning immune mechanism to deal with destroyed bacteria. A therapeutic antibiotic should also be bactericidal and preferably excreted in bile. It is an advantage if the agent is weakly bound to protein since penetration of abscess is facilitated if the antibiotic is freely diffusible (Wise 1981). It is also desirable to use an antibiotic with a narrow spectrum of activity provided the pathogen is known or can be accurately predicted.

It is necessary to prescribe a therapeutic antibiotic for a number of days (usually at least five) so that there is complete penetration of the infective process, allowing repair to occur without further bacterial invasion. The duration of the antibiotic will need to be longer if host defences are impaired, as for instance in a neutropaenic patient. Prolonged antibiotic therapy may also be necessary if the infective process is walled off and where surgical drainage is contraindicated.

The therapeutic agent should be non toxic and have minimal side effects. It is particularly important to avoid agents like the first generation cephalosporins which may lead to renal failure when used with a diuretic, since jaundiced patients are at risk from developing renal damage. By the same token, aminoglycosides are to be avoided, not only because of the risks of toxicity to the kidney and VIII cranial nerve but also because they may interfere with non-depolarising muscle relaxants.

Finally, it is desirable to choose an antibiotic which may be precribed by the systemic as well as the oral route since parenteral therapy may not be necessary for more than a few days, whereas the antibiotic may need to be continued for longer.

b) Prophylaxis

The term prophylaxis is applicable only if there is no preoperative infection by micro organisms in tissues. For this reason only a single dose of antibiotic is generally necessary, since the aim of prophylaxis is to provide high serum levels of antibiotic during endogenous bacterial contamination from the bile (Keighley & Burdon 1979). Since only a single or two doses of antibiotic are necessary, it is possible to prescribe very high doses of an agent without the fear of toxicity.

Since the purpose of antibiotic prophylaxis is to prevent the colonisation of bacteria liberated into the circulation or the operation site, it is mandatory that blood and tissue antibiotic levels are sufficient when the operation is being performed. Furthermore, as septicaemia is the complication which is most feared by biliary surgeons operating on the jaundiced patient, it is crucial that the serum antibiotic concentration should be at least five times greater than the minimum inhibitory concentrations for most biliary pathogens.

There are a variety of routes of antibiotic administration which may be used. Oral antibiotics like neomycin and metronidazole may be given for two or three days before operation in an attempt to suppress faecal flora (Arabi et al 1978). Such a regime is popular in colorectal surgery and it has a theoretical application in operations for obstructive jaundice. It has been suggested that endotoxaemia and renal failure may be due to abnormal absorption of endotoxin from the colon due to the absence of intraluminal bile salts (Bailey 1976). Attempts to suppress the faecal flora might therefore reduce the risk of endotoxin release in jaundiced patients. Unfortunately this practice has not been widely accepted, and it is probably of dubious clinical benefit. An alternative and possibly a more attractive approach is to replace intestinal bile salts. Oral antibiotics are therefore not advised for prophylaxis since the aim is to provide high blood levels at operation.

The intravenous route is to be preferred to intramuscular injection since this achieves much higher blood levels. It is also an advantage to use an antibiotic with a long half-life since the use of an antibiotic rapidly excreted by the kidney will be associated with insufficient serum levels after three to four hours. These considerations are particularly important for patients requiring prolonged operations, and it is generally advised that if the procedure takes more than 4 hours a second dose of antibiotic should be used. There are some people who still consider that topical antibiotics have a place in biliary surgery. Topical agents may be used in the peritoneal cavity or in the incision. Antibiotic irrigation in the peritoneal cavity may be dangerous since some agents are rapidly absorbed and can reach toxic levels in the serum (Ericsson et al 1978). Intra incisional antibiotics are certainly extremely effective at reducing wound sepsis (Finch et al 1979). However, since the antimicrobial is administered too late they do not protect against septicaemia and intra-abdominal abscess (Hares et al 1981). Furthermore, topical antimicrobials encourage the development of bacterial resistance.

In summary, therefore, the following policy of antibiotic prophylaxis is advised. Choose a safe intravenous antibiotic with low protein binding and with a short half-life. Give the antibiotic intravenously in the anaesthetic room just before the operation and repeat the antibiotic if the operation takes more than 4 hours. No further antibiotics are recommended, since single dose prophylaxis has been shown to be as good as (if not a little better than) 5-day cover. Use a big dose of antibiotic. If someone has forgotten to give the antibiotic it is pointless giving postoperative antibiotics, since their use will not protect patients from postoperative sepsis (Stone et al 1976). Having said this, antibiotics cannot be expected to provide a bad surgeon with good results. Every effort must therefore be made to prevent spillage of infected bile: the operative field should be packed away from the rest of the abdomen, there must be efficient haemostasis to avoid haematoma, tissues should be handled gently, non absorbable suture materials should be avoided whenever possible, and if gross contamination occurs, it is advisable to leave the skin and subcutaneous tissues open.

Choice of antibiotic

It is beyond the scope of this chapter to discuss the relative merits of one antimicrobial against another, since the choice of available antimicrobial agents changes each year and their relative merits become apparent only after extensive clinical usage. Clinicians are bombarded by detailed in vitro microbiological data claiming advantages of one drug against another but with little clinical support for claims of superiority. Fortunately the choice of a prophylactic agent is not crucial, provided that the drug is active against the organisms likely to be encountered in bile. More care will need to be exercised in the choice of therapeutic agents, and a failure to respond indicates either an incorrect choice of antibiotic, the need for surgical drainage of pus or decompression of an obstructed biliary tract.

a) Antibiotic sensitivities

In elective surgery amongst patients who have never had a previous biliary operation the principal pathogens which are likely to be encountered are *Escherichia coli*, *Klebsiella* sp, *Streptococcus faecalis* and staphylococci. Many clinicians do not consider that *Streptococcus faecalis* is a pathogen since it is rarely isolated from blood culture and is never associated with monomicrobial post-operative sepsis. Staphylococci certainly play an important role in the pathogenesis of wound sepsis amongst diabetic patients. If on the other hand the patient requires an emergency operation for acute cholecystitis, cholangitis or an abscess, or if there is a past history of previous biliary surgery (particularly with an anastomosis between the bile ducts and the small bowel), then other important pathogens are likely to be encountered. These include: *Proteus* sp, *Peptostrepto-coccus* sp, *Clostridium perfurigens* and occasionally *Bacteroides fragilis*.

Four groups of antimicrobials are potentially useful in biliary surgery: penicillins, cephalosporins, aminoglycosides and the sulphonamides. Most early penicillins had a narrow spectrum of activity, and with the exception of fluxcloxacillin were unstable to β-lactamase. The newer agents such as mecillinam, mezlocillin, piperacillin and ticarcillin are active against most of the aerobic Gram negative organisms likely to be encountered in bile, but they are not suitable for all coagulase positive staphylococci. The earlier cephalosporins such as cephaloridine or cephazolin have a wide range of activity and most aerobic biliary pathogens are sensitive, including staphylococci. The newer third generation cephalosporins such as cefuroxime, cephamandole, cephotoxeme and moxa-lactam are very active against Gram negative aerobes but are less active against staphylococci. In addition most of the agents are effective against the anaerobes likely to be isolated from infected bile. hence these are valuable agents for the management of the high risk biliary problems already referred to. The aminoglycosides such as gentamicin, tobramycin and amikacin are no longer recommended for prophylaxis, and should be reserved for life-threatening aerobic Gram negative infections since they are nephrotoxic unless carefully monitored. Furthermore, they have no activity against anaerobes. The sulphonamides have been popular in Scandinavia and their combination with trimethoprin in compounds like cotrimoxazole provide a useful safe agent for prophylaxis in routine elective operation (Morran et al 1978).

b) Pharmacokinetics

Reference has already been made to certain desirable pharmacokinetic properties such as low protein binding, long half-life, rapid bactericidal activity and good tissue penetration, but the question of biliary excretion has not been considered. Clearly it is desirable, particularly in patients with cholangitis or those undergoing an operation, to have therapeutic levels of antibiotic in the bile, both to eliminate bacteria from the bile and to minimise post-operative sepsis (Bevan & Williams 1971). However the majority of patients with infected bile have obstructive biliary disease and in these patients it is unlikely that adequate biliary levels of antibiotic can be achieved.

To determine the influence of biliary excretion on prophylactic antibiotic therapy we performed a controlled trial in 150 consecutive patients undergoing biliary operations (Keighley et al 1976a). Patients were allocated to one of three antibiotic groups: gentamicin, (an antibiotic with high serum but low bile levels), no antibiotic or rifamide, (an antibiotic excreted almost entirely into the bile). Samples of the bile and blood were collected at operation for antibiotic assay and the concentration of gentamicin or rifamide necessary to inhibit each biliary isolate was determined. The concentration of gentamicin sufficient to inhibit over 80% of organisms in the bile was 2.0 mg/l. Therefore, twice this figure (4 mg/l) was considered to provide 'adequate' levels of gentamicin in patients with biliary disease. 'Adequate' levels of gentamicin were found in the bile in only two cases (4%) whereas 'adequate' serum concentrations were present in almost 90% of patients.

Table 14.6 Results of prophylactic antibiotic therapy in biliary surgery

	Gentamicin (50)	Controls (50)	Rifamide (50)
Bacteria in bile	12 (24%)	19 (38%)	10 (20%)
Wound sepsis	3 (6%)*	11 (22%)	5 (10%)
Bacteraemia	1 (2%)*	7 (14%)	4 (8%)

* $p < 0.05$ compared with controls

Conversely over 80% of the organisms in the bile were inhibited by 31.25 mg/l of rifamide, so twice the level (62.5 mg/l) was regarded as an 'adequate' concentration for patients with biliary disease. Serum levels of rifamide were invariably too low to be of therapeutic value, and although extremely high bile levels were achieved in most patients in whom there was no evidence of obstruction to the biliary tract, 'adequate' levels were present in only two of 12 patients with obstructive biliary disease (17%). Hence although high concentrations of rifamide are normally achieved in the bile, for patients with biliary obstruction in whom there is a high risk of infection both serum and bile levels of the antibiotic were too low to be of therapeutic value. It is hardly surprising, therefore, that recovery of organisms in bile was not influenced by either antibiotic, and that a significant reduction in post-operative sepsis was demonstrated only in the patients receiving the antibiotic (gentamicin) with satisfactory serum levels (Table 14.6). Hence antibiotics which achieve satisfactory serum levels are more reliable in patients with obstructive biliary disease, than those which are excreted almost entirely into the bile. For most clinical situations it is desirable to use an antibiotic which provides both a high serum as well as high bile l,evels. Cephazolin is a good example of such an agent and one in which clinical trials have confirmed its efficacy (Strachan et al 1977).

Selection of patients requiring antibiotics in biliary surgery

It has been argued that it is both inappropriate and undisciplined to give antibiotics to all patients having a biliary tract operation, since the bile contains organisms in only a third of patients. Abuse of antibiotics will inevitably lead to emergence of resistant strains. These arguments seemed appropriate until it became clear that a single dose of antibiotic is sufficient for prophylaxis. The problems of resistance using only a single high dose of antibiotic seem remote, and a case could therefore be made for the use of a single antibiotic infusion for all patients. Nevertheless there are those who would wish to confine prophylaxis to patients with bacterbilia.

The clinical factors associated with infected bile have been well described. When we undertook a multivariate analysis (Keighley et al 1976b) eight factors were significantly more common in the patients with infected bile (Table 14.7). Using these criteria only 40% of patients were given an antibiotic and the overall rate of post-operative sepsis was only 5%. Other methods of detecting the presence

Table 14.7 Factors significantly associated with infection in bile: results of a multivariate analysis

Preoperative:	Patients over 70 years
	Obstructive jaundice
	Recent cholangitis
	Reoperations on the biliary tract
	Emergency operation
	Operation within one month of acute cholecystitis
Operative:	Bile duct obstruction
	Choledocholithiasis

and type of organisms in the bile include Gram stains on material aspirated from the gallbladder at the beginning of the operation or pre-operative duodenal aspirates after cholecystokinin. Gram stains on bile may be accurate in 77% of patients (McLeish et al 1980) but it is technically demanding, and if an antibiotic policy is based upon these findings most patients will receive their first dose of antibiotic near the completion of the operation, which is after potential bacterial inoculation and therefore too late. Similarly, duodenal aspirates are unpleasant for the patient, and results may be confused by the presence of the normal duodenal flora (Chetlin & Elliott 1973).

Results of controlled trials
It would be an impossible task to review all of the antibiotic trials (Keighley & Burdon 1978, Chetlin & Elliott 1973) in biliary surgery, but a variety of studies confined to patients having biliary surgery are reviewed in Table 14.8. The cephalosporins have been universally successful provided they are given preoperatively.

Future problems of infection in biliary surgery

It seemed appropriate to review the persistent morbidity and mortality from infection in a consecutive group of 118 patients having an operation for obstructive jaundice, all of whom had received single dose prophylaxis with cephazolin and oral mannitol during their operation (Table 14.9). We were somewhat surprised to find a high rate of wound sepsis, particularly in patients with malignant obstructive jaundice (13%). Many of these patients were diabetic and developed staphylococcal infections. More alarming was the 7% incidence of septicaemia, with three fatal cases, two of whom were having an operation for stones. I now believe that in jaundiced patients, and particularly in the compromised host, such as the patient with diabetes or malignant disease, it would seem wise to prolong antibiotic cover for five days. The clinical trials quoted earlier (Table 14.8) consist largely of patients having elective cholecystectomy, for whom single dose prophylaxis appears to be eminently satisfactory.

Table 14.8 Antibiotic prophylaxis in biliary operations (results of controlled trials)

Agent	Reference	Patients	Duration	Administration	Number	% Sepsis Treated	% Sepsis Control
Rifamide	Bevan & Williams 1971	All	3 days	Pre-op IM	61	3	19
Cephaloridine	Chetlin & Elliott 1973	All	5 days	Pre-op IM	84	4	27
Gentamicin	Keighley et al 1975	All	5 days	Pre-op IM	98	7	22
Cephazolin	Stone et al 1976	All	1 dose	12 hrs pre-op IM	131	5	22
				1 hour pre-op IM		4	
				1–4 hrs post-op IM		17	
Cephazolin	Strachan et al 1977	All	1 dose	Pre-op IM	201	3	17
			5 days	Pre-op IM		5	
Cotrimoxazole	Morran et al 1978	All	1 dose	Pre-op iv	95	4	21

Table 14.9 Morbidity of biliary surgery in jaundiced patients all of whom received preoperative cephazolin and mannitol (1975–1979)

	Total 118	Cancer 55	Non Malignant 63
Wound sepsis	12	7 (13%)	5 (8%)
Septicaemia	7	3 (6%)	4 (6%)
Abscess	2	0	2 (3%)
Mortality (all causes)	10	6 (11%)	4 (6%)
Mortality from sepsis	3	1	2

Conclusions

Sepsis is an important complication of operations and interventional endoscopic or radiographic procedures in biliary disease. The majority of infections originate from organisms in the bile and the predominant pathogens are *Escherichia coli*, *Klebsiella* sp and *Staphylococcus*, through *Proteus* sp, *Peptostreptococcus* sp, *Clostridium perfurigens* and occasionally *Bacteroides fragilis* may be identified in patients with acute cholecystitis, cholangitis or after previous biliary operations. For routine elective biliary surgery, systemic administration of a single dose of cephazolin to all patients before operation has been shown to reduce morbidity. For jaundiced patients and those with established infection, five-day antibiotic therapy should be employed using a newer broad spectrum cephalosporin such as moxalactam or cefotaxime. There are serious problems from colonisation of tubes used for decompression of the biliary tract, which might detract from their routine use for preoperative drainage of jaundiced patients.

References

Anderson R E, Priestley J T 1951 Observations on the bacteriology of choledochal bile. Annals of Surgery 133: 486–489

Arabi Y, Dimock F, Burdon D W, Alexander-Williams J, Keighley M R B 1978 Influence of bowel preparation and antimicrobials on colonic microflora. British Journal of Surgery 65: 555–559

Bailey M E 1976 Endotoxin, bile salts and renal function in obstructive jaundice. British Journal of Surgery 63: 774–778

Bevan P G, Williams J D 1971 Rifamide in acute cholecystitis and biliary surgery. British Medical Journal 3: 284–287

Chetlin S H, Elliott D W 1973 Preoperative antibiotics on biliary surgery. Archives of Surgery 107: 319–323

Edlund V A, Mollstedt B O, Onchterlony O 1959 Bacteriological investigations of the biliary system and liver in biliary tract disease correlated to clinical data and microstructure of the gallbladder and liver. Acta chirurgica scandinavica 116: 461–476

Elkeles G and Mirrizi P L 1942 A study of the bacteriology of the common bile duct in comparison with other extra hepatic segments of the biliary tract. Annals of Surgery 116: 360–366

Elliott D W 1980 Prevention of sepsis in biliary surgery. In: Controversies in surgical sepsis. Ed: Karran Praeger, Sussex pp 285–291

Engstrom J, Hellstrom K, Hogman L, Lonngvist B 1971 Microorganisms of the liver, biliary tract and duodenal aspirates in biliary diseases. Scandinavian Journal of Gastroenterology 6: 177–182

Ericsson C D, Duke J, Pickering L K 1978 Clinical pharmacology of intravenous and intraperitoneal aminoglycoside antibiotics in prevention of wound infection. Annals of Surgery 188: 66–69

Finch D R A, Taylor L, Morris P J 1979 Wound sepsis following gastrointestinal surgery: a comparison of topical and two dose systemic cephradine. British Journal of Surgery 66: 580–582

Flemma R J, Flint L M, Osterhunt S, Shingleton W W 1967 Bacteriological studies of biliary tract infection. Annals of Surgery 166: 563–572

Hares M M, Hegarty M A, Warlow J, Malms D, Youngs D, Bentley S, Burdon D W, Keighley M R B 1981 A controlled trial to compare systemic and intraincisional cefuroxime prophylaxis in high risk gastric surgery. British Journal of Surgery 68: 276–280

Keighley M R B 1977 Microorganisms in the bile. Annals of the Royal College of Surgeons of England 59: 329–334

Keighley M R B, Burdon D W 1978 Identification of bacteria in the bile by duodenal aspiration. World Journal of Surgery 2: 255–259

Keighley M R B, Burdon D W 1979 In: Antimicrobial Prophylaxis in Surgery. Pitman Medical, Tunbridge Wells

Keighley M R B, Graham N G 1971 Infective complications of choledochotomy with T-tube drainage. British Journal of Surgery 58: 764–769

Keighley M R B, Baddeley R M, Burdon D W, Edward J A, Quoraishi A H, Oates G D, Watts G T, Alexander-Williams J 1975 A controlled trial of parenteral prophylactic gentamicin therapy in biliary surgery. British Journal of Surgery 62: 275–279

Keighley M R B, Drysdale R B, Quoraishi A H, Burdon D W, Alexander-Williams J 1976a Antibiotics in biliary disease: the relative importance of antibiotic concentrations in the bile and serum. Gut 17: 495–500

Keighley M R B, Flinn R, Alexander-Williams 1976b Multivariate analysis of clinical and operative findings associated with biliary sepsis. British Journal of Surgery 63: 528–531

McLeish A R, Keighley M R B, Bishop H M, Burdon D W, Quoraishi A H, Dorricott N J, Oates G D, Alexander-Williams J (1980) Selecting patients requiring antibiotics in biliary surgery by immediate Gram stains of bile at operation. Surgery 81: 473–477

McPherson G A D, Blenkharn I, Nathanson B, Bowley N B, Benjamin I S, Blumgart L H 1982 The significance of bacteria in external biliary drainage systems. A possible role for antisepsis. Journal of Clinical Surgery 1: 22–26

Maddocks A C, Hilson G R F, Taylor R 1973 The bacteriology of the obstructed biliary tract. Annals of the Royal College of Surgeons of England 52: 316–319

Mason G R 1968 Bacteriology and antibiotic selection in biliary surgery. Archives of Surgery 97: 533–537

Morran G, McNaught W, McArdle C S 1978 Prophylactic cotrimoxazole in biliary surgery. British Medical Journal 2: 462–464

Stone H H, Hooper C A, Kolb L D, Geheber D E, Dawkins EZ J 1976 Antibiotic prophylaxis in gastric, biliary and colonic surgery. Annals of Surgery 184: 443–450

Strachan C J, Black J, Powis S J, Waterworth T A, Wise R, Wilkinson A R, Burdon D W, Severn M, Mitra B, Norcott H 1977 Prophylactic use of aphazolin against wound sepsis after cholecystectomy. British Medical Journal 1: 1254–1256

Watson J F 1969 The role of bacterial infection in acute cholecystitis, a prospective clinical study. Military Medicine 134: 416–426

Wise R 1981 Pharmacokinetics and tissue fluid penetration: the relevance to elective surgical prophylaxis. In: Herfarth C, Horn J, Daschner F (eds) Aktuelleprobleme in Chirurgie und Orthopadie. Verlag Hans Heuber, Bern, p 15–20

15 *Biliary disease in the tropics*

D. A. LLOYD and J. A. M. WHITE

Biliary ascariasis

Introduction

The round worm *Ascaris lumbricoides* infests more than a quarter of the world's population and is particularly common in Asia, Africa and Central America where ecologic factors favour maturation of excreted ova. In endemic regions poor socioeconomic conditions, notably inadequate sanitation, lead to heavy faecal contamination of soil around dwellings and 70%–90% of the population harbour the worm.

In man the adult worm lives in the small intestine where the female, when fertilised, lays approximately 200 000 eggs a day. The eggs, or ova, are excreted in the host's faeces and are able to survive adverse environmental conditions. Ova deposited in warm moist soil undergo maturation and are infective if swallowed by man. The mature ovum hatches in the host's duodenum, releasing larvae which penetrate the mucosa of the proximal intestine to enter the portal venous blood in which they are carried through the liver and the right side of the heart to the pulmonary capillary beds. Here the larvae develop further before penetrating the alveoli to travel up the trachea, enter the oesophagus and return to the intestine. In the ileum they mature to adulthood reaching a length of 20–30 cm and have a life-span of one to two years.

Pathology

The tendency for *Ascaris lumbricoides* to enter the common bile duct, especially when there is heavy duodenal infestation, is well known. Usually only one or two worms enter the common bile duct, but massive infestation by more than 60 worms may occur. A worm in the ampulla of Vater stimulates spasm of the sphincter of Oddi and causes biliary colic. The severity of pain depends on the activity of the migrant worm and symptoms may resolve if the worm dies within the biliary tree. The presence of the worm, plus sphincter spasm and papillitis, results in partial biliary obstruction; complete obstruction with jaundice is uncommon. Prolonged biliary infestation leads to ascending cholangitis which may in turn result in necrosis and perforation of the common bile duct, empyema of the gallbladder, or multiple small hepatic abscesses. Dead worms in the biliary

236

tree provoke an inflammatory reaction producing granulomatous strictures of the bile ducts, and calculi may form around skeletal debris. Worms migrating into the intrahepatic bile ducts may invade the liver parenchyma, where they die. The resulting granulomatous reaction may heal without complications or secondary pyogenic infection may result in a liver abscess. Small liver abscesses usually resolve with medical treatment, but untreated abscesses may enlarge and rupture into the peritoneal cavity or into adjacent organs. Obstruction of the pancreatic duct by biliary worms may cause pancreatitis.

The major cause of morbidity and mortality in biliary ascariasis is secondary biliary and hepatic infection leading to septicaemia. Rarely, erosion of an hepatic artery in the wall of a liver abscess causes haemobilia with severe gastrointestinal haemorrhage.

Incidence

Over a four year period 487 children were hospitalised with abdominal ascariasis. Biliary ascariasis was identified in 57 patients of whom 23 (40%) had biliary and hepatic complications and four had acute pancreatitis (Table 15.1). This is a higher incidence of complications than previously reported by Chang & Han (1966) and Louw (1974) who found that fewer than 7% of their patients had complications. We attribute this to a high incidence of massive biliary infestation (Lloyd 1981). During the same period only six adults were treated for biliary ascariasis; all had complications.

Table 15.1 Complications of biliary ascariasis.

	Children	Adults
Biliary ascariasis: all patients	57	6
Hepato-biliary complications	23 (40%)	6 (100%)
Ascending cholangitis	19	4
Empyema of the gall bladder	0	2
Biliary stricture	0	1
Biliary calculi	0	4
Clinical jaundice	4	4
Liver worms	11	1
Liver abscesses	17	3
Haemobilia	1	0
Pancreatitis	4	0

Clinical features

Biliary ascariasis occurs most commonly in children between the ages of two and eight years with a history of vomiting worms or passing worms in the stools (Table 16.2). Acute biliary infestation is characterised by colicky upper abdominal pain with tenderness localised to the right upper quadrant or epigastrium. There may be muscle guarding in the same area and the gallbladder or a mass may be palpable. Some patients have transient fever.

With the development of ascending cholangitis the patient becomes ill, apathetic, irritable and pyrexial. The abdominal colic persists and there may in addition be constant abdominal pain. There is pronounced right upper quadrant tenderness, guarding and rebound tenderness extending towards the epigastrium.

Rarely these signs may be minimal, which can be misleading. The liver may become enlarged and tender; less common findings are a palpable gallbladder, an inflammatory mass in the right upper quadrant and jaundice. Persistent pyrexial illness and increasing hepatomegaly may indicate enlarging liver abscesses. A ruptured liver abscess results in an acute grave illness with peritonitis, although in one patient an abscess ruptured into the stomach with minimal clinical signs.

Table 15.2 Biliary ascariasis in children: clinical features

	Uncomplicated	Hepatobiliary Complications
Number of patients	30	23
Evidence of intestinal worms	25	22
Upper abdominal pain	27	20
Right upper quadrant tenderness	26	22
Right upper quadrant guarding	10	20
Right upper quadrant mass	2	2
Tender hepatomegaly	3	7
Palpable gallbladder	1	3
Clinical jaundice	0	4
Pyrexial illness	2	18

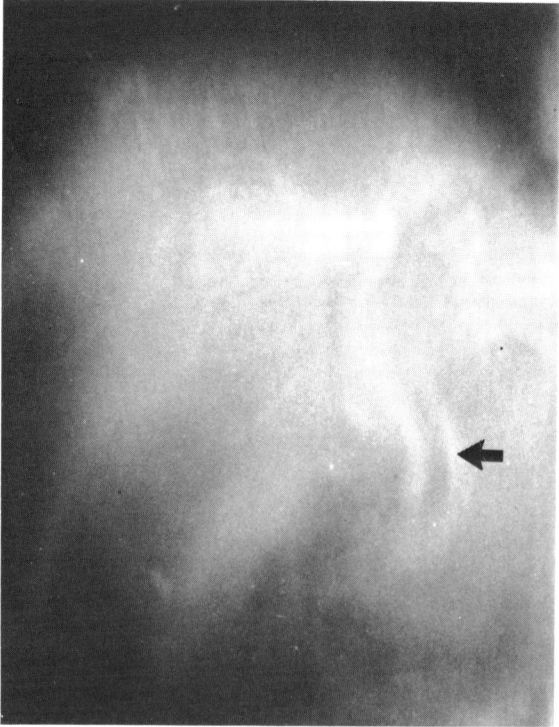

Fig. 15.1 Intravenous cholangiogram showing a tubular filling defect in the common bile duct due to the presence of a round worm (arrow).

Biliary strictures and biliary calculi are late complications usually encountered in adults (Table 15.1). Suppurative cholangitis is common and patients are typically extremely ill with right upper quadrant peritonitis and obstructive jaundice (Pillay et al 1978). There may be no clinical evidence of ascariasis if the complications become manifest long after the precipitating infestation.

Diagnosis
Laboratory studies
Stool microscopy may demonstrate ascaris ova or remnants of dead worms. This is of value in the absence of a firm history of intestinal infestation.

Peripheral blood count. In uncomplicated biliary ascariasis the peripheral white cell count is usually normal. A leucocytosis greater than 12 000 cells/mm^3 is associated with biliary and hepatic complications. The eosinophil count is seldom elevated above 5% and is not of diagnostic value.

Biochemical investigations. Moderate elevation of the serum bilirubin level may occur in uncomplicated biliary ascariasis; hyperbilirubinaemia greater than 70 mm/l indicates biliary or hepatic complications. Elevation of serum alkaline phosphatase and liver enzyme levels may also occur with complicated disease. The serum amylase level is usually normal or moderately elevated but may rise as high as 5000 units/100 ml in patients with otherwise uncomplicated biliary ascariasis.

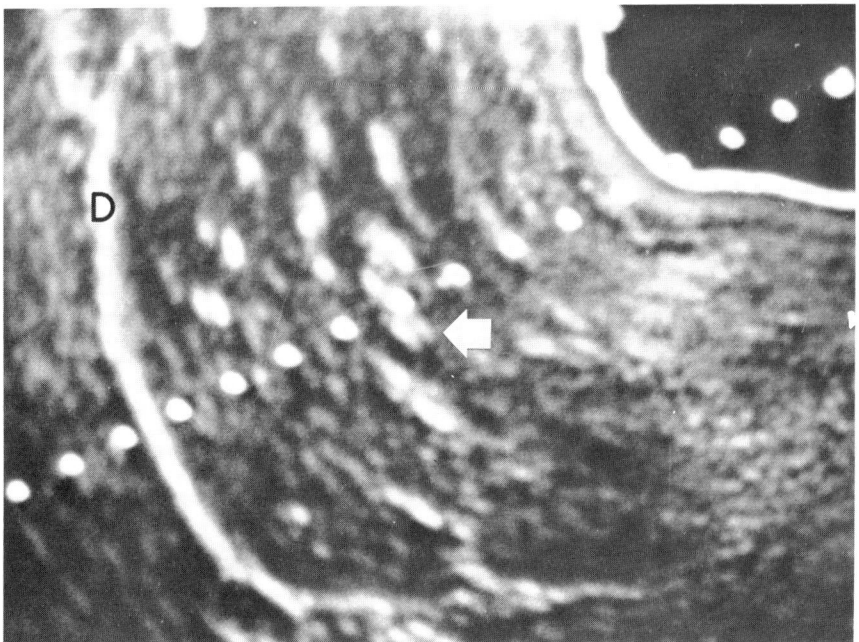

Fig. 15.2 Longitudinal ultrasonic scan of the liver 5 cm to the right of the midline showing multiple linear and rounded areas of increased echogenity distributed throughout the liver parenchyma, representing intrahepatic worms (arrow). D = diaphragm.

Diagnostic imaging

Abdominal radiographs will confirm the presence of intestinal worms in 90% of patients. Rarely, air is seen in the biliary tree or in hepatic or subphrenic abscesses.

Intravenous cholangiography (IVC) is diagnostic in 75% of patients with uncomplicated biliary ascariasis, showing tubular filling defects in the bile ducts representing worms (Fig. 15.1). A dilated common bile duct without a filling defect may be seen in biliary ascariasis and requires further investigation.

The IVC fails to opacify the biliary tree in 10% of patients with uncomplicated biliary ascariasis and in 68% of those with biliary and hepatic complications, even when the serum bilirubin is normal. The reason for this is not known. With massive biliary infestation the incidence of non-opacification is 80% and we regard the 'failed' cholangiogram as strongly suggestive of massive infestation if the clinical features are compatable with a diagnosis of biliary ascariasis.

Ultrasonic scanning. Static B-mode grey-scale ultrasonography will demonstrate a dilated biliary system containing round worms. A distended gallbladder or swollen pancreas may sometimes be seen. Ultrasonic scanning is particularly valuable for identifying intra-hepatic worms and abscesses and is a safe method of

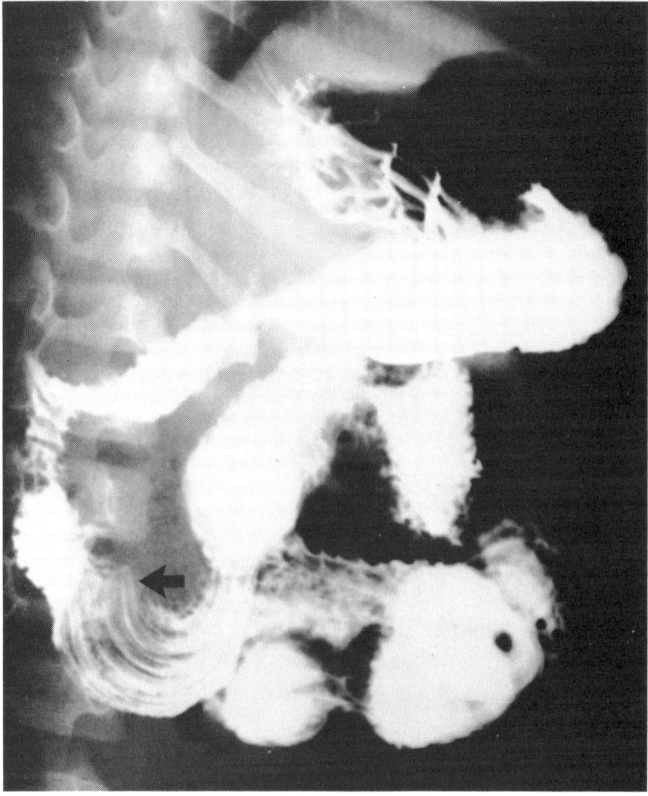

Fig. 15.3 Barium meal examination showing linear filling defects representing a mass of worms in the third part of the duodenum entering the ampulla of Vater (arrow), the 'ampullary cut-off' sign. (Reproduced with permission from the British Journal of Surgery 1981.)

monitoring the response of these lesions to treatment (Fig. 15.2). Ascaris liver abscesses are more echogenic compared to other types of liver abscesses, probably because they contain worm debris. Experience is necessary if subjective errors in interpreting the ultrasound scan are to be avoided.

Barium meal examination is useful when the intravenous cholangiogram fails to opacify the biliary tree. The presence of worms in the duodenum supports the diagnosis of biliary ascariasis. Worms in the second part of the duodenum may be seen to enter the ampulla of Vater, beyond which the part of the worm within the common bile duct is not visible. This is the 'ampullary cut-off sign' (Fig. 15.3).

Endoscopic retrograde cholangiography (ERCP). Fibre-optic endoscopy is used when the above investigations fail to provide a firm diagnosis. A vermifuge is given before the examination to eliminate worms from the duodenum. Worms found protruding from the ampulla of Vater may be removed by the endoscopist. ERCP will demonstrate worms in the biliary, hepatic and pancreatic ducts and may opacify hepatic abscesses (Fig. 15.4). We have not encountered infective complications following endoscopic cannulation, but broad spectrum antibiotic cover may be advisable.

Percutaneous trans-hepatic cholangiography (PTHC). In adults with obstructive jaundice resulting from late complications of biliary ascariasis PTHC has been

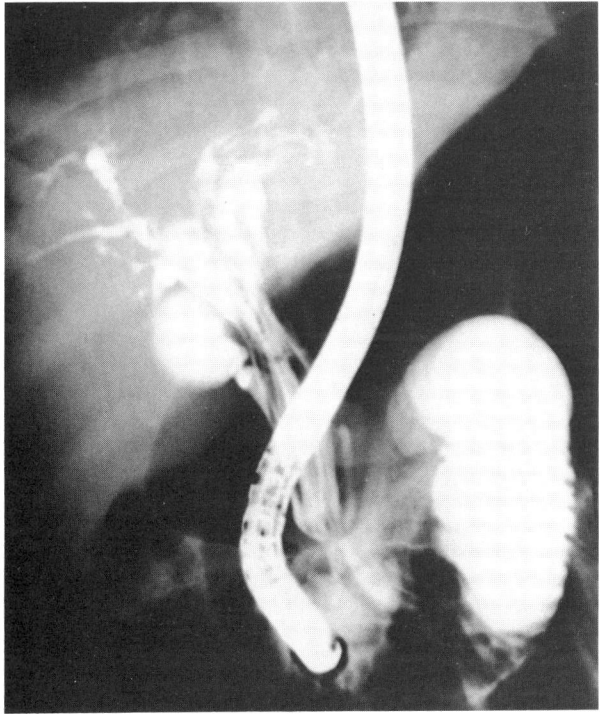

Fig. 15.4 Endoscopic retrograde cholangiogram of the same patient as Fig. 15.3 after anthelminthic therapy. Note numerous filling defects in the biliary tree representing round worms, and dilated intrahepatic ducts. (Reproduced with permission from the British Journal of Surgery 1981.)

used successfully to demonstrate the biliary tree (Fig. 15.5). We have not used PTHC in children, preferring less invasive investigations.

Radioisotope liver scanning may demonstrate a cold area representing an intrahepatic abscess, but most ascaris liver abscesses are too small to be identified by this method. A distended gallbladder may produce a cold area mimicking a right lobe liver abscess.

Selective hepatic arteriography is required for the rare patient with haemobilia due to major haemorrhage into an ascaris liver abscess. It may be possible to combine this with selective arterial embolisation.

Computerised axial tomography may be of value in diagnosing complicated hepatobiliary ascariasis. A disadvantage in children is the relatively high dose of radiation emitted.

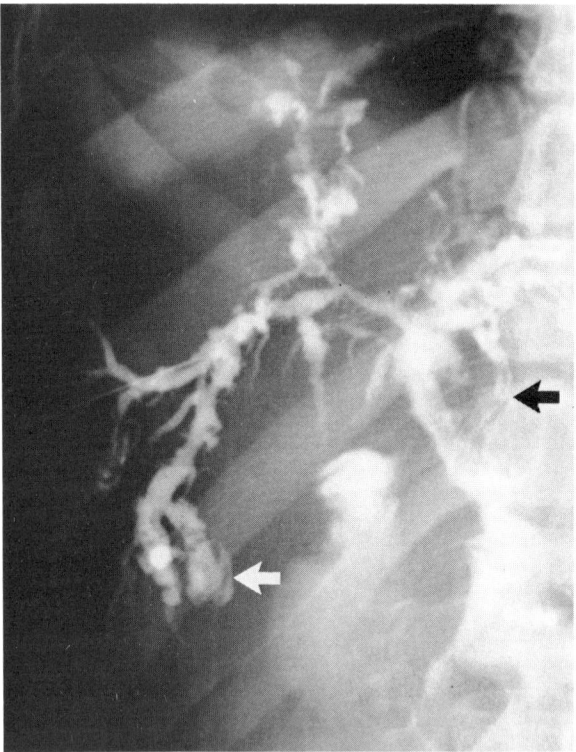

Fig. 15.5 Percutaneous transhepatic cholangiogram showing irregularities throughout the biliary tree due to extensive ascariasis and pyogenic infection. Filling defects representing worms are seen in a liver abscess (white arrow) and the common bile duct (black arrow).

Management

Chang & Han (1966) and Louw (1966) showed that in over 90% of patients with uncomplicated acute biliary ascariasis the worm will spontaneously leave the common bile duct if appropriate medical treatment is given. In our own experience 83% of patients with uncomplicated biliary ascariasis recovered without operation (Table 15.3).

Table 15.3 Biliary ascariasis in children: management

	Uncomplicated	Hepatobiliary complications	Pancreatitis
Number of patients	30	23	4
Conservative	25	8	2
Endoscopic removal	1	0	1
Operation	4*	15	1†

*Indications: persistent filling defect on cholangiography (1), unremitting symptoms (3).
†Extraction of biliary worms and drainage of pancreatic abscess.

The medical management of biliary ascariasis aims to relax the sphincter of Oddi with parenteral antispasmodics, thus relieving the biliary colic and enabling the worm to return to the intestine. Occasionally analgesia is required for severe pain. Intravenous fluids and naso-gastric drainage are advised during the acute stage, which usually lasts from two to four days. Anthelminthics are not given until after the acute symptoms have resolved to avoid killing worms in the biliary tree and because of the risk of precipitating intestinal obstruction by killing worms packed into the proximal small intestine.

Follow-up intravenous cholangiography is recommended to confirm that the worm has evacuated the common bile duct. The acute symptoms resolve when the worm withdraws from the sphincter of Oddi and the worm may lie within the biliary tree without producing symptoms.

The role of surgery
Indications for operation have been defined by Chang & Han (1966) and Louw (1966), namely a persistent filling defect in the biliary tree on follow-up cholangiography, persistent severe symptoms not controlled by adequate conservative therapy, and clinical evidence of biliary or hepatic complications. These principles pertain today, but the role of surgery has been modified by advances in ultrasonic scanning and fibre-optic endoscopy. Biliary and hepatic lesions can be accurately identified and monitored, and in some patients worms can be removed from the bile ducts endoscopically.

Following the operative removal of biliary worms troublesome complications may occur because of worms left in inaccessible intrahepatic ducts or as a result of re-infestation of the bile ducts by intestinal worms. Surgery is therefore not necessarily the ultimate cure and conservative management is preferred whenever possible.

Management of persistent uncomplicated biliary infestation
Follow-up IVC is done on all patients with uncomplicated biliary ascariasis ten days after symptoms have resolved. If the worm is still in the biliary tree a second course of anthelminthics is given. The IVC is repeated two weeks later, by which time the worms have usually left the biliary tree. Should worms persist in the bile ducts fibre-optic endoscopic removal is attempted. A worm protruding from the ampulla of Vater can be removed with biopsy forceps. When the worm is completely within the common bile duct it may be possible to flush it out with

saline or extract it with a Dormia basket (Höchter et al 1980). If this fails, surgical removal is required (Table 15.3). Worms should not be allowed to remain in the biliary tree longer than six weeks, since by this time they are likely to be dead and may disintegrate, provoking a granulomatous inflammatory reaction and becoming difficult to remove.

Management of persistent symptoms

When there is severe unremitting pain without evidence of complications, an anthelminthic is given to eliminate the duodenal worms and thus encourage the biliary worms to return to the intestine. In persistent cases endoscopic removal is recommended. Surgery should rarely be necessary provided medical management has been adequate.

Management of complicated biliary ascariasis

Uncomplicated biliary ascariasis is a benign condition which usually resolves spontaneously, but when complications develop the condition becomes serious and potentially fatal and it is essential that complications be recognised and treated early. The risk of complications increases when there is massive biliary infestation (Lloyd 1981).

Urgent operation is indicated when there is severe toxaemia and localised or generalised peritonitis. A limited period of conservative management with preoperative antimicrobial and anthelminthic therapy is recommended, depending on the clinical condition of the patient.

Patients who have signs of complications but who are not severely ill are initially managed conservatively and broad spectrum antimicrobials are administered. This allows time for:

(a) urgent investigations to define the nature and extent of the disease. In most patients with complicated biliary ascariasis the intravenous cholangiogram fails to opacify the biliary tree and additional investigations are required to establish the diagnosis.

(b) adequate anthelminthic therapy to eradicate the intestinal worms and prevent postoperative re-infestation of the biliary tree. Eliminating duodenal worms may aid spontaneous recovery in some patients by encouraging the biliary worms to return to the intestine. When the intestine is heavily laden with worms the vermifuge should be given cautiously because of the risk of precipitating intestinal obstruction, but this has not occurred in our experience.

Conservative management is continued as long as there is clinical improvement. We recommend operation if a satisfactory response is not being maintained after treatment for ten days, as the risk of serious septic complications increases after this. Patients treated conservatively must be monitored closely and operation is undertaken urgently if there is evidence of deterioration. The danger signs are worsening toxaemia and right upper quadrant peritonism, progressive tender enlargement of the liver, and increasing jaundice with a serum bilirubin level greater than 70 mmol/l.

In our series 8 (35%) of 23 patients with hepatobiliary complications responded to conservative management (Table 15.3). These included 2 with tender hepatomegaly; two with jaundice and a serum bilirubin level greater than 60 mmol/l; and three with ultrasonic evidence of liver abscesses. Of 17 patients with massive biliary infestation, 14 required operation.

Haemobilia due to haemorrhage into a liver abscess is a rare complication of biliary ascariasis. The diagnosis is made by hepatic angiography. Refractory haemorrhage may be controlled by selective arterial embolisation or surgical intervention; in our single patient the bleeding ceased spontaneously.

Surgical aspects

In acute biliary ascariasis the common bile duct is oedematous and distended and worms are palpable as thickened cords within the duct. Worms may be found in the cystic duct, but rarely in the gallbladder. Operative cholangiography via the gallbladder or common bile duct may be useful.

The common bile duct is explored through a longitudinal choledochotomy and worms are removed. A careful search is made for worms in the hepatic ducts and compression of the superior surface of the liver will help to move intrahepatic worms towards the common bile duct. We have removed up to 65 worms from the biliary tree. With prolonged infestation dead worms, purulent bile and calculi may be encountered. The biliary tree is irrigated with saline and closed with T-tube drainage. Peroperative cholangiography will confirm patency of the common bile duct and detect residual biliary and intrahepatic worms. Fibre-optic choledocho-scopy may be of value. When a biliary stricture is present choledocho-jejunostomy-en-Y is recommended. Cholecystectomy is not necessary unless the gallbladder contains worms or is abnormal.

The liver may contain nodules or abscesses and worms may be seen under the liver capsule. The worms are removed and prominent nodules are explored by blunt dissection, yielding worms, granulation tissue or pus. Large worm nests and abscesses are not common, but one of our patients had 78 live worms in a cavity in the right lobe of the liver. We recommend biliary decompression after draining ascaris liver abscesses, either by T-tube if the common duct is explored or by cholecystostomy. As well as draining the biliary tree this provides access for postoperative cholangiography.

Toxaemia is common after operation and broad spectrum antimicrobials and supportive therapy are required. Postoperative anthelminthic therapy is administered when intestinal function has returned. T-tube cholangiography is performed eight to ten days after operation to confirm patency of the biliary tree.

Re-infestation of the bile duct

There have been many reports of this complication, which is serious in that a second operation may be required to remove the biliary worms. Although re-infestation may be due to worms overlooked in the intrahepatic biliary tree at operation, in most patients it results from migration of intestinal worms into the common bile duct. Re-infestation is best prevented by preoperative anthelmin-thic therapy but this is not always possible. When intestinal worms are encountered in large numbers at operation, removal through an enterostomy is the most reliable way of preventing biliary re-infestation. Milking worms from the proximal small intestine to the colon is time consuming and traumatic and does not always prevent re-infestation (Lloyd 1981). Anthelminthics administered in the immediate postoperative period do not reach the small intestine in time to prevent biliary re-infestation. Re-infestation of the bile ducts is treated expectantly as the worm may spontaneously return to the intestine. Failing this, endoscopic removal or re-operation will be required. If a T-tube is *in situ* the worm may have become stuck in or around the tube and may be removed by applying suction to the tube and gently withdrawing it.

Pancreatitis

Invasion of the pancreatic duct by worms is rare in our experience. Acute pancreatitis may be associated with biliary ascariasis and is suspected when the abdominal pain and tenderness involve the epigastrium, left upper quadrant or left lumbar area (Louw 1974). The serum amylase level is elevated and swelling of the pancreas may be identified on ultrasonic scanning. Treatment is directed at the biliary worms and the pancreatitis resolves spontaneously once the worms have left the biliary tree. Conservative management is usually successful, but endoscopic or operative removal of the worm may be required (Table 15.3). Cyst-gastrostomy is recommended for a peristent pseudocyst (Louw 1974) and a pancreatic abscess will require drainage.

Prognosis

Full recovery is usual in uncomplicated biliary ascariasis. With careful selection of patients for operation the prognosis is good, and in Chang & Han's (1966) series of 788 patients treated selectively the mortality rate was 0.25%. The single death in our series was a patient with massive hepatobiliary infestation who developed a right subphrenic abscess following evacuation of a large nest of worms in the right lobe of the liver. The biliary tree was not drained. The subphrenic abscess ruptured through the diaphragm resulting in a broncho-pleural fistula and multiple lung abscesses, and the patient died of septicaemia.

Conclusions

The frequency with which uncomplicated intestinal ascariasis is encountered in endemic areas has led to a casual and indifferent attitude on the part of clinicians, many of whom are unaware of the natural history and potential hazards of biliary infestation. We would emphasise the following:

1. Acute minimal biliary ascariasis due to infestation of the bile ducts by one or two worms is usually an uncomplicated disease in childhood and is treated conservatively.

2. In adults, biliary ascariasis is uncommon and is frequently complicated by calculi, biliary strictures and suppurative cholangitis.

3. Massive hepatobiliary ascariasis, characterised by infestation of the biliary tree by large numbers of worms and non-opacification of the bile ducts on intravenous cholangiography, does not readily respond to conservative manage-ment and is commonly associated with biliary and hepatic complications, in children as well as adults.

4. Fibre-optic endoscopy is playing an increasing role in the management of biliary ascariasis. Endoscopic retrograde cholangiography is useful when other investigations have failed to provide a firm diagnosis. We recommend endoscopic removal of worms under the following circumstances: unremitting symptoms of biliary ascariasis; persistent radiological evidence of biliary infestation after conservative treatment; and postoperative re-infestation of the bile ducts.

5. Operation is indicated when attempts at endoscopic clearance are unsuccessful or when there is evidence of progressive complications with toxaemia and peritonitis.

6. A trial of conservative management is warranted for patients with signs of complications who are not severely ill because some will recover without operation. An accurate diagnosis and careful monitorng are essential.

7. Preoperative anthelminthics may prevent the vexing post-operative complication of biliary re-infestation.

8. Prevention of biliary infestation is impossible in endemic areas. The risk of biliary invasion is proportional to the degree of intestinal infestation and regular anthelminthic therapy to reduce the intestinal load may discourage migration of worms into the biliary tree.

Biliary hydatid disease

Echinococcus granulosus is a small tape worm infesting dogs, jackals and other carnivores. Eggs passed in the faeces are ingested by sheep, cattle and occasionally man, resulting in the formation of hydatid cysts at various sites, predominantly the liver and lungs.

The wall of a hydatid cyst consists of three layers. The inner (germinal) layer gives rise to brood capsules which, with freed scolices, form 'hydatid sand'. The intermediate layer is a tough laminated membrane and an outer fibrous capsule separates the cyst from the surrounding host tissues. A fertile cyst contains clear fluid, daughter cysts and 'hydatid sand', but cysts may be parasitologically sterile and contain no brood capsules. Secondary bacterial infection of an hepatic hydatid cyst renders the cyst sterile and leads to the formation of a liver abscess which may rupture.

A large hepatic hydatid cyst may compress and obstruct the intrahepatic bile ducts. If a cyst ruptures into a bile duct, the biliary system may be blocked by extrusion of parts of the intermediate layer of the cyst wall or by hydatid sand and daughter cysts. Obstruction of the common bile duct leads to progressive obstructive jaundice with cholangiohepatitis. Even in highly endemic areas this is a rare complication of hydatid liver disease and we have treated only two such cases over a 20 year period. A high incidence of intrabiliary rupture (16%) has been reported from Iraq (Kattan 1975).

Clinical features
There is a history of residence in an endemic area. Biliary obstruction is manifest by acute colicky right hypochondrial pain, increasing pyrexia and malaise with rigors and obvious jaundice. There is diffuse hepatomegaly and marked upper

abdominal tenderness and rigidity. The clinical picture mimics an empyema of the gallbladder with incipient perforation, but there are atypical features suggesting that the liver is the primary site of the pathology. The jaundice tends to be progressive with evidence of cholangiohepatitis that does not respond to antimicrobal drugs.

Diagnosis

Laboratory investigations: Peripheral blood examination shows a polymorph leucocytosis but eosinophilia has little significance in countries with a high incidence of other parasitic diseases. Biochemical examination shows rapidly escalating serum bilirubin levels up to 200 mmol/l with other features of obstructive jaundice and hepatocyte damage. Serum amylase values are normal or slightly raised. Serological tests are unreliable and are seldom used. Stool examination may be non-contributory but is routinely performed to exclude other parasitic diseases.

Diagnostic imaging: Plain abdominal and chest radiographs may show associated hydatid lung disease, calcification of the wall of hepatic hydatid cycts, mass lesions in the liver and gas in the biliary tract. Intravenous cholangiography and excretory radioisotope biliary scanning were not feasible in our patients because of the high serum bilirubin levels. Ultrasonic scanning of the liver shows a well defined transonic area in which multiple septae are seen when daughter cysts are present. Echoes consistent with amorphous debris are associated with secondly infection. Fibreoptic endoscopy may be used to exclude coincidental gastro-duodenal pathology but retrograde biliary cannulation with cholangiography is not advised in these heavily infected patients.

Aspiration of an hepatic hydatid cyst may cause leakage of hydatid fluid, dissemination of hydatid material and an acute allergic reaction. These problems do not arise in grossly infected cysts that have ruptured into the biliary system. Examination of the aspirate permits accurate diagnosis of the cause of the hepatic abscess and isolation of aerobic and anaerobic bacteria. In our patients hydatid debris was identified but complete drainage could not be achieved because the wide-bore needles used were repeatedly blocked by debris. Injection of contrast material into the abscess cavity gave accurate delineation of its extent but did not demonstrate communication with the biliary tract. Masses of hydatid material within the cavity were outlined to give the characteristic 'soap-bubble' appearance.

Management

In these gravely ill patients an initial conservative approach is advised in an attempt to control the secondary bacterial infection. Management includes aspiration-drainage of the abscess cavity coupled with antimicrobial therapy.

Intractable biliary obstruction with severe secondary infection is an indication for early biliary decompression and evacuation of the liver cyst. In patients with a large right lobar hepatic abscess, access to the gallbladder and bile ducts is severely restricted and is not greatly improved by formal drainage of the abscess because the whole hepatic parenchyma is swollen. Following full duodenal mobilisation and intraoperative cholangiography, supraduodenal choledochotomy is performed and hydatid debris is extracted from the ducts by manipulation and lavage, aided by fibre-optic choledochoscopy. The gallbladder is removed if abnormal and clearance of the duct system confirmed by fractionated control cholangiography.

Rapid improvement follows drainage of the hepatic abscess, continuing antimicrobial therapy and T-tube drainage of the duct system. Mebendazole is used in the recovery period to aid resolution of the underlying hepatic disease (Kayser 1980).

Fascioliasis

Humans are an incidental definitive host of the sheep liver fluke *Fasciola hepatica* in moist highly endemic areas of the tropics, where infestation may deciminate flocks due to progressive liver destruction (Fripp 1979).

The adult form of *F. hepatica* is a large (20 x 10 mm) flat, leaf-shaped fluke which inhabits the bile ducts and gallbladder of the host. Eggs laid in the bile ducts enter the intestine and, after being passed in the faeces, hatch to form a motile miracidium that enters snails of the Lymnae species. These excrete encysted metacercaria which contaminate riverside vegetation and irrigated crops and are ingested by the host, liberating larvae which penetrate the intestinal wall and reach the biliary tree by eating through the liver. The adults develop in the bile ducts and have a life-span of three to four years. Heavy biliary infestation in man causes focal hepatic necrosis and abscess formation, hepatic and biliary fibrosis, cholangiohepatitis, impaired nutrition and death.

Severe *Fasciola* infestation is not amenable to surgical treatment and may respond poorly to the many drugs used in conservative management (Chloroquin 150 mg twice daily for 14 days is recommended). Significant biliary obstruction is rare and has been seen only twice in 20 years. In both patients intermittent biliary obstruction was shown on intravenous cholangiography to be due to flukes impacted in the distal common bile duct and the characteristic eggs were found on stool examination. The flukes were removed by supraduodenal choledochotomy without difficulty.

Clonorchiasis (opisthorchiasis)

Infestation by the liver fluke *Clonorchis sinensis* is common in eastern Asia, particularly in China, Taiwan, Korea and Japan. The adult worms inhabit the intrahepatic bile ducts and with massive infestations may be found throughout the biliary tree. The eggs are laid in the bile ducts and reach the intestine to be excreted in the faeces. The life-cycle continues in fresh water where certain species of snail and fish are consecutive intermediate hosts. Human infestation occurs from eating inadequately cooked contamined fish (Muller 1975).

Clonorchiasis results in inflammation of the biliary epithelium. The inflammatory reaction extends through the wall of the bile ducts and long-standing infestation leads to periductal fibrosis and destruction of adjacent liver parenchyma. Stones form around worm debris and there is an increased incidence of carcinoma of the bile duct in endemic areas. Other late complications include cirrhosis of the liver and portal hypertension with splenomegaly and ascites.

In 75% of patients the infestation is symptomless. The presence of more than 100 worms in the bile ducts results in diarrhoea and abdominal discomfort. Heavy infestation by thousands of worms causes biliary colic and pyogenic cholangitis leading to cholecystitis and hepatitis. These are manifest by fever, right upper quadrant pain and tenderness, and hepatomegaly. Jaundice occurs in 8% of patients. Chronic relapsing suppurative cholangitis is common and severe infection may be fatal.

The diagnosis is made by identifying eggs in the faeces or duodenal aspirate, and an intradermal test with purified antigen is available. Radiological investigations will demonstrate biliary pathology (Baker et al 1974).

There is no satisfactory medical treatment for clonorchiasis and operation is necessary for complications. Choledochotomy with T-tube drainage is required for obstruction of the common bile duct by stones and worms, with or without cholangitis. Sphincteroplasty or choledochoduodenostomy may also be required (Sullivan & Koep 1980).

Opisthorchis viverrini infests 90% of the population of Thailand. Over 80% of those infested have no symptoms but long-standing biliary infestation may result in chronic biliary and hepatic lesions.

Hepato-biliary amoebiasis

Entamoeba histolytica infestation is highly endemic in the moist areas of many countries lying in the tropical and sub-tropical zones and is a common cause of hepatic abscess formation. We admit approximately 40 children annually with amoebic liver abscesses. Hepatic amoebiasis may be insidious in its presentation and is usually a progressive liquefactive necrosis of one or more areas of liver tissue. Secondary infection may occur, especially after repeated aspiration of large abscess cavities. In an already ill patient, it causes increasing toxaemia, deepening jaundice and signs of cholangiohepatitis.

In 80% of patients the diagnosis of amoebic liver abscess is confirmed by ultrasonic scanning. Treatment is by percutaneous needle aspiration and oral metronidazole, with antimicrobial agents when there is secondary bacterial infection. Surgery is reserved for abscesses which do not respond to aspiration or which are not easily accessible for safe aspiration, and for left lobar abscesses which may rupture into the thoracic cavity causing cardiac tamponade.

The response to formal drainage is good but a biliary-cutaneous fistula may follow removal of the drain. This will usually close spontaneously but occasionally becomes chronic. A rare but grave complication is persistence of a residual fibrous cavity in the liver communicating with a major bile duct; this may be the source of recurrent cholangiohepatitis and septicaemia. The cavity can be accurately localised by sinography and other imaging methods. Recurrent cholangiohepatitis may persist in spite of apparently adequate drainage of the tract, curettage of the cavity and continued drug therapy. Under these circumstances elective formal resection of the cavity and adjacent liver tissue is indicated. In our experience the results of such a limited resection are good but the procedure is technically difficult.

Typhoid fever

Large-scale migration from poverty-stricken rural areas into the cities in search of industrial employment in many tropical countries has been followed by the development of periurban slums with poor social services. Reliable purified water supplies are not available and faecal contamination of surface water is common. In such areas typhoid fever is endemic and periodic outbreaks affect both children and adults (Mandal 1979).

Acute cholecystitis occurring as a complication of overt typhoid is seen in only 1% of cases and is associated with excretion of bacilli in the bile during the septicaemic phase of the disease. A more common presentation in adults is acute cholecystitis occurring without a previous history of typhoid fever in an otherwise healthy patient. The gallbladder is recognised as a common reservoir in persistent carriers of the disease.

Gallstones are rare among the poorer classes in tropical countries because the high carbohydrate, low fat and low protein content of the diet does not favour the formation of lithogenic bile. In these population groups acute cholecystitis is seldom associated with gallstones and *S. typhi* should be remembered as one of the organisms causing acalculous cholecystitis. Appropriate steps should be taken to isolate the organism from stools, urine and blood and to perform serological tests.

Emergency surgery is rarely indicated in this condition and the response to conservative management using a modern synthetic penicillin or chloramphenicol is good. In tropical countries latent biliary infestation may cause serious complications following major hepatic trauma.

References

Baker M S, Baker B H, Woo R 1979 Biliary clonorchiasis. Archives of Surgery 114: 748
Chang C-C, Han C-T 1966 Biliary ascariasis in childhood. A clinical analysis of 788 cases. Chinese Medical Journal 85: 167–171
Fripp P J 1979 An introduction to human parasitology. Macmillan, Johannesburg, p 57–61
Höchter W, Weingart J, Dofel W, Stölzle K, Ottenjann R 1980 Endoskopische transpapilläre extraktion eines Ascaris lumbricoides. Deutsche Medizinisches Wochenschrift 48: 1685–1686
Kattan Y B 1975 Intrabiliary rupture of hydatid cyst of the liver. British Journal of Surgery 62: 885–890
Kayser H J S 1980 Treatment of hydatid disease with mebendazole at Frere Hospital, East London. South African Medical Journal 58: 560–563
Lloyd D A 1981 Massive hepato-biliary ascariasis in childhood. British Journal of Surgery 68: 468–473
Louw J H 1966 Abdominal complications of Ascaris lumbricoides infestation in children. British Journal of Surgery 53: 510–521
Louw J H 1974 Biliary ascariasis in childhood. South African Journal of Surgery 12: 219–225
Mandal B K 1979 Typhoid and para-typhoid fever. Clinics in Gastroenterology 8: 715–735
Pillay S P, Baker L W, Angorn I B 1978 Ascaris lumbricoides producing obstructive jaundice. Annals of the Royal College of Surgeons of Edinburgh 23: 25–29
Sullivan W G, Koep L J 1980 Common bile duct obstruction and cholangiohepatitis in clonorchiasis. Journal of American Medical Association 243: 2060–61

16 Diseases of the bile ducts in the paediatric age group

P. G. JONES

Diseases of the bile ducts in infants and children can be divided into two groups:

(a) Those due to developmental anomalies or destructive perinatal inflammation (biliary atresia)

(b) those occurring most commonly in adult life (cholelithiasis, cholecystitis, traumatic injuries etc) which may nevertheless arise in the paediatric age group. Those to be described in this chapter are as follows:

I   Developmental anomalies
    1. Duodenal obstruction and related anomalies of the bile ducts
    2. Cystic dilatations: choledochal cysts
    3. Coexistant or associated malformations

II Acquired biliary disease
    1. Atresia of the extrahepatic bile ducts
    2. Cholelithiasis
    3. Acute acalculous cholecystitis

III Tumours of the liver and bile ducts

IV Traumatic injuries

Developmental anomalies

While some anomalies do not in themselves cause any disturbance of function, and other malformations may not give rise to symptoms until adult life, a few aberrations of the complex embryology of duodenal region, including the extrahepatic bile ducts, are responsible for an important group of malformations presenting in the neonatal period. The following conditions, and their importance in diagnosis and management, will be described.

Duodenal obstruction: septum, 'atresia' or stenosis (with or without an annular pancreas) invariably associated with some abnormality of the terminal segment of the common bile duct.

Cystic dilatation(s) of the bile ducts, intra- or extrahepatic or both, i.e. choledochal cysts.

Co-existant or associated malformations, e.g. preduodenal portal vein; anomalous rotation and fixation of the duodenum; variations in the number, origin, course and branches of the hepatic artery; accessory bile ducts; anomalies of the gallbladder and cystic duct and the intramural ducts forming the ampulla. These anatomical variations are generally well known as hazards to be anticipated and avoided in biliary surgery (Lilly & Chandra 1974), and with the exception of ampullary anomalies, will not be considered further.

Duodenal obstruction

Although not necessarily causing biliary obstructive disease, a group of duodenal malformations associated with ductal anomalies present as intestinal obstruction in the newborn (Gourevitch 1971, Grosfeld 1975. Lynn 1979, Merrill & Raffensperger 1976). A knowledge of the variations in the number and probable sites of opening of the bile duct(s) is essential to avoid injury to them during operative relief of some forms of duodenal obstruction. Some of the entities which have been identified are shown in Figure 16.1, but the practical solution is to bypass the obstruction without attempting to determine the nature of any latent biliary anomalies. As bypass operations are usually successful, the precise anatomy is delineated only infrequently, in autopsy material.

An *annular pancreas* covering or surrounding the duodenum (usually the second part), originally thought to contribute to or cause the duodenal obstruction, is now recognised as incidental, although covering the real cause of obstruction in the duodenal wall (Gilroy & Adams 1960). The occasional incidental discovery of an asymptomatic annular pancreas at laparotomy in later life confirms this view. The exact anatomy of duodenal obstruction associated with an annular pancreas probably varies from one example to another, but what appears to be the commonest pattern found in autopsy material, is shown in Figure 16.1b.

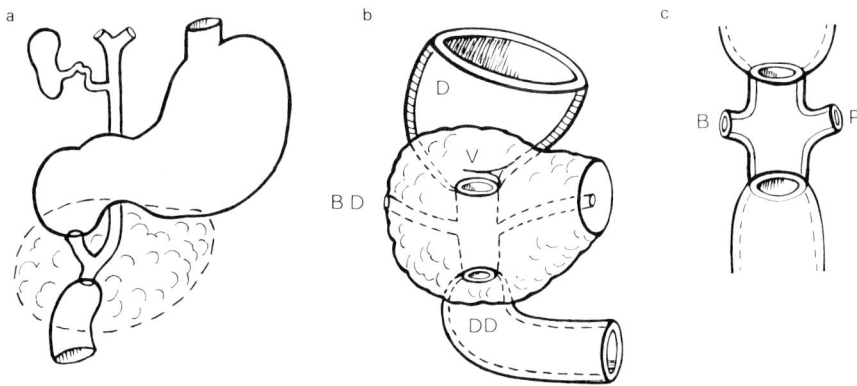

Fig. 16.1 Atresia of the duodenum: a. There is discontinuity of the wall; the bifid common duct opens into both segments, and the outline of the overlying pancreas is indicated (Jona & Belin 1976); b. A common arrangement seen in autopsy material. Continuity between the proximal duodenum (D) and the distal segment (DD) is provided by a short segment of bile duct into which opens (schematically) the 'common' bile duct (BD) and at least one pancreatic duct (P). Continuous continuity is limited by the presence of a mucosal flap (V) which can act as a valve; c. Diagramatic detail of b. (After Noblett & Paton 1970).

Estimates of the incidence of anomalous bile ducts in infants with duodenal obstruction range from 19% to 78% (Gourevitch 1971, Gross 1953, Noblett & Paton 1970); the lowest figures are derived from operative rather than autopsy findings.

Treatment
The associations of supra-ampullary duodenal obstruction and Down's syndrome should be remembered, and a thorough examination for sometimes far from obvious external markers should be made, and also for evidence of a cardiovascular malformation. As in any neonate with suspected intestinal obstruction, a nasogastric tube to decompress the stomach and duodenum and prevent the inhalation of vomitus is a matter of urgency, especially when the infant is to be transported to a paediatric surgical centre.

Preservation of normal body temperature, and restoration of fluid and electrolyte losses are essential before surgical treatment. Plain films of the abdomen typically show the 'double-bubble' of duodenal obstruction and delayed, or incomplete, aeration of the distal bowel. Contrast studies with barium or Gastrografin® are not required and better omitted when careful positioning reveals the typical findings.

At laparotomy the obstruction is relieved by an appropriate 'bypass' anastomosis, e.g. duodenoduodenostomy or duodenojejunostomy. In centres with the full complement of paediatric facilities and skills the prognosis is good and in the absence of serious coexistant anomalies, prematurity, etc, most infants should survive.

Whether the associated biliary anomalies are likely to cause complication in later life, is as yet uncertain, but there have already been reports of cholelithiasis in such cases, and as more survivors reach adolescence and adult life, the true incidence will become apparent.

Duodenal septum

A complete septum, or more commonly, an incomplete septum with an eccentric deficiency, are recognised as causes of duodenal obstruction, in which the associated anomalous openings of the bile ducts, similar to those in duodenal 'atresia-stenosis', suggest that both conditions are part of one spectrum of anomalies. Some of the common forms of incomplete duodenal septum are illustrated in Figure 16.2. In one type the septum is elongated, ab initio or as the result of peristaltic distension, with an eccentric defect (Fig. 16.3) prone to intermittent obstruction. This type can cause symptoms of obstruction (a) in the newborn; (b) when solid foods are introduced; (c) in the toddler age group; or (d) later in childhood. Occasionally symptoms first appear when a foreign body becomes impacted in the orifice. The membranous 'wind sock' type of septum poses technical difficulties in identifying its site of attachment to the duodenal wall, and a gastrotomy, or one or two duodenotomies may be required to introduce a Foley catheter or urethral sounds to demonstrate the precise anatomy.

As the common bile duct probably opens via one or two orifices into the septum, or into the duodenal wall just above and below it, usually in the left or posterior

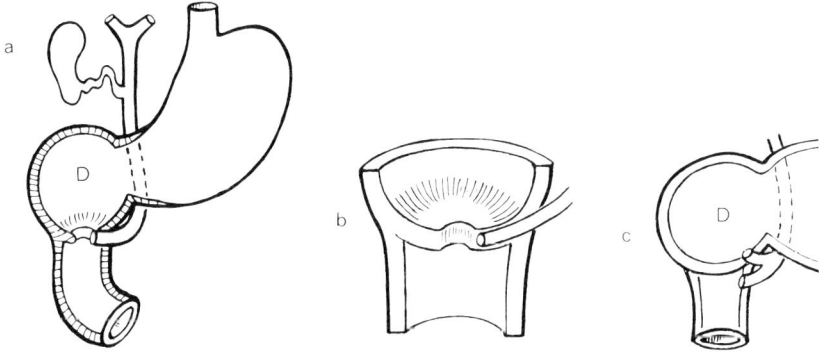

Fig. 16.2 Duodenal septum: a. The septum is complete and short; the common bile duct opens into its free edge usually in the left posterior quadrant; b. Detail of a.; c. In this example the septum is complete and a bifid duct system opens above and below it.

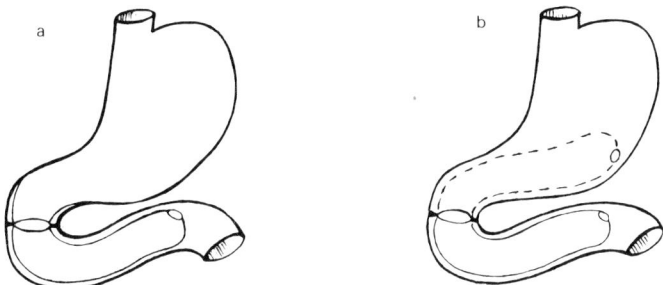

Fig. 16.3 'Wind-sock' septum: In the example illustrated the septum is attached at the junction of second and third parts of the duodenum, but the free end, with a stenotic eccentric orifice, may reach the duodenojejunal flexure or well into the stomach.

quadrants of the septum, these quadrants should be carefully avoided when septal tissue is excised. The anomalous ducts and orifices are difficult or impossible to identify at operation, and undetected damage to them can lead to postoperative complications such as biliary peritonitis, an external biliary fistula or ductal obstruction and jaundice.

Choledochal cysts
Cystic dilatations of the intraheptatic and extrahepatic bile ducts often present their first symptoms in childhood (Fonkalsrud & Boles 1965).

Collected series of choledochal cysts in children show that the lower third of the common bile duct (Alonso-Lej Type 1) is the commonest site of dilatation (Alonso-Lej 1959). The etiology is obscure, and the two longest standing theories: deficient musculature and neuromuscular incoordination, remain speculative (Flanigan 1975).

A third theory, recently revived by Miyano and others (Arima & Akita 1979, Miyano et al 1979, Kato 1980), rests upon anomalous conjunctions of the biliary and pancreatic ducts. The findings revealed by dissection, serial microscopic sections and experimental studies, summarised in Figure 16.4, indicate the possibility that reflux of pancreatic secretations into the lower reaches of the common bile duct might weaken its wall, causing dilatation extending distoproximally. As a corollary, reflux of bile into the pancreatic duct(s) has been postulated as a cause of acute haemorrhagic pancreatitis, possibly precipitated or aggravated by a strategically impacted biliary calculus. Confirmation of this theory will depend upon demonstrating the precise anatomy of the two ducts in the ampulla, and lack of separation (i.e. a septum). As this situation is regarded as a variant of the normal anatomy, present in perhaps as many as 30% of the population, an element of distal obstruction is a necessary part of the theory (Kato 1980).

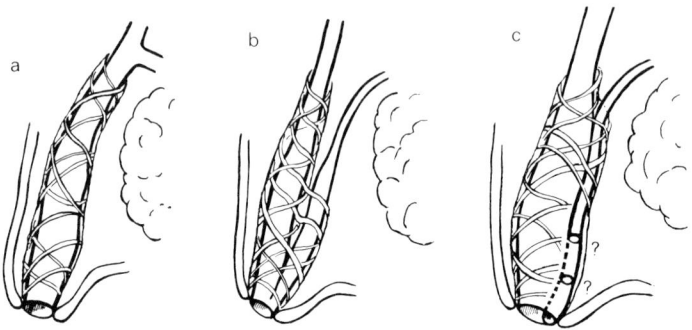

Fig. 16.4 Distal common bile duct: a. a long common channel when the pancreatic duct is short; b. parallel ducts with little or no common channel; c. intermediate types with variations in the length of the pancreatic duct and 'septum'. (After Miyano et al 1979).

Symptoms and signs
The typical triad, abdominal pain, jaundice and a palpable abdominal mass seldom occur together, in only about one-third of the patients. A history of brief episodic attacks, and a low index of suspicion of biliary disease in the paediatric age group, tend to delay diagnosis. The appearance of jaundice, present in only 30% of cases, is a valuable pointer in directing attention to the bile ducts.

Diagnosis
The diagnosis has been greatly facilitated by the introduction of ultrasonography. Previously, demonstration of a choledochal cyst depended chiefly on contrast studies showing typical displacement of the duodenum, downwards, forwards and to the left (Fig. 16.5). The displacement may be mainly or only detectable during an episodic increased tension in the cyst, usually giving rise to symptoms

Complications
Secondary changes, such as hepatic fibrosis and portal hypertension, can occur if diagnosis is delayed, and perforation, spontaneously or resulting from abdominal trauma, is also a rare complication.

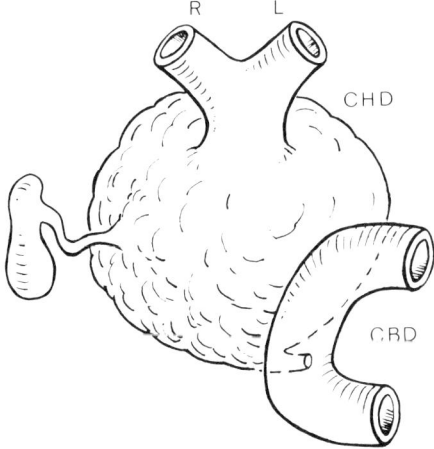

Fig. 16.5 Choledochal cyst: the common findings showing absorption of the cystic duct into the wall. bulging extensions upwards behind the common hepatic duct, and behind the duodenum displacing it to the left.

Presentation

In our experience symptoms usually commence at about 5 years of age, and the average age at diagnosis in paediatric patients is less than 10 years (Clarke 1961). Exceptions are a small number of infants presenting with a choledochal cyst and jaundice in the first few months of life, raising the possibility of confusion with biliary atresia.

A fully developed choledochal cyst can occur within three months of birth and the surgical treatment is along the same lines as in older children and adults. The superficial resemblance of one type of biliary atresia to a choledochal cyst is described below.

Treatment

An operative cholangiogram is an essential first step in delineating the extent of the dilatation, the size of the intrahepatic ducts, and the relations of the cyst to neighbouring structures. The operative treatment has changed over the years, and drainage of the cyst, by an anastomosis to the adjacent duodenum or a Roux-en-Y choledochocystojejunostomy, long considered the operation of choice, has been superseded by total excision of the cyst whenever technically feasible.

In children there is usually a plane of areolar tissue surrounding the cyst, which allows dissection and excision of the cyst in toto, followed by anastomosis of the proximal common hepatic duct to the end, or side of a Roux loop of jejunum (Kasai et al 1970). This has been found to have the lowest incidence of recurrent symptoms, an important desideratum in paediatric patients, with the added advantage of removing the site of a potential and occasional carcinoma arising in a retained choledochal cyst. One technical problem is closure of the lower extremity of the cyst or duct after excision, and uncertainty as to the site of the pancreatic duct. In our experience this is solved by leaving a 'cuff' of 4–5 mm of the cyst, closing it flush with the wall of the duodenum (Fig. 16.6) thus avoiding any damage to the pancreas or its duct. Sometimes in children, and probably more frequently in adults, the plane around the cyst is fibrotic, or chronically inflamed and hyperaemic so that total excision may not be technically easy. In such cases an alternative technique is to remove the lining of the cyst (Fig. 16.7) by developing a plane between the lining and the adventitia, thus avoiding or reducing the risk of injury to the hepatic artery and portal vein during dissection.

The unacceptably high operative mortality predicted to follow total excision of a choledochal cyst has been proven to be unfounded, given high standards of anaesthesia, resuscitation and replacement of blood loss, and above all, an accurate preoperative diagnosis supported by information provided by an operative cholangiogram (Jones & Shreeve 1970).

A previous drainage procedure, following by recurrence of symptomatic attacks

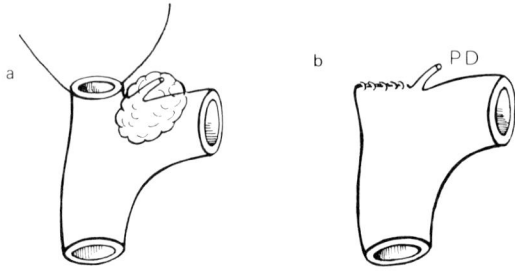

Fig. 16.6 Closure of the lower end of a choledochal cyst after excision: a. conjectural relationships of pancreas and pancreatic duct; b a 'cuff' of the wall of the cyst is retained and closed without disturbing the adjacent pancreas or its duct.

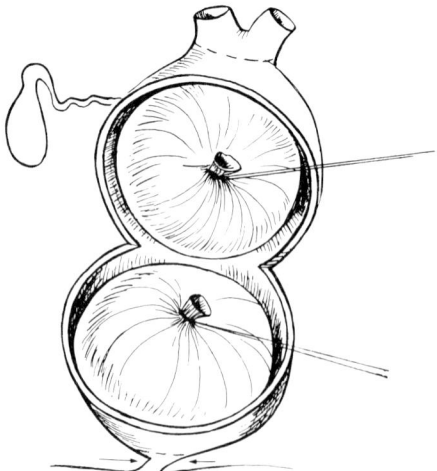

Fig. 16.7 Choledochal cyst: The anterior fibrous wall has been transsected horizontally; after developing a plane between adventitia and the lining mucosa, the mucosa is doubly ligated and removed by dissecting upwards and downwards within the intact posterior adventitia (after Lilley 1979).

of inflammation, is not a contraindication to total excision (Filler & Stringel 1980, Jones et al 1971).

Coexistent developmental malformations

Congenital dilatation of the intra-hepatic bile ducts (Caroli's disease) in our experience, is confined to a few children who also had a choledochal cyst. However, some cases of Caroli's disease (Caroli et al 1958), may be an isolated variant of the malformation seen in a choledochal cyst, causing cavernous ectasia of the intrahepatic ducts with a normal or relatively normal extra-hepatic duct system (Mittelstaedt et al 1980). Hepatic lobectomy has been suggested for those in whom gross dilatations are confined to one lobe, but the prognosis is influenced by the coexistence of renal dysplasia (medulla sponge kidney), congenital hepatic fibrosis and, very rarely, the occurrence of cholangiocarcinoma.

The embryological errors leading to the occurrence of a preduodenal portal vein have been clarified, and while it may cause duodenal obstruction (Makey and Bowen 1978, Esscher 1980) it is more often encountered as an asymptomatic finding at laparotomy. For no known reason, there is an association with biliary atresia, as noted by Wakayama et al 1976, who found that 10 out of 55 cases of preduodenal portal vein collected from literature also had biliary atresia. In such cases the abnormal vein poses significant difficulties in dissection, and prevents location of the probable site of any remaining intra-hepatic ducts.

Spontaneous perforation of the bile ducts is a rare occurrence (Lilley et al 1974) in infants less than 3 months of age. The fact that there is a typical site, the junction of the cystic and common hepatic ducts, suggests the possibility of a congenital defect. The onset and clinical course are, surprisingly, chronic rather than acute, leading to abdominal distension, 'ascites', jaundice, a low fever and mild jaundice (Prévot & Babut 1971). When suspected following paracentesis yielding bile-stained fluid, the diagnosis can be confirmed by intravenous cholangiography and an 131 I-rose Bengal scan, both showing leakage of bile into a fibrinous pseudocyst and/or the peritoneal cavity. An operative cholangiogram via the gallbladder shows the site and size of the perforation; misleading appearances suggesting obstruction at the lower end of the common bile duct should be anticipated and discounted. Cholecystostomy and simple drainage of the area of perforation is all that is required, for spontaneous closure of the perforation can be expected. Antibiotics, and drainage, until a cholangiogram via the cholecystostomy shows a normal flow of bile into the duodenum, are required. Spontaneous rupture of a choledochal cyst should be carefully distinguished, for an intestinal anastomosis to the wall of a fibrinous pseudocyst has a high mortality rate.

Acquired diseases of the bile ducts

Biliary atresia

The etiology is still unknown, but the nature and course of pathological changes suggest that this condition is the result of an inflammatory or ischaemic destruction of variable segments of the extrahepatic bile ducts, possibly viral in origin, although neither a bacterial or a viral agent can be identified (Landing 1972).

Jaundice developing in the second or subsequent weeks of life can be the result of a long list of conditions, including for example, septic infections, hypothyroidism, and alpha$_1$ amino-trypsin deficiency. Having excluded these by appropriate investigations, there remains a small group of infants in whom the diagnosis lies between severe neonatal hepatitis and biliary atresia. A preponderance of conjugated bilirubin in a jaundiced infant suggests an obstructive (ductal) cause rather than a 'parenchymatous' (metabolic) hepatitis which typically causes high levels of unconjugated bilirubin. Unfortunately, fluctuations in the level of serum bilirubin, and the proportion conjugated, do not permit a clear distinction between hepatitis and atresia on these findings alone. Other investigations purported to make this distinction have often been found to have unacceptably high rates of false positive or/and false negative results. A prospective study of patients at the Royal Children's Hospital over 20 years has led to reliance on the histology of percutaneous needle biopsies of the liver to distinguish those with biliary atresia requiring exploration. When the findings are equivocal and uncertain, biopsy is repeated at intervals of 2–3 weeks, ideally commencing at the age of 2–3 weeks, so that a final decision can be made before the age of 5–6 weeks, which we regard as the optimum age for exploration. In most infants with hepatitis the jaundice will eventually disappear, but when the jaundice is due to atresia this waiting period is unacceptable because of progressive intrahepatic fibrosis in the portal tracts. The results of surgical correction of atresia after the age of 100–120 days, even when a remediable abnormality is found, are invariably poor.

Terminology
Until relatively recently, survival of infants with biliary atresia depended upon the presence of a 'correctable' situation, i.e. a patent portion of the extrahepatic ducts which communicated with the intrahepatic ducts; all other cases were termed 'uncorrectable'. Since the Kasai operation (Kasai et al 1968, Kasai 1974, 1980) was introduced, 'uncorrectable' cases are 'operable', but the earlier terminology has persisted.

Correctable biliary atresia
The incidence of this type in reported series varies from 4–40%, with an average of approximately 10%. Theoretically an anastomosis between the patent proximal segment to a Roux-en-Y loop of jejunium (choledochojejunostomy, Fig. 16.8) should consistently lead to an adequate flow of bile and clearance of jaundice. In practice this is not always the case, because of hepatic fibrosis before operation, progressive biliary (nodular reparative) cirrhosis after operations, and episodes of 'ascending' cholangitis with additional hepatic fibrosis, all of which are prone to occur after operation in both correctable (Arima et al 1974) and uncorrectable types of biliary atresia (Lilley & Altman 1979).

Uncorrectable biliary atresia

This is the situation in approximately 90% of all infants with biliary atresia; by definition, no patent portion of the extrahepatic ducts communicates with the intrahepatic ducts. Many anatomical variations have been described (Fig. 16.9d, e) and the crucial structures are the right and left hepatic ducts and the common hepatic duct. Any patency below the common hepatic duct is irrelevant, for it cannot influence the surgery or the outcome (Fig. 16.9d).

The rationale of the operation devised for 'uncorrectable' atresia by Kasai, also described as hepatic portojejunostomy, theoretically depends upon the presence of multiple minute ducts within a conical fibrous mass, 4–10 mm in circumference and up to 1 cm in height, which represents the site of the right and left hepatic

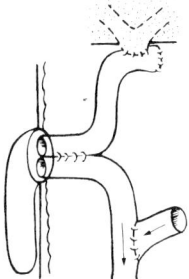

Fig. 16.8 Choledochojejunostomy: The operation performed for 'correctable' biliary atresia, joining patent ducts in the porta to a Roux loop of jejunum long enough to allow a cutaneous jejunostomy, over which a urine collecting bag is placed.

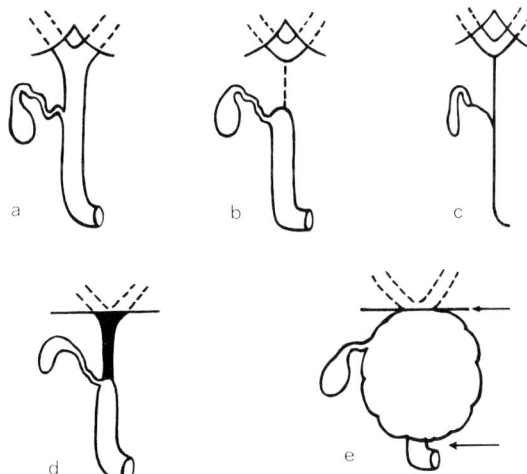

Fig. 16.9 Biliary atresia: a. normal; b. and c. 'correctable' types in which the right and left hepatic ducts are patent; d. a common 'uncorrectable' type, the black area indicating complete absence or persistence as a fibrous cord with no lumen; e. a rare form of uncorrectable atresia in which a large non-communicating cystic segment superficially resembles a choledochal cyst, except that it contains only 'white' bile, i.e. mucus containing a variable amount of bilirubin derived from its blood supply.

ducts. There is evidence that the prognosis following portojejunostomy is related to the size and number of ductal spaces in the fibrous mass, that they are larger and more numerous in patients aged 1–2 months, and thereafter diminish progressively, so that in most cases they have disappeared completely by the age of 4–5 months, leaving a 'fibrous mass' containing only fibrous tissue.

Diagnosis
Although other investigations may be helpful in reaching a firm pre-operative diagnosis of biliary atresia, in our experience reliance is placed on evidence in optimum needle biopsies interpreted by an experienced paediatric histo-pathologist.

Operation
As in other rare paediatric conditions, the best results are obtained in centres where experience has accumulated and misconceptions concerning intraoperative findings have consequently been dispelled. An upper right transverse incision is used to approach the gastrohepatic ligament and the porta. An operative cholangiogram via the gallbladder is the first objective; and if the entire biliary duct system fills completely, the diagnosis is either severe neonatal hepatitis or one of the obscure group of cholestatic conditions. Apart from a further 'open' liver biopsy, no further surgery is indicated.

If, as is not unusual, there is no lumen in the gallbladder, or only an isolated loculus a few millimetres in length, cholangiography is impossible, and dissection of the porta is commenced. In some patients with biliary atresia cholangiography shows a flow of contrast material from the gallbladder into the cystic duct, common bile duct and into the duodenum, without any flow upwards into the common hepatic duct. In such cases a second injection, after occluding the common bile duct with a non-crushing clamp, is required to confirm that there is no demonstrable lumen in the common hepatic duct before commencing dissection.

The gallbladder is mobilised and the remains of the cystic duct, if any, traced to the site of its junction with the common hepatic duct which is usually represented by a strand of fibrous tissue running upwards to attach to the liver, in the form of a conical 'fibrous mass' (Fig. 16.10). Because of the wide variations in the hepatic artery and its branches, it is only prudent to clear and identify all structures encountered in the gastro-hepatic ligament. The posterior aspect of the fibrous mass is cleared from the closely related portal vein (Fig. 16.11) dividing one or two very small vessels running between the two structures. The portal vein is then retracted posteriorly and downwards, following the fibrous mass over the top of its bifurcation. This is the point where the fibrous mass is attached to the capsule of the liver, and the fibrous mass is detached at this plane (Fig. 16.12) leaving a roughly elliptical area which represents the site of the right and left hepatic ducts (Kimura et al 1979). A Roux-en-Y loop of jejunum is selected and prepared, with the distal arm long enough to reach the porta and sufficient extra length to make a double-barrelled jejunostomy (Fig. 16.8). An anastomosis is then made between the area in the porta and the antimesenteric border of the jejunal loop, having closed its cut end. A jejunojejunostomy is performed to restore continuity.

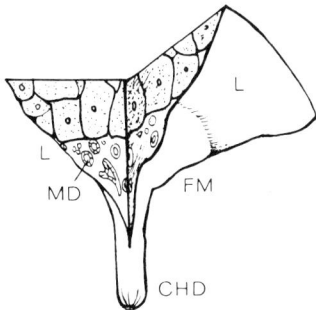

Fig. 16.10 Biliary atresia: diagram indicating a fibrous remnant of the common hepatic duct (CHD) attached to a 'fibrous mass' (FM) representing remnants of the right and left hepatic ducts, cut away to show minute duct-like structures (MD) embedded in fibrous tissue (after Kumura et al 1979).

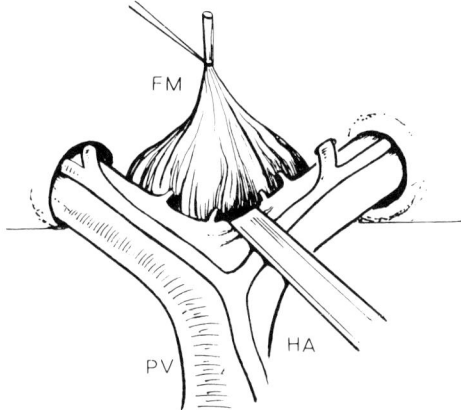

Fig. 16.11 Biliary atresia: dissection of the fibrous mass (FM) from the hepatic artery (HA) and portal vein (PV), assisted by downward retraction on the bifurcation of the portal vein.

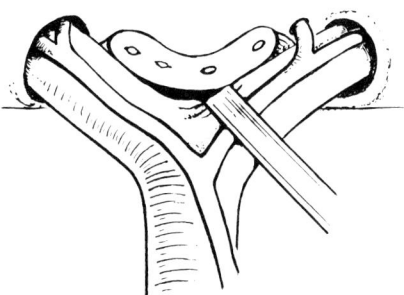

Fig. 16.12 Biliary atresia: the fibrous mass has been excised flush with the capsule of the liver. The elliptical area represents the hepatic side of the hepatic portojejunostomy which follows. The ductal structures indicated diagrammatically are not visible at operation.

Nasogastric suction, intravenous fluids and antibiotics (penicillin and gentamicin) are instituted, and urine-collecting bag is placed to collect and measure bile from the cutaneous jejunostomy.

Results
Some guide to the likelihood of success can be obtained from number and size of small duct-like space in histological sections of the base of conical 'fibrous mass' but the first indication of a successful operation is the appearance of real bile (as distinct from bile-stained mucus) from the jejunostomy. Bile may appear at any time after three days, but may not commence for several days or weeks. The volume of bile is measured daily, and an adequate flow (100–350 ml/day), accompanied by return of the serum bilirubin to normal levels, can be expected in 60–65% of patients, and possibly in 70–75% of those operated on before the age of 4–6 weeks and who have 'favourable' histological findings.

Postoperative complications e.g. fibrous stenosis and obliteration of the hepatic stoma are common, because it is not possible to construct an epithelium-to-epithelium anastomosis; recurrent attacks of 'ascending' cholangitis causing progressive hepatic fibrosis; and nodular (reparative) cirrhosis leading to portal hypertension (Altman et al 1975). The long-term success rate (five-year survivors free of jaundice) is consequently reduced to approximately 25–30%, i.e. approximately 40–50% of those in whom a satisfactory flow of bile is obtained initially (Kasai et al 1975, Odièvre 1980).

Cholelithiasis
Although biliary calculi are not commonly seen in childhood the true incidence depends upon the ethnic background and dietary customs of the particular community (Söderlund & Zetterstrom 1962). The low expectation of gallstones as a cause of abdominal pain in children tends to delay diagnosis, and the clinical picture may also differ somewhat from adults. Pain is epigastric rather than subcostal, and jaundice very rarely occurs. Differential diagnosis is complicated by the high incidence of psychosomatic and non-calculous causes of abdominal pain in children. There is a misapprehension that pigment stones, due to haemolysis, are more common than metabolic calculi in childhood, but data from the Royal Children's Hospital (Table 16.1) show that this is not our experience, in accord with most 'western' populations (Bates & Brown 1952).

The role of congenital malformations in the etiology of biliary calculi in children is still uncertain. Forshall & Rickham (1954) found latent abnormalities in all of three cases in which the operative specimen was submitted to detailed and

Table 16.1 Cholelithiasis in children, Royal Children's Hospital, Melbourne, 1952–1976: 47 cases (Solomon 1979)

'Non haemolytic' calculi		32
Haemolytic calculi		
Spherocytosis	6	
Thalassaemia	9	15
		47

microscopic examination, e.g. a stenotic or bifid cystic duct, or multiple minute channels in place of a single cystic duct.

Biliary calculi are occasionally found in a choledochal cyst, and the late appearance in adolescence of calculi in the common bile duct in patients operated on successfully in the neonatal period for a duodenal anomaly (atresia-stenosis) has already been reported. In children, non-haemolytic calculi are two or three times more common in girls than in boys in keeping with with greater incidence in adult females.

The paediatric stereotype is an intra- or postpubertal girl,–13 years of age, slightly overweight, of central or southern European origin and one parent, usually the mother, whose gallbladder was removed for calculous disease before the age of 35 years.

Once the diagnosis is suspected, investigation and treatment are along the same lines as in adults including the indications for operative exploration of the duct system for calculi. The one debatable point in children is whether cholecystostomy is preferable to cholecystectomy when (a) the calculi are pigment stones due to excess haemolysis, e.g. congenital spherocytosis (b) when the cause can be or has been removed e.g. by splenectomy (c) when the gallbladder and bile ducts are free of secondary pathological changes.

Acute acalculous cholecystitis

This is a very uncommon occurrence in childhood, but in the paediatric age group it is more common than acute cholecystitis as a complication of cholelithiasis (Arnspiger et al 1960, Brenner & Stewart 1964, Brown & Zimenes 1968).

The correct diagnosis is seldom made before operation, for symptoms are usually referred to the periumbilical region. Fever, toxaemic malaise and the white cell count are frequently high, and jaundice is also more common than might be expected in the absence of calculi. No associated or causative malformations have been identified as part of the etiology (Crystal & Fink 1971).

Cholecystectomy, whenever feasible, is considered to be the appropriate surgical treatment in most cases, and although it rarely leads to the discovery of a calculus in paediatric patients, an operative cholangiogram should probably be performed to exclude an underlying calculus or other cause.

Cholecystostomy should be considered as an alternative to cholecystectomy when indicated by the local pathology, the general condition of the patient, and the age.

Tumours of the liver and bile ducts

Primary tumours of the liver are relatively uncommon in children, the hepatoblastoma being the most frequently occurring (Keeling 1971) almost exclusively in the first four or five years of life. Jaundice is exceptionally rare, even with a massive tumour.

Hepatoblastomas tend to remain localised to the primary site, and excellent results can be obtained by hepatic lobectomy, without adjuvant chemotherapy or radiotherapy, when confined to one lobe, and completely removed.

Hepatocarcinoma is much less common and occurs in an older age group as multicentric tumours, in a cirrhotic liver. There is a much greater tendency to obstruct or grow into the lumen of major biliary ducts, and jaundice is therefore a common symptom. Major excisional surgery is rarely possible and the prognosis is very poor.

Rhabdomyosarcoma of the bile ducts (Davis et al 1969) is virtually the only primary tumour of the ducts in children, in who cholangiocarcinoma is exceedingly rare.

The typical clinical features of a rhabdomyosarcoma are malaise, fever, pain and jaundice, in a child who may have an ill-defined tender mass in the right hypochondrium or epigastrium. Barium studies usually show displacement of the duodenum and stomach to the left, while ultrasonography confirms the presence of a mass, and would probably show areas of variable echogenicity.

The diagnosis can only be made at laparotomy, and the potentially misleading paucity of malignant cells in the 'cambium' layer of the usual botryoid type of rhabdomyosarcoma may be misleading in frozen sections. This, and the rarity of the condition, are sufficient grounds for some form of temporary biliary drainage, to gain time for paraffin sections and a definitive histological diagnosis.

Radical surgical excision may be indicated if metastases can be excluded, but more often the diagnosis is made at a late stage and the general condition of the patient does not favour pancreaticoduodenectomy and Roux-en-Y hepatico-dochojejunostomy.

Biliary drainage initially, followed by intensive cytotoxic chemotherapy is more commonly the treatment employed, and while the prognosis is very poor, an occasional long-term survivor has been reported (Akers & Needham 1971).

Traumatic injuries

Trauma to the extra-hepatic ducts occasionally occurs with penetrating injuries of the upper abdomen involving the liver, but there are particular hazards from blunt (closed) abdominal trauma because of the bizarre and practically inexplicable injuries which can affect the gallbladder and its associated ducts, with or without injury to the liver (Stone & Astley 1977).

Ahmed (1976) collected 45 such cases from the literature and classified them as follows (Table 16.2):

1. *Transection* or complete rupture of one of the ducts
2. *Incomplete rupture* or a perforation

The clinical picture is also divided into two types:

1. Presenting as an 'acute abdomen' soon after the injury with signs prompting early exploration and the opportunity for early diagnosis. However, injury to the gallbladder or ducts may not be detected, and only discovered later at a second operation for complications, e.g. biliary peritonitis or external biliary fistula through the laparotomy wound.

2. Diagnosis may be delayed by apparent recovery during initial observation, with symptoms and signs appearing weeks or even months later. This is more likely

Table 16.2 Closed abdominal injury to gallbladder and bile ducts — 45 cases collected from the literature (Ahmed 1976)

Complete rupture:		
Rupture of the gallbladder		12
Complete rupture (transsection) of a bile duct		
Common bile duct	13	
Left hepatic duct	3	16
Incomplete rupture:		
Common bile duct	6	
Common hepatic duct	7	
Left hepatic duct	1	
Unidentified site	1	17
		45

with lacerations or perforation of a duct, rather than avulsion or complete transection.

In children with a suspected intra-abdominal injury, the development of fever, ileus, jaundice and tenderness, with an indefinite mass in the upper abdomen, suggests the possibility that closed abdominal trauma has caused some injury to the bile ducts. The potentially misleading variability of the clinical signs of biliary 'ascites' or peritonitis are well known; the diagnosis of a mass in a child with acholic stools may be the first indication of a ruptured or perforated bile duct.

A partial transection or perforation can be closed by local repair and the area drained. More severe and complex injuries may require a complicated surgical reconstruction such as re-implantation of an avulsed common bile duct, or anastomasis of a bile duct or a continuing leak of bile from a hepatic laceration, to a Roux-en-Y loop of jejunum.

References

Ahmed S 1976 Bile duct injuries from non-penetrating abdominal trauma in childhood. Australian and New Zealand Journal of Surgery 46: 209

Akers D R, Needham M E 1971 Sarcoma botryoides (rhabdomyosarcoma) of the bile ducts with survival. Journal of Pediatric Surgery 6: 474

Alonso-Lej F, Rever W B, Pessagno D J 1959 Congenital choledochal cyst with a report of two and an analysis of 94 cases. International Abstracts of Surgery 108: 1

Altman R P, Lilly J R 1975 Technical details in the surgical correction of extrahepatic biliary atresia. Surgery, Gynecology and Obstetrics 140: 952

Altman R P, Chandra R, Lilly J R 1975 Ongoing cirrhosis after successful portico-enterostomy in infants with biliary atresia. Journal of Pediatric Surgery 10: 685

Arima E, Akita H 1979 Congenital biliary tract dilatation and anomalous junction of the pancreatico-biliary duct system. Journal of Pediatric Surgery 14: 9

Arima E, Fonkalsrud E W, Neerhout R C 1974 Experiences in the management of surgically correctable biliary atresia. Surgery 75: 229

Arnspiger L A, Martin J G, Krempin H O 1960 Acute noncalculous cholecystitis in children: report of a case in a 17 day old infant. American Journal of Surgery 100: 103

Brenner R W, Stewart C F 1964 Cholecystitis in children. Review of Surgery 327

Brown H W, Ximenes J O 1968 Cholelithiasis and cholecystitis in childhood. Case reports of sisters and review of literature. International Surgery 49: 547

Caroli J, Soupault R, Kassabowski J 1958 La dilatation polykystique conénitale des voies biliaire intrahépatique; essai de classification. Semaine des hôpitaux de Paris 34: 488

Clarke A M 1961 Choledochal cyst. Medical Journal of Australia 2: 669

Crystal R F, Fink R L 1971 Acute acalculous cholecystitis in childhood. Clinical Pediatrics 10: 423

Davis G L, Kissane J M, Ishak K G 1969 Embryonal rhabdomyosarcoma (sarcoma botryoides) of the biliary tree. Cancer 24: 333

Esscher T 1980 Preduodenal portal vein: a cause of intestinal obstruction? Journal of Pediatric Surgery 15: 609

Filler R M, Stringel G 1980 Treatment of choledochal cyst by excision. Journal of Pediatric Surgery 15: 437

Flanigan D P 1975 Biliary cysts. Annals of Surgery 182: 635

Fonkalsrud E W, Boles E T 1965 Choledochal cysts in infancy and childhood. Surgery, Gynecology and Obstetrics 121: 733

Forshall I, Rickham P P 1954 Cholecystitis and cholelithiasis in childhood. British Journal of Surgery 42: 161

Gilroy J A, Adams A B 1960 Annular Pancreas. Radiology 75: 568

Gourevitch A 1971 Duodenal atresia in the newborn. Annals of the Royal College of Surgeons of England 48: 141

Grosfeld J L 1975 Alimentary tract obstruction in the newborn. In: Current problems in pediatrics. Year Book Medical Publishers, Chicago

Gross R E 1953 The surgery of infancy and childhood. Saunders, Philadelphia

Jona J Z, Belin R P 1976 Duodenal anomalies and the ampulla of Vater. Surgery, Gynecology and Obstetrics 143: 565

Jones A W, Shreeve D R 1970 Congenital dilatation of the intrahepatic biliary ducts with cholangiocarcinoma. British Medical Surgery 2: 277

Jones P G, Smith E D, Clark A M, Kent M 1971 Choledochal cyst: experience with radical excision. Journal of Pediatric Surgery 6: 112

Kasai M 1974 Treatment of biliary atresia with special reference to hepatic portoenterostomy and its modifications. Progress in Pediatric Surgery 6: 5

Kasai M 1980 Hepatic portoenterostomy and its modifications. In: Cholestasis in infancy. University Press, Tokyo, p 337–344

Kasai M, Asakura Y, Taira Y 1970 Surgical treatment of choledochal cysts. Annals of Surgery 172: 844

Kasai M, Kimura K, Asakura Y, Suzuki H, Ohashi E 1968 Surgical treatment of biliary atresia. Journal of Pediatric Surgery 3: 665

Kasai M, Watanabe I, Ohi R 1975 Follow up studies of long-term survivors after hepatic portoenterostomy for non-correctable biliary atresia. Journal of Pediatric Surgery 10: 173

Keeling J W 1971 Liver tumours in infancy and childhood. Journal of Pathology 103: 69 Kimura K, Tsugawa C, Kubo M, Matsumoto Y, Itoh H 1979 Technical aspects of hepatic portal dissection in biliary atresia. Journal of Pediatric Surgery 14: 27

Landing B 1972 Considerations of the pathogenesis of neonatal hepatitis, biliary atresia cholangiopathy and choledochal cyst: the concept of infantile obstructive cholangiopathy. University Park Press, Baltimore

Lilly J A, Altman R P 1975 Hepatic portoenterostomy (the Kasai operation) for biliary atresia. Surgery 78: 76

Lilly J R, Chandra R S 1974 Surgical hazards of coexisting anomalies in biliary atresia. Surgery, Gynecology and Obstetrics 139: 49

Lilly J R, Weintraub W H, Altman R P 1974 Spontaneous perforation of the extrahepatic bile ducts and bile peritonitis in infancy. Surgery 75: 664

Lynn H B 1979 Duodenal obstruction: atresia, stenosis and annular pancreas. In: Ravitch M M, Welch K J (eds) Pediatric surgery. Year Book Medical Publishers, Chicago, Vol 1: 902

Makey D A, Bowen J C 1978 Preduodenal portal vein; its surgical significance. Surgery 84: 689

Merrill J R, Raffensperger J G 1976 Pediatric annular pancreas; 20 years experience. Journal of Pediatric Surgery 11: 921

Mittelstaedt C A, Volberg F M et al 1980 Caroli's disease: sonographic findings. American Journal of Roentgenology 134: 585

Miyano T, Suruga K, Suda K 1979 Abnormal choledocho-pancreatic ductal junction related to etiology of infantile obstructive jaundice diseases. Journal of Pediatric Surgery 14: 16

Noblett R N and Paton C 1970 Intrinsic duodenal obstruction associated with interposition of the pancreas. Proceedings of an International Paediatric Surgical Congress, Melbourne 2: 392

Odièvre M 1980 Late complications after surgery for biliary atresia. In: Cholestasis in infancy. University Press, Tokyo, p 397

Prévot, Babut J M 1971 Spontaneous perforations of the biliary tract in infancy. Progress in Pediatric Surgery 3: 187

Söderlund S, Zetterstrom B 1962 Cholecystitis and cholelithiasis in children. Archives of Disease in Childhood 37: 174

Solomon J R 1979 Royal Children's Hospital. Unpublished data

Stone H, Astley J D 1977 Management of liver trauma in children. Journal of Pediatric Surgery 12: 3

Wakayama M 1976 Preduodenal portal vein associated with congenital biliary atresia. Japanese Journal of Pediatric Surgery and Medicine 8: 229

17 Economic aspects of gallstone disease and its management

S. BENGMARK, B. LINDGREN and R. SÖRBRIS

Introduction

In 1977 the number of discharges from the Swedish hospitals (national population approx 8 million) for cholelithiasis and cholecystitis was about 29 000, making a total of more than 277 000 bed-days or 1.3% of the total number of bed-days for all diseases. About 17 400 operations were performed, and the mean length of stay for patients operated on was 10.1 days; around 4.6% of the bed-days in surgical departments were occupied by cholecystitis and cholelithiasis patients (estimates based on data from the Swedish National Board of Health and Welfare (Socialstyrelsen), various years). The number of lost productive man-years due to short-term illness for cholelithiasis and cholecystitis was over 3500 in 1970, i.e. about 1.3% of the total loss of man-years due to work absenteeism (estimates based on statistics from the Swedish National Social Insurance Board (Riksförsäkringsverket) 1974).

Together with duodenal ulcer, appendicitis, inguinal hernia and other diseases of the digestive system (except for dental diseases) included in the ninth main category according to the international (WHO) classification of diseases, cholelithiasis and cholecystitis accounted for about 4% of the health care consumption in Sweden in 1975. Moreover, at the same time, this category accounted for slightly more than 5% of the indirect costs of illness, i.e. the loss of production due to short-term illness, permanent disability, and premature death (Lindgren 1981).

In Sweden as in most Western industrialized countries, considerable resources are used for the treatment of gallstone disease. It is hence understandable that great efforts have been made to decrease the total costs of this disease. Theoretically a number of possibilities always exist as to how to deal with the costs of any disease in a society. The disease may be prevented if a suitable and cheap prophylaxis is available. Early detection of a disease might lead to cheaper treatment costs. Cheaper and more accurate diagnostic aids may be developed. Finally, the indication for treatment and the choice of method for treatment can be altered.

Gallstone disease is an example of a very common disease about which we know little concerning prevention. Nor do we know the optimum surgical treatment of

270

Table 17.1 Regional differences in cholecystectomy rate, based on cholecystectomies per 10 000 population

Location or Country	Year	Rate	Reference
England and Wales	1967	4.9	Vayda, 1973
England and Wales	1966	6.1	Bunker, 1970
West Midlands, England	1976–78	6.3	McPherson et al, 1981
Luton, England	1971	7.0	Plant et al, 1973
Rennes, France	1965	8.0	Plant et al, 1973
Norway	1977	8.6	McPherson et al, 1981
United States	1971	18.5	Bunker, 1970
Sweden	1977	21.0	Socialstyrelsen
Maine, Rhode Island and Vermont, USA	1974–76	23.8	McPherson et al 1981
Sweden	1973	31.1	Socialstyrelsen
Canada	1968	31.1	Vayda, 1973
Sweden	1964	37.0	Socialstyrelsen
Sweden	1969	43.0	Socialstyrelsen
Kapuskasing, Canada	1971	43.7	Plant et al, 1973
Windsor, Canada	1971	45.8	Plant et al, 1973

those affected by the disease. It is clear that there are great variations between countries as to the relative frequency of cholecystectomy (Table 17.1). For a given treatment, in this case surgery, it is relatively easy to calculate the benefits of all the measures involved in the procedure. It is also simple to compare different diagnostic procedures and different treatments. Minor changes in the diagnostic routine and/or in the policy of treatment may alter the total costs of the disease.

In the etiology of gallstones, factors influencing the balance between the bile acids, cholesterol and phospholipids of the bile seem to be of great importance (Bennion & Grundy 1978). Most probably diet plays a major role. No single dietary factor is known to result in or prevent gallstone formation. Theoretically bran and other dietary fibers may prevent gallstones by increasing the relative proportion of bile acids in the bile. Even if it is true that dietary fibre could prevent gallstone formation, it is not at all certain that people would eat fibre daily to avoid future trouble. We know from experience that prophylaxis by single dose vaccination is relatively successful, but the opposite is true for preventive measures requiring daily 'sacrifice' (for instance giving up smoking in order to avoid cancer of the lungs).

Should all patients with gallstones be treated? Two extreme views prevail, one claiming that all patients with gallstones must be treated because sooner or later substantial numbers will develop severe side effects, the other saying that only people with repeated attacks of pain or complications should be treated since the treatment in itself has obvious side effects. The first view relies very much on natural history data (Newman et al 1968, Wenckert & Robertson 1966) which are probably based on patients that have been selected in one way or the other. The second view is based on the fact that only a proportion of all patients with gallstones are treated and that therefore the condition is benign. In the USA Way & Dunphy (1981) claimed that one third of all patients with gallstones undergo surgery. Until we have data available on the 'true' natural history of gallstone disease our calculations as to the efficiency of different strategies must be based on a mixture of available data and guesswork.

Several new tools in the diagnosis of the biliary tree have been introduced during the last decade. Among the most important is the development of ultrasonography which in the near future probably will replace oral cholecysto-graphy as the primary method of detecting gallstones (Cooperberg et al 1979, Deitch & Engel 1980). It is cheaper, and the fact that no X-rays are used makes it a useful method to screen populations. There is a substantial risk, however, that the availability of this method will lead to an increased diagnosis of 'asymptomatic' patients and to unnecessary operations.

The major treatment of gallstones is by cholecystectomy. The specific limitations of the medical treatment by chenodeoxycholic acid (Weis 1980) makes it impossible to replace surgical treatment. A number of cost-saving improve-ments in surgical therapy have been made during the last 20 years. It seems clear that long-term postoperative stay in the hospital is not needed, and most patients can be sent home 3–5 days postoperatively. The early surgical treatment of acute cholecystitis seems to be equally safe and definitely cheaper than the delayed surgical treatment (van der Linden & Sunzel 1970, Fowkes & Gunn 1980, Järvinen & Hästbacka 1980). The claimed advantages of routine intraoperative cholangiography have been questioned. A substantial number of retained gallstones in the common duct no longer need surgical exploration but can be removed endoscopically. It is also possible that in some cases endoscopic elimination of common duct stones may be enough without subsequent cholecystectomy. Most of the questions concerning the optimum treatment and optimum number of treatments could be answered if the likely pattern of the disease without and with various treatments were available. Unfortunately there are many lacunae in our knowledge, so definite answers cannot be given to these questions. There have been some attempts to evaluate costs and benefits of various approaches to the management of gallstones based on our present knowledge. Some of these attempts will be summarized in the following. The object is not to present any final conclusions but to show the applicability of economic analysis.

Silent gallstones

In a world of limited resources only those activities should be performed where benefits outweigh costs. This is a rule to follow also for health-care management and decisions concerning strategy in treating cholelithiasis and cholecystitis.

Removing a gallbladder is fairly expensive. In Sweden, the estimated total hospital costs (surgery included) were SEK (Swedish crowns) 6620 (around $1325) for an uncomplicated cholecystectomy in 1977 (Holmin et al 1980). The estimated costs for all the 17 400 operations in Sweden in 1977 were SEK 115–130 million.

Where gallstones become clinically symptomatic, causing cholecystitis, cholangitis or jaundice, there is no doubt of the benefits of surgery. Often the relief of severe pain implies benefits to the patient sufficient to defend the claim on resources. Where gallstones are asymptomatic or produce only minimal symptoms the benefits of removing the gallbladder prophylactically are not obvious.

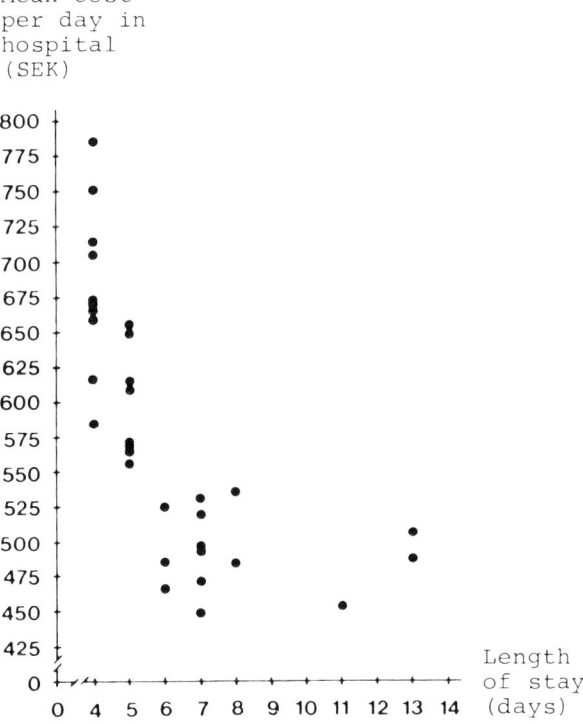

Fig. 17.1 Mean cost per day in hospital, distributed according to the length of stay, for 32 gallstone patients in the surgical department at Lund University Hospital, 1975 (from Lindgren et al 1979). Comment: Length of stay refers to the net length, i.e. the day of admission and the day of discharge have each been counted as a half-day.

Certainly the operative mortality rate is low for elective cholecystectomy, when carried out in relatively healthy, young patients, but the risk is substantially higher for older patients, perhaps in poor physical conditions and perhaps requiring an exploration of the common duct. Before concluding that elective cholecystectomy for silent stones is to be preferred, in order to avoid the increased risks of later emergency surgery, one must take into account the expected course and risk of the disease in the absence of surgery at an early stage. The crucial question regards the probability that surgery will be required at a later stage.

The cost-effectiveness of surgical versus symptomatic medical treatment of silent gallstones has been studied by Fitzpatrick et al (1977). Due to lack of data on morbidity and convalescence, the analysis was restricted to the outcome of death under the two options of 1 'operate now' and 2 'wait and see'. The number of expected days of life saved following the two options was calculated for patients of different age, sex, and anesthetic risk. Some of the results are reproduced in Table 17.2.

It appears that good-risk men and women will lose two weeks of their lives if a 'wait and see' policy is chosen. Poor-risk men and women will gain as much as one month by choosing this option. The gains with the two strategies seem, in terms of

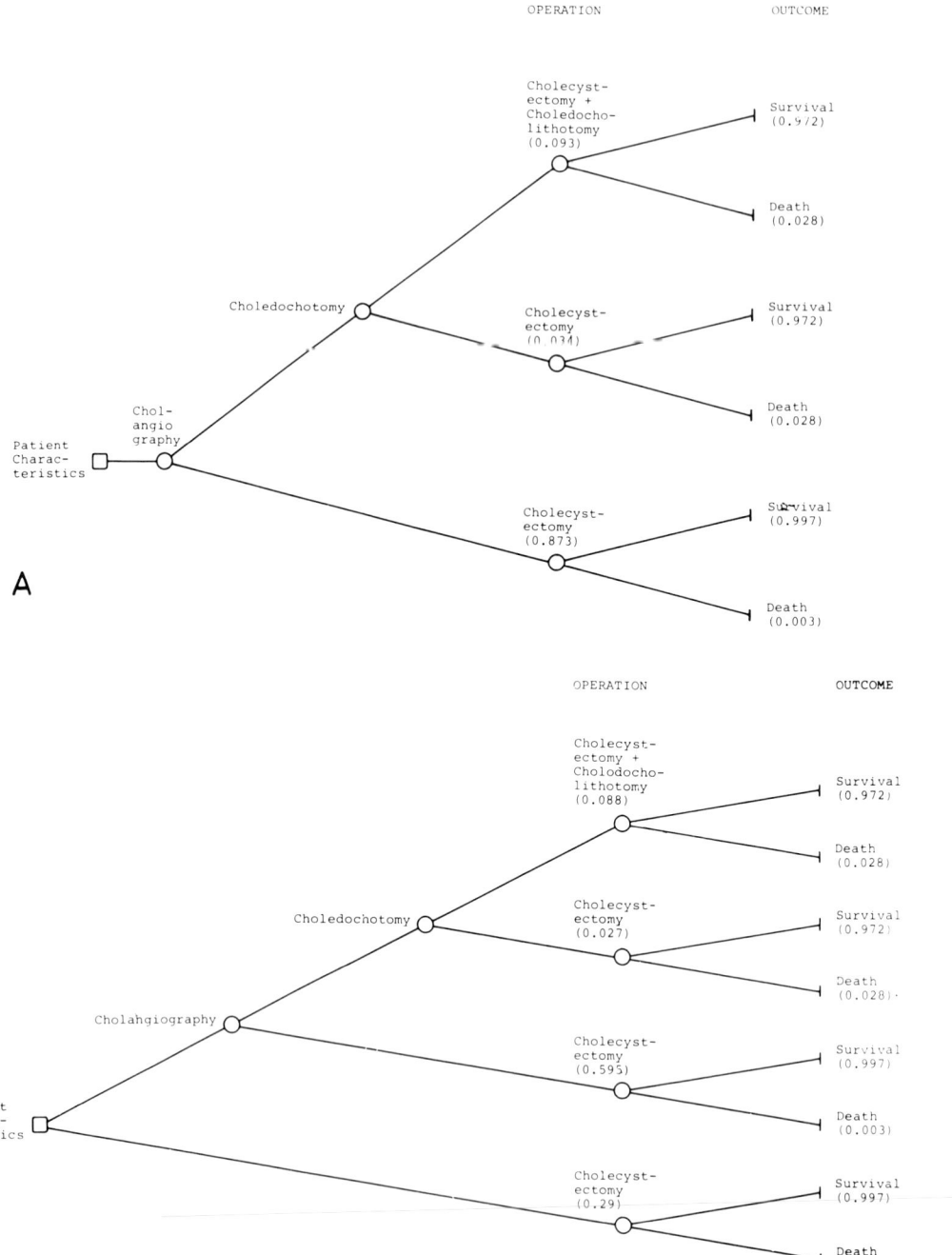

Fig. 17.2 Decision tree for patients under suspicion for stones in the common bile duct. A. Strategy 1: Routine intraoperative cholangiography performed on all patients undergoing operation for gallstones. B. Strategy 2: Selective intraoperative cholangiography, performed only when at least one of four criteria is present. (From Holmin et al 1980.)

Key: □ denotes decision point
     ○ denotes chance point

Table 17.2 Days of life expectancy gained by surgery or by a 'wait and see' policy for minimally symptomatic gallstones. (From Fitzpatrick et al 1977.)

	Age	Good Risk	Poor Risk
Men	49	S 16*	W 33**
	60	S 7	W 37
Women	49	S 15	W 4
	60	S 11	W 14

*S = Surgery is preferred
**W = Waiting is preferred

quantity of life, to be small, at the largest in the order of one month. However, no conclusions can be drawn as to the quality of the remaining life. It is obvious that most people care much more about the present than about the future, so the benefit of the possibility of getting one or two more weeks added to the expected lifetime may be valued low.

Fitzpatrick et al made calculations of the cost of removing silent gallstones from low-risk patients. If, for instance, all 50-year-olds and all 60-year-olds in the USA were screened every year, the stones at age 50 and the stones that had appeared over the following decade of very high incidence would hopefully be found. Some 4 million Americans would thus receive a cholecystogram each year in this screening programme. According to the authors, this would cost $200 million a year. Some 368 000 cases would be found, and if all were operated on, this would cost another $1100 million. As the authors conclude 'considerations of an investment of this magnitude in order to prolong life by one or two weeks should of course take into account the many other demands on medical resources'. As Fitzpatrick et al point out, their analysis cannot be definitive. They restricted their analysis to the outcome of death under two options. However, there are more than two options to consider. Moreover, data on morbidity and convalescence were lacking, which explains why life expectancy was chosen as the sole outcome measure. In view of the very small gains and losses in quantity of life, the decision to operate for a silent gallstone cannot be based on life expectancy but more on the risk of morbidity, the patient's preferences, and similar factors. It should be added that many estimates of the probabilities are uncertain. If the 'true' probability were higher than the estimated probability, then surgery at an early stage would seem more attractive. Secondly, probabilities change over time. If the fatality rate for complicated cholecystectomies decreases over time, the 'wait and see' strategy will become more attractive.

Early discharge and changes in the costs of cholecystectomies

According to inpatient statistics published by the Swedish National Board of Health and Welfare, the mean length of stay for cholelithiasis and cholecystitis in the surgical departments in Sweden decreased from 11.8 days in 1964 to 10.1 days in 1977. It is evident that almost two days per hospital stay have been saved, but it is in no way clear that a corresponding decrease in the costs of a hospital stay for cholelithiasis and cholecystitis has occurred.

In the present hospital accounting system used in Swedish hospitals, the hospital department is the basic accounting unit. This means that it is only possible to obtain data on mean cost per bed-day (including costs of physicians, surgeons, anaesthetists, nurses, drugs, X-ray examinations etc) from the hospital accounts. However, using the mean cost of a bed-day would overestimate the changes in costs due to shorter hospital stays. These will automatically raise the average cost per day for most treatments, since the very first days in hospital are very expensive; the cost of one day in hospital towards the end of a patient's stay consists mainly of expenses for board and lodging and is considerably lower than the average cost. This is evident from those studies which do not rely on per-day-cost accounting data but which attempt to estimate the actual resource use caused by a particular hospital stay.

An example may be found in the work of Lindgren et al (1979) (Fig. 17.1). Shorter hospital stays are accompanied, as expected, by a higher average day cost. Furthermore, sometimes it is only possible to reduce the length of stay by increasing the use of resources during the remaining days of hospital treatment. This explains why shorter stays may well result in unchanged or even higher cost per hospital stay.

So the answer to the question that was put forward at the beginning of this section is not easily available. However, the present authors made an attempt to estimate the changes in the costs of an uncomplicated elective cholecystectomy at Lund University Hospital between 1955 and 1965 and from 1965 to 1975. In order to exclude the effects of changed age or sex distribution we chose to examine women, aged 45–59. All the records of patients who satisfied these criteria and who were treated in the Surgical Department of Lund University hospital were examined. 59, 54 and 33 patients from 1955, 1965 and 1975 respectively satisfied the criteria. A few patients had to be excluded due to lack of information about the length of operations.

In order to obtain the cost per hospital stay we need to know all the various services which were provided to the patient and also the cost of each service. If patient bills were being generated routinely, as in the USA, this would not pose any problem. However, in Sweden such patient bills are not produced even for accounting purposes, since the hospital department and not the patient is the basic accounting unit. Therefore, it was necessary to abstract data on service use from the patients' medical records. We then calculated the costs of hospital treatment for each patient in fixed prices, (i.e. the effects of inflation were allowed for). Because of the absence of markets in public health care, data on the costs of providing a particular service are not readily available. So these 'prices' were to be calculated indirectly; we made no such imputations of our own, but used the 'prices' calculated for 1971 in a study by Spek & Thorburn (1976).

Our main results are summarized in Table 17.3. The mean cost for a cholecystectomy decreased by 18% between 1955 and 1965 and by further 7% between 1965 and 1975. The 7% decrease between 1965 and 1975 is not statistically significant. When we tested the hypothesis that the observations from

Table 17.3 Mean cost (and standard deviation) expressed in 1971 level of cost (SEK) for a cholecystectomy*. (From Lindgren et al 1979.)

Year	N	Total		Pre-operatively	Per-operatively	Post-operatively
		Mean	SD			
1955	57	4391	153	962	910	2519
1965	54	3585	129	746	970	1869
1975	32	3340	169	677	1303	1360

*Total surgical procedure and divided into preoperative, peroperative and postoperative costs.

1965 and 1975 are samples of the same population, it appeared that the variation within each sample is great in comparison with the differences between them. The null hypothesis that they belong to the same population was accepted (F = 1.35; $V_1 = 2$, $V_2 = 86$ DFR). It appears from Table 17.3 that the cost of peroperative measures increased while the cost of postoperative measures decreased. The rise in the peroperative costs is mainly explained by increased length of operation, while the reduced number of postoperative bed days is a main factor contributing to the decrease in the postoperative costs (Table 17.4). The mean length of operation increased by 12% from 1955 to 1965 and by a further 22% from 1965 to 1975. More than compensating for this rise in the length of operation, there is a sharp decline in the average duration of hospital stay. The mean length of stay decreased by about 27% between 1955 and 1965 and by the same amount between 1965 and 1975.

Not only the length of operation but also several other factors changed between the three years studied. Such preoperative investigations as X-rays of the heart and lung increased from 1965 to 1975. Second, every gallbladder was examined in 1975 by a pathologist, which was not the case in 1955, nor in 1965. Finally, in the postoperative treatment the use of postoperative parenteral nutrition was much more extensively used in 1955 than in 1965 or in 1975. The actual cost for the parenteral solutions given (mainly glucose) was low per se. It was, however, not possible to estimate the extra labour used, which might be of some importance. Nor was it possible to estimate the activity of the physiotherapists during the years studied, but it can be assumed that this activity increased from 1955 to 1975. It is

Table 17.4 Cholecystectomies. Mean length of operation in minutes and the mean number of bed days, totally and divided preoperatively and postoperatively in 1955, 1965, and 1975. (From Lindgren et al 1979.)

Year	Mean length of operation in minutes	Mean number of bed days		
		Total	Pre-operatively	Post-operatively
1955	65	11.6	2.0	9.6
1965	72	8.4	1.3	7.1
1975	89	6.1	1.1	5.0

Note: The day of admission and the day of discharge counted as half a day each.

impossible to determine the influence of these tendencies in the postoperative treatment, since no data are available.

The results of our study show that reductions in the number of bed-days per hospital stay cannot be used as indicators of saved resources within the hospital. For instance, despite the fact that the mean number of bed days declined by 27% from 1965 to 1975, the cost per hospital stay did not decrease significantly. While contributing to the decrease in hospital costs between 1955 and 1965, early discharge now seems to have reached the limit beyond which it is no longer possible to save hospital resources.

Selective or routine intraoperative cholangiography

One of the many difficult decisions with which the surgeon is faced during cholecystectomy is whether or not to perform a choledochotomy. Under ideal conditions he would restrict choledochotomy to patients with common bile duct stones, and to these patients only. However, for lack of perfectly discriminating diagnostic tools, the surgeons must in fact weigh the benefit of detecting a stone against the risk of making an unnecessary exploration of the common bile duct as a result of a positive, but false, diagnostic finding.

Intraoperative cholangiography is one of the diagnostic methods available, and routine intraoperative cholangiography is performed in 96% of the surgical units in Sweden. In a retrospective analysis, the present authors compared the cost-effectiveness of 1. the present strategy of routine use in all cases, versus 2. the selective use of intraoperative cholangiography on patients satisfying at least one of four common clinical criteria (Holmin et al 1980). The criteria used were (a) history of at least three attacks of biliary colic; (b) history of past or present pancreatitis; (c) history of past or present cholecystitis; and (d) history of past or present jaundice.

The choice between the two strategies is illustrated by the two decision trees shown in Figure 17.2. In strategy 1 all patients would have undergone intraoperative cholangiography. On the basis of this cholangiography, simple cholecystectomy would have been performed in 87.3% of cases, and exploration of the common bile duct would have been added in 12.7% of the cases. As a result of the common duct exploration, choledocholithotomy would have been performed in 9.3% of all patients. In strategy 2, only patients with at least one of the four criteria would have undergone intraoperative cholangiography. Accordingly, patients with no criterion present (29%) would have had cholecystectomy without intraoperative cholangiography. On the basis of cholangiography, a further 59.5% of patients would have undergone simple cholecystectomy without common duct exploration. A stone would have been found in the common duct in 8.8% of all patients, while 2.7% would have been explored without any stone being found. These calculations were based on a projection of data obtained in a retrospective review of the medical records of the 590 patients electively cholecystectomized from 1975 through 1977 in the Department of Surgery at the University Hospital of Lund. Of the 590 patients 55 had stones removed from the common duct; three

Table 17.5 Relative distributions of the patients between the two strategies. (From Holmin et al 1980.)

	Cholecystectomy	Cholecystectomy + cholangiography	Cholecystectomy + cholangiogaphy + choledochotomy + no stone	Cholecystectomy + cholangiography + choledochotomy + stone
Strategy 1: Routine intraoperative cholangiography	0	0.873	0.034	0.093
Strategy 2: Cholangiography when 1 or more criteria are met	0.29	0.595	0.027	0.088

of these patients showed none of the four criteria and therefore would not have undergone common duct explorations under strategy 2.

For the sake of simplicity, the distribution of patients according to each strategy is shown in Table 17.5 Table 17.6 shows for each strategy the predicted financial costs of treatment in the hospital and the expected mortality rates for an elective cholecystectomy. The predicted hospital cost would be $0.873 \times 6620 + (0.034 + 0.093) \times 13\,000 = SEK^* 7430$ for strategy 1, and $0.290 \times 5730 + 0.595 \times 6620 + (0.027 + 0.088) \times 13\,000 = SEK\ 7095$ for strategy 2. The predicted cost of an elective cholecystectomy would be SEK 335, or about 4.5%, lower in strategy 2.

The expected mortality rate would be $0.873 \times 0.003 + (0.034 + 0.093) \times 0.028 = 0.006175$ for strategy 1 and $(0.290 + 0.595) \times 0.003 + (0.027 + 0.088) \times 0.028 = 0.005875$ for strategy 2. The mortality rate would be about 5% lower in strategy 2.

Routine intraoperative cholangiography, compared with no intraoperative cholangiography at all, has been analysed by Barnes & Barnes (1977). They found relatively small differences in costs and mortality rates between the two strategies. Similarly, we found the differences between our two strategies to be relatively small. The results of these two studies indicate, however, that no cholangiography is worse than routine cholangiography, but that performing cholangiography on

*SEK = Swedish kronor

Table 17.6 Expected hospital costs and mortality rates (index) for each of the two strategies. (From Holmin et al 1980.)

	Expected hospital cost (SEK)	Expected mortality (index)
Strategy 1: Routine intraoperative cholangiography	7430	100
Strategy 2: Cholangiography when 1 or more criteria are met	7095	95

selected patients is better than performing it as a routine measure. This conclusion is also supported by Skillings et al (1979).

Our analysis on the cost-effectiveness of intraoperative cholangiography has the same kind of weaknesses as the study on silent gallstones referred to earlier. For instance, the analysis did not include morbidity and convalescence nor recurrencies or re-explorations. Furthermore, all the probabilities used are subject to some uncertainty. Finally, it is by no means certain that intraoperative cholangiography is the ultimate method of detecting stones in the common bile duct. There is a great need for studies comparing other techniques with routine or selective intraoperative cholangiography. Clearly, a safe and immediate pre-exploratory investigation of the biliary tree would be preferable, since the surgeon would also find it easier to plan the coming operation if he knew something of the anatomy of the biliary tract in advance. New radiographic techniques and fibroendoscopy provide hope of safer techniques and lower costs for the detection of stones in the common bile duct.

Future aspects

Although it is not always recognized, management of biliary stones and its complications is under constant development. Several major alterations in policy will be expected during the 1980s. The availability and the spreading of the endoscopic technique will have a great impact on the field. Complications like common duct stones will probably be recognized and treated before cholecystectomy. This is in line with the development in other fields of surgery, where the complications of the disease are treated separately and the final operation of the disease is performed later and under optimal conditions. In elderly patients with non-functioning gallbladders and occluded connection between the gallbladder and the common duct, endoscopic papillotomy and extraction of the stones will probably be the only procedure performed.

The oral cholecystogram is slowly disappearing as the routine tool for preoperative work-up. Instead, ultrasound is taking its place. The peroperative cholangiography, from which biliary surgery has benefitted enormously during the last three decades, will probably disappear as a routine in every patient during the 1980s. It will be replaced by preoperative exploration of the common duct with injection or infusion cholangiography or, in jaundice cases, endoscopic retrograde cholangiography. The advantage of this will be, that it will be known, ahead of time, whether a simple cholecystectomy or a common duct exploration is to be performed and the strategy planned according to that. As mentioned above, surgical common duct explorations will probably be less common, as it is expected that the stones are taken out through endoscopic approach earlier. If necessary, choledochoscopy will be more used than peroperative cholangiography.

Chemical dissolution of biliary stones is at present not economically defendable as a routine. The finding that only smaller doses of the drug can keep the stones away might lead to a combined surgical-medical approach, i.e. the stones are taken out through simpler cholecystotomy and the patient then is kept on a low dose of long-term treatment with the drug to prevent formation of new stones.

However, we cannot take advantage of all these new techniques in the treatment of gailstone disease. Since economics is the science of how to make the best choice within limited resources, economic analysis should be routinely used for evaluating new as well as old techniques.

References

Barnes B A, Barnes A B 1977 Evaluation of surgical therapy by cost-benefit analysis. Surgery 82: 21–33

Bennion L J, Grundy S M 1978 Risk factors for the development of cholelithiasis in man (2 parts). New England Journal of Medicine 299: 1161–1167, 1221 1227

Bunker J P 1970 Surgical manpower. A comparison of operations and surgeons in the United States and in England and Wales. New England Journal of Medicine 282: 135–144

Cooperberg P L, Pon M S, Wong P, Stoller J L, Burhenne H J 1979 Real-time high resolution ultrasound in the detection of biliary calculi. Radiology 131: 789–790

Deitch E A, Engel J M 1980 Ultrasound in elective biliary tract surgery. American Journal of Surgery 140: 277–283

Fitzpatrick G, Neutra R, Gilbert J P 1977 Cost-effectiveness of cholecystectomy for silent gallstones. In: Bunker J P, Barnes B A, Mosteller F (ed) Costs, Risks and Benefits of Surgery, Oxford University Press, New York, p 246–261

Fowkes F G R, Gunn A A 1980 The management of acute cholecystitis and its hospital cost. British Journal of Surgery 67: 613–617

Holmin T, Jönsson B, Lindgren B, Olsson S-Å, Petersson B G, Sörbris R, Bengmark S 1980 Selective or routine intraoperative cholangiography: a cost-effectiveness analysis. World Journal of Surgery 4: 315–322

Järvinen H J, Hästbacka J 1980 Early cholecystectomy for acute cholecystitis. Annals of Surgery 191: 501–505

van der Linden, W, Sunzel H 1970 Early versus delayed operation for acute cholecystitis. A controlled clinical trial. American Journal of Surgery 120: 7–13

Lindgren B 1981 Costs of illness in Sweden 1964–1975. Liber, Lund, p 4–163

Lindgren B, Petersson B G, Sörbris R, Bengmark S 1979 Changes in the costs of elective cholecystectomies 1955–1965–1975. Annals of Surgery 189: 447–454

McPherson K, Clifford P, Wennberg J F, Hovind O B 1981 Small area variations in the use of discretionary surgery. An international comparison between New England, England and Norway. Mimeography. Oxford Department of Community Medicine and General Practice

Newman H F, Northup H F, Rosenblum M, Abrams H 1968 Complications of cholelithiasis. American Journal of Gastroenterology 50: 476–496

Plant J C D, Percy J, Bates T 1973 Incidence of gallbladder disease in Canada, England and France. Lancet 2: 249–254

Riksförsäkringsverket (Swedish National Social Insurance Board) 1974 Sjukdomsorsaker inom den allmänna sjukförsäkringen år 1970 (Short-term illness distributed by disease categories in 1970). Statistisk Rapport No 1974: 1, Stockholm

Skillings J C, Williams J S, Hinshaw J R 1979 Cost-effectiveness of operative cholangiography. American Journal of Surgery 137: 26–31

Socialstyrelsen (Swedish National Board of Health and Welfare) Various years Patientstatistik (In-patient statistics)

Spek J E, Thorburn T 1976 Analys av kostnadsförhållanden inom utomlänssjukvården (Analysis of the costs of treating patients at hospitals with regional specialities). Memorandum 63 from the Department of Economics, University of Gothenburg

Vayda E 1973 A comparison of surgical rates in Canada and in England and Wales. New England Journal of Medicine 289: 1224–1229

Way L W, Dunphy J E 1981 In: Current surgical diagnosis and treatment, 5th edn. Lange Medical Publications, Los Altos, Cal

Weis H J 1980 Indikationen zur medikamentösen Gallenstein-Auflösung 33: 1235–1239

Wenckert A, Robertson B 1966 The natural course of gallstone disease: Eleven-year review of 781 nonoperated cases. Gastroenterology 50: 376–382

Index